Atlas of
DIABETES

THIRD EDITION

Editor

Jay S. Skyler, MD

Professor of Medicine, Pediatrics, and Psychology
Division of Endocrinology Diabetes and Metabolism
Associate Director, Diabetes Research Institute
University of Miami Miller School of Medicine
Miami, Florida

With 31 contributors

Developed by Current Medicine LLC
Philadelphia

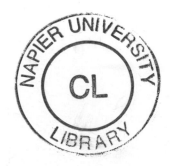

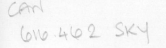

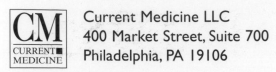

Current Medicine LLC
400 Market Street, Suite 700
Philadelphia, PA 19106

Developmental Editor . . . . Anthony Mirra
Commissioning Supervisor . . . . Annmarie Piacentino
Cover Design. . . . . Kim Broadbent
Design and Layout . . . . William C. Whitman, Jr.
and Andrea Penko
Illustrator . . . . Maureen Looney
Assistant Production Manager. . . . . Margaret LaMare
Indexer . . . . Holly Lukens

Library of Congress Cataloging-in-Publication Data

Atlas of diabetes / editor, Jay S. Skyler ; with 31 contributors.-- 3rd ed.
    p. ; cm.
  Includes bibliographical references and index.
  ISBN 1-57340-222-2
  1. Diabetes--Atlases.
  [DNLM: 1. Diabetes Mellitus--Atlases. WK 17 A8808 2006] 1. Title: Diabetes. II. Skyler, Jay S.
  RC660.A87 2006
  616.4'62--dc22

                         2005053769

ISBN 1-57340-222-2

For more information, please call 1-800-427-1796 or email us at inquiry@phl.cursci.com
www.current-science-group.com

Although every effort has been made to ensure that drug doses and other information are presented accurately in this publication, the ultimate responsibility rests with the prescribing physician. Neither the publishers nor the authors can be held responsible for errors or for any consequences arising from the use of information contained herein. Products mentioned in this publication should be used in accordance with the prescribing information prepared by the manufacturers. No claims or endorsements are made for any drug or compound at present under clinical investigation.

Printed in Hong Kong by Paramount Printing Co. LTD

10 9 8 7 6 5 4 3 2 1

Diabetes mellitus is increasing in incidence, prevalence, and importance as a chronic disease throughout the world. In the United States, the burden of diabetes is enormous, whether one considers the magnitude of the population afflicted, the impact on the lives of people affected by diabetes, the morbidity rendered by diabetes, or the economic toll it takes. Over 18 million Americans, 6.3% of the population, have diabetes. Over 1 million Americans, or over 2800 people each day, develop diabetes each year. Among those under 20 years of age, the disease pattern is changing rapidly. One of every 400 to 500 children and adolescents has type 1 diabetes. The striking thing, however, is that the incidence of type 2 diabetes among adolescents has increased 15-fold since 1982. In some pediatric diabetes clinics, the number of patients with type 2 diabetes now equals the number with type 1 diabetes. Indeed, the average age of onset of type 2 diabetes is dropping. With more people developing the disease in their teens, 20s, and 30s, their lifetime potential for complications increases.

Strikingly, although type 2 diabetes is increasing among the young, its burden on older patients is growing as well. The prevalence among people 60 years of age or older now exceeds 18%, with diabetes afflicting 8.6 million Americans in this age group. In fact, 20% of the Medicare population has diabetes, but 30% of the Medicare budget is spent on diabetes, an indication of the disproportionate share of the health care budget that diabetes consumes. Diabetes accounts for 14% of total health care costs.

There are a number of paradoxes in terms of complications. Diabetic retinopathy is the leading cause of blindness in adults of working age, yet the National Eye Institute estimates that 90% of vision loss caused by diabetic retinopathy is preventable. Diabetic nephropathy is far and away the leading cause of endstage renal disease, accounting for 43% of all new cases, yet the National Institute of Diabetes, Digestive, and Kidney Diseases estimates that most future endstage renal disease from diabetes is probably preventable. Diabetes accounts for 60% of all nontraumatic lower extremity amputations, with diabetes imposing a 15- to 40-fold increased risk of amputation compared with the nondiabetic population, yet the American Diabetes Association and the Centers for Disease Control estimate that more than 85% of limb loss is preventable. The presence of type 2 diabetes imposes a risk of coronary events equal to that of a previous myocardial infarction in the nondiabetic population, yet people with diabetes are not as likely to be prescribed cardioprotective medication. Although in the United States the incidence and mortality rates from heart disease and stroke are decreasing in the nondiabetic population, patients with diabetes are two- to sixfold more likely to develop heart disease and two- to fourfold more likely to suffer a stroke. Optimal glycemic control is critical for reducing the risk of long-term complications associated with diabetes. The Diabetes Control and Complications Trial provided strong evidence of the importance of achieving near-normal blood glucose levels in type 1 diabetic patients by means of intensive insulin therapy programs. The United Kingdom Prospective Diabetes Study suggested similar beneficial effects of improved glycemic control in type 2 diabetes, yet diabetes patients are still not achieving recommended target blood glucose values. Data from the Third National Health and Nutrition Examination Survey of 1988–1994 showed that approximately 60% of patients with type 2 diabetes had A_{1c} values greater than 7% and that 25% had A_{1c} values greater than 9%. In the 1999–2000 update, over 37% had A_{1c} values greater than 8%.

The bottom line is that neither physicians nor patients are paying enough attention to diabetes. Diabetes is underrepresented in medical school curricula compared with the burden of the disease. This is particularly the case when it is appreciated that this disease impacts virtually all medical specialties. Our health care system fails to adequately meet the needs of patients with chronic diseases in general, diabetes in particular. Referrals of patients with diabetes to diabetes specialist teams (which include medical nutrition therapists and certified diabetes educators, as well as diabetologists/endocrinologists) are infrequent, and there are not enough of these teams or the specialists who constitute them.

Meanwhile, treatment options are expanding dramatically. As recently as 1995, the only classes of medications available in the United States to lower glycemia were sulfonylureas and insulins. Now we have added biguanides, α-glucosidase inhibitors, glitazones (PPARγ activators), glinides (rapid-acting insulin secretagogues), amylin analogues, incretin mimetics, rapid-acting insulin analogues, and long-acting basal insulin analogues. Several additional classes of agents are in development. The use of insulin pumps has increased more than tenfold since 1985. Pancreatic transplantation has become a routine procedure in the company of kidney transplantation.

There has been an exciting explosion of knowledge about fundamental mechanisms related to diabetes. We have gained insights into the pathogenesis both of type 1 and type 2 diabetes, and with that, the prospect of implementing prevention strategies to delay or interdict the disease processes. Great progress has been made in islet transplantation, which offers the potential of reversing diabetes. The major challenge has become finding sources of islets sufficient to meet potential needs, given that there are annually only about 4000 organ donors nationwide. Whether diabetes prevention will come from advances in understanding the processes of islet neogenesis and proliferation, from genetic engineering, or from protecting xenoislets from attack remains unclear. All are potential avenues of pursuit.

It is with this background that we have asked leading authorities to contribute their thoughts and images concerning various aspects of diabetes. Their input makes this Atlas possible.

Jay S. Skyler, MD

Contributors

Lloyd Paul Aiello, MD, PhD
Associate Professor
Department of Ophthalmology
Harvard Medical School
Assistant Director
Beetham Eye Institute
Investigator and Head, Eye Research
Joslin Diabetes Center
Boston, Massachusetts

Rodolfo Alejandro, MD
Professor of Medicine
Department of Medicine
University of Miami Miller School
  of Medicine
Miami, Florida

Mark A. Atkinson, PhD
Sebastian Family Eminent Scholar
Department of Pathology
University of Florida College
  of Medicine
Gainesville, Florida

Bruce W. Bode, MD, FACE
Medical Director
Atlanta Diabetes Associates
Atlanta, Georgia

Susan Bonner-Weir, PhD
Associate Professor
Department of Medicine
Harvard Medical School
Senior Investigator
Joslin Diabetes Center
Boston, Massachusetts

Michael Brownlee, MD
Professor of Medicine and Pathology
Department of Medicine
Albert Einstein College of Medicine
  of Yeshiva University
Bronx, New York

Veronica M. Catanese, MD
Senior Associate Dean for Education
Associate Professor
Department of Medicine and
  Cell Biology
New York University School
  of Medicine
New York, New York

Daina Dreimane, MD
Assistant Professor
Department of Pediatrics
Keck School of Medicine of University
  of Southern California
Childrens Hospital Los Angeles
Los Angeles, California

Ele Ferrannini, MD
Professor of Medicine
Department of Internal Medicine
University of Pisa Medical School
Professor of Internal Medicine
Ospedale Santa Chiara
Pisa, Italy

Tracey L. Fisher, BA
Graduate Student
Joslin Diabetes Center
Boston, Massachusetts

John E. Gerich, MD
Professor of Medicine
Department of Medicine
University of Rochester School
  of Medicine and Dentistry
Strong Memorial Hospital
Rochester, New York

Robert R. Henry, MD
Professor
Department of Medicine
University of California, San
  Diego School of Medicine
Chief, Diabetes/Metabolism Section
VA San Diego Healthcare System
San Diego, California

Irl B. Hirsch, MD
Professor
Department of Medicine
University of Washington School
  of Medicine
Medical Director
Diabetes Care Center
University of Washington Medical
  Center
Seattle, Washington

Susanna Hofmann, MD
Department of Pathology and
  Laboratory Medicine
Center for Lipid and
  Atherosclerosis Studies
Genome Research Institute
University of Cincinnati
Cincinnati, Ohio

Lois Jovanovic, MD
Clinical Professor
Department of Medicine
Keck School of Medicine of University
  of Southern California
Los Angeles, California
Director of Research
Chief Scientific Officer
Sansum Diabetes Research Institute
Santa Barbara, California

Francine Ratner Kaufman, MD
Professor
Department of Pediatrics
Keck School of Medicine of University
  of Southern California
Head, Division of Endocrinology
Childrens Hospital of Los Angeles
Los Angeles, California

Abbas E. Kitabchi, MD, PhD
Professor
Departments of Medicine and
  Molecular Sciences
University of Tennessee College
  of Medicine
Consult
Regional Medical Center at Memphis
Veterans Affairs Medical Center
Methodist Healthcare
Baptist Memorial Hospital
Memphis, Tennessee

Eleftheria Maratos-Flier, MD
Associate Professor of Medicine
Department of Medicine
Harvard Medical School
Staff Physician
Beth Israel Deaconess Medical Center
Boston, Massachusetts

Jennifer B. Marks, MD, CDE, FACP
Professor
Department of Medicine
University of Miami Miller School
  of Medicine
Section Chief, Endocrinology, Diabetes,
  and Metabolis
Miami VAMC
Miami, Florida

**Sunder Mudaliar, MD,
MRCP(UK), FACE**
Associate Clinical Professor
Department of Medicine
University of California, San Diego
  School of Medicine
Staff Physician
VA San Diego Healthcare System
San Diego, California

**Mary Beth Murphy, RN, MS,
CDE, MBA**
Research Nurse Director
Department of Medicine
University of Tennessee College
  of Medicine
Memphis, Tennessee

Antonello Pileggi, MD
Research Assistant Professor
  of Surgery
Department of Surgery and the
  Diabetes Research Institute
University of Miami Miller School
  of Medicine
Miami, Florida

Camillo Ricordi, MD
Stacy Joy Goodman Professor
  of Surgery
Diabetes Research Institute
University of Miami Miller School
  of Medicine
Miami, Florida

F. John Service, MDCM, PhD
Professor of Medicine
Department of Medicine
Mayo Medical School
Rochester, Minnesota

Arun Sharma, PhD
Assistant Professor
Department of Medicine
Harvard Medical School
Investigator, Islet Transplantation and
  Cell Biology
Joslin Diabetes Center
Boston, Massachusetts

Jay S. Skyler, MD
Professor of Medicine, Pediatrics, and
  Psychology
Division of Endocrinology Diabetes
  and Metabolism
Associate Director, Diabetes
  Research Institute
University of Miami Miller School
  of Medicine
Miami, Florida

Robert C. Stanton, MD
Assistant Professor of Medicine
Department of Medicine
Harvard Medical School
Chief, Renal Section
Joslin Diabetes Center
Boston, Massachusetts

Ervin Szoke, MD
Assistant Professor
Department of Medicine
University of Rochester School
  of Medicine and Dentistry
Rochester, New York

Aaron I. Vinik, MD, PhD
Professor of Medicine
The Strelitz Diabetes Institutes
  at Eastern Virginia Medical School
Norfolk, Virginia

Gordon C. Weir, MD
Professor
Department of Medicine
Harvard Medical School
Head, Islet Transplantation and
  Cell Biology
Joslin Diabetes Center
Boston, Massachusetts

Morris F. White, PhD
Associate Professor
Department of Biological and
  Biomedical Sciences
Harvard Medical School
Associate Investigator
Howard Hughes Medical Institute
Children's Hospital Boston
Boston, Massachusetts

Contents

REGULATION OF INSULIN SECRETION AND ISLET CELL FUNCTION

Gordon C. Weir, Susan Bonner-Weir, and Arun Sharma

1

The β cells of the islets of Langerhans are the only cells in the body that make a meaningful quantity of insulin, a hormone that has evolved to be essential for life, exerting critical control over carbohydrate, fat, and protein metabolism. Islets are scattered throughout the pancreas; they vary in size but typically contain about 1000 cells, of which approximately 80% are β cells located in a central core surrounded by a mantle of non–β cells. A human pancreas contains about one million islets, which comprise only about 1% of the mass of the pancreas. Insulin is released into the portal vein, which means the liver is exposed to particularly high concentrations of insulin.

Insulin secretion from β cells responds very precisely to small changes in glucose concentration in the physiologic range, thereby keeping glucose levels within the range of 70 to 150 mg/dL in normal individuals. β cells have a unique differentiation that permits linkage of physiologic levels of glucose to the metabolic signals that control the release of insulin. Thus, there is a close correlation between the rate of glucose metabolism and insulin secretion. This is dependent on the oxidation of glucose-derived acetyl-coenzyme A and also NADH generated by glycolysis, which is shuttled to mitochondria to contribute to adenosine triphosphate (ATP) production. Insulin secretion is also regulated by various other physiologic signals. During eating, insulin secretion is enhanced by not only glucose but also by amino acids and the gut hormones glucagon-like peptide-1 (GLP-1) and gastric inhibitory peptide. Free fatty acids can also modulate insulin secretion, particularly to help maintain insulin secretion during prolonged fasting. The parasympathetic nervous system has a stimulatory effect exerted by acetylcholine and probably the peptidergic mediator vasoactive intestinal polypeptide (VIP), which may also contribute to enhanced insulin secretion during eating. With epinephrine from the adrenal medulla and norepinephrine from nerve terminals, the sympathetic nervous system acts on α-adrenergic receptors to inhibit insulin secretion. This suppression of insulin is particularly useful during exercise. Important drugs include sulfonylureas, which have a stimulatory influence useful for the treatment of diabetes, and diazoxide, with an inhibitory effect used for treatment of hypoglycemia caused by insulin-producing tumors.

Type 1 diabetes is caused by reduced β-cell mass resulting from autoimmune destruction of β cells, which leads to profound insulin deficiency that can progress to fatal hyperglycemia and ketoacidosis. The non–β cells of the islet are spared, with glucagon secretion actually being excessive, which accounts for some of the hyperglycemia of the diabetic state. The situation is more complicated in type 2 diabetes, which has a strong genetic basis that predisposes individuals to obesity and insulin resistance, a problem greatly magnified by our Western lifestyle with its plentiful food and lack of physical activity. Diabetes, however, only develops when β cells are no longer able to compensate for this insulin resistance. Indeed, most people with insulin resistance never develop diabetes, but as our population ages, more β-cell decompensation occurs and the prevalence of diabetes increases. Pathology studies indicate that β-cell mass in type 2 diabetes is about 50% of normal and that islet cells often are infiltrated with amyloid deposits that may have a toxic effect on β cells.

In all forms of diabetes, whether type 2 diabetes, early type 1 diabetes, or failing pancreas or islet transplants, insulin secretory abnormalities are found that seem largely secondary to exposure of β cells to the diabetic milieu and that are reversible if normoglycemia can be restored. The most prominent abnormality is an impairment of glucose-induced insulin secretion, which is more severe for early release (first phase) than the longer second phase of secretion. In contrast, β-cell responses to such nonglucose secretagogues as arginine, GLP-1, isoproterenol, or sulfonylureas are more intact. The cause of these β-cell secretory abnormalities is not fully understood, but β cells exposed to abnormally high glucose concentrations lose the differentiation that normally equips them with the unique metabolic machinery needed for glucose-induced insulin secretion. Marked abnormalities are found at the level of gene expression that appear to have a crippling effect on the metabolic integrity of the β cell.

Abnormalities of glucagon secretion are also found in both forms of diabetes, with secretion not being appropriately suppressed by hyperglycemia or stimulated by hypoglycemia, which is problematic because glucagon is an important counterregulatory hormone for protection against hypoglycemia. This failure of glucagon to respond makes people with type 1 diabetes more vulnerable to the dangers of insulin-induced hypoglycemia.

Anatomy, Embryology, and Physiology

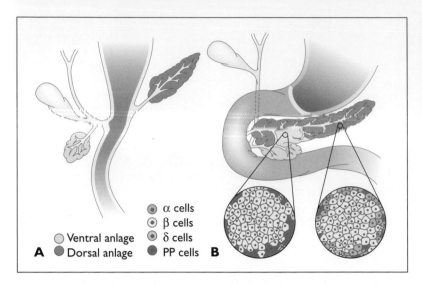

A ○ Ventral anlage
● Dorsal anlage

◉ α cells
◉ β cells
◉ δ cells
● PP cells

B

FIGURE 1-1. Embryologic origin of the pancreas and islet cells. A dorsal anlage and one or two ventral anlagen form from the primitive gut (**A**) and later fuse (**B**) [1]. The ventral anlage forms part of the head of the pancreas and has pancreatic polypeptide-rich islet cells with few, if any, α cells. The dorsal anlage forms the major portion of the pancreas, that being the tail, body, and part of the head; here the islets are glucagon rich and pancreatic polypeptide poor. Roughly, the α and PP cells substitute for each other in number (15% to 25% of the islet cells), the percentages of β cells (70% to 80%) and δ cells (5%) remain the same.

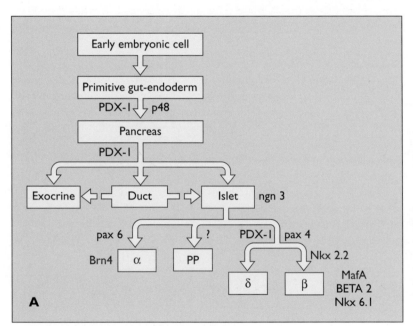

A

B. UNIQUE β-CELL DIFFERENTIATION

Increased Expression	Decreased Expression
GLUT2	Glucose-6-phosphatase
Glucokinase	Hexokinase
mGPDH	Lactate dehydrogenase
Pyruvate carboxylase	PEPCK
Insulin	c-myc
IAPP	
PDX-1	
Nkx 6.1	

FIGURE 1-2. Pancreatic and islet cell differentiation. The complex control of differentiation of the pancreas and its three major components (exocrine acinar cells, ducts, and islets of Langerhans) is being elucidated by genetic analysis (**A** and **B**) [1–5]. At present, only some of the transcription factors that are involved in the transition from endoderm to pancreas and then to final mature pancreatic cell types are known; several of them (BETA 2, Nkx 2.2, Nkx 6.1, and ngn 3) are also involved in the development of the nervous system. One that is clearly necessary, but not sufficient, is PDX-1 (ipf-1, stf-1, idx-1); without it, no

pancreas is formed, and later it seems to be needed for β-cell differentiation. Exocrine and islets differentiate from the pancreatic ductal epithelium, but whether they arise from the same precursor pool or even whether all the islet cells share a cell lineage remains unanswered. GLUT2—glucose transporter 2; IAPP—islet amyloid polypeptide; mGPDH— mitochondrial glycerol phosphate dehydrogenase; PEPCK— phosphoenolpyruvate carboxykinase; PP—pancreatic polypeptide. (*Adapted from* Edlund [1].)

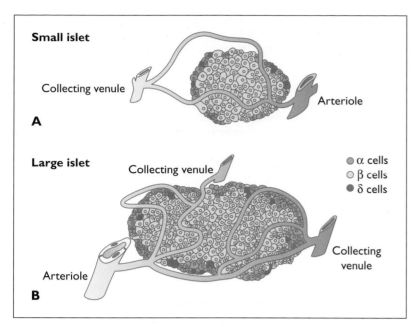

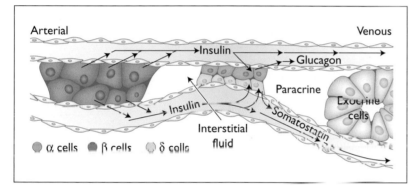

Small islet

Collecting venule

A

Arteriole

Large islet

Collecting venule

- ● α cells
- ○ β cells
- ● δ cells

Arteriole

B

Collecting venule

FIGURE 1-3. Islet vasculature and core/mantle relations. A diagrammatic summary of combined data from corrosion casts and the serial reconstructions of rat islet cells [6]. In small and large islets, β cells make up the central core, and the non–β cells (α, pancreatic polypeptide [PP], and δ cells) form the surrounding mantle. The α cells containing glucagon are found mainly in islets of the dorsal lobe of the pancreas, PP cells are found mainly in ventral lobe islets, and δ cells containing somatostatin are found in the islets of both lobes of the pancreas.

Short arterioles enter an islet at discontinuities of the non–β-cell mantle and branch into capillaries that form a glomerular-like structure. After traversing the β-cell mass, capillaries penetrate the mantle of non–β -cells as the blood leaves the islet. **A,** In small islets (< 160 μm in diameter), efferent capillaries pass through exocrine tissue before coalescing into collecting venules. **B,** In large islets (> 260 μm diameter), capillaries coalesce at the edge of the islet and run along the mantle as collecting venules.

Arterial

Venous

Insulin

Glucagon

Paracrine

Exocrine cells

Insulin

Somatostatin

Interstitial fluid

● α cells ● β cells ○ δ cells

FIGURE 1-4. The relationship between islet core and mantle, indicating potential intraislet portal flow and paracrine interactions. This formulation is based on the known vascular anatomy and studies with passive immunization [6,7]. These relationships suggest that β cells, being upstream, are unlikely to be very much influenced by the glucagon and somatostatin produced by the α cells and δ cells of the islet mantle, respectively. The downstream α cells, however, may be strongly influenced by insulin from the upstream β cells, which have a suppressive influence on glucagon secretion. This helps explain why glucagon secretion cannot be suppressed by the hyperglycemia of diabetes, which means that glucagon is secreted in excessive amounts, thus further contributing to the hyperglycemia of diabetes. This vascular pattern is known as the islet-acinar portal circulation, which means that islet hormones are released downstream directly onto exocrine cells; insulin in particular is thought to have a trophic effect on the exocrine pancreas.

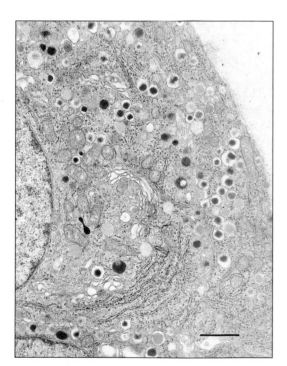

FIGURE 1-5. Electron micrograph of a β cell. The four major endocrine cell types in mammalian islet cells are the insulin-producing β cell, the glucagon-producing α cell, the somatostatin-producing δ cell, and the pancreatic polypeptide (PP)-producing PP cell. Recently, the ε cell expressing ghrelin has been identified as a consistent small population of cells in the islet [8]. Ultrastructural and immunocytochemical techniques are used to distinguish these cell types. β cells are polyhedral, being truncated pyramids about 10 X 10 X 8 μm, and are usually well granulated with about 10,000 secretory granules. The two forms of insulin granules (250 to 350 nm in diameter) are 1) mature ones with an electron-dense core that is visibly crystalline in some species and a loosely fitting granule-limiting membrane giving the appearance of a spacious halo and 2) immature granules with little or no halo and moderately electron-dense contents. Immature granules have been shown to be the major, if not the only, site of proinsulin to insulin conversion [9]. In each granule besides insulin, there are at least 100 other peptides, including islet amyloid polypeptide ([IAPP], amylin) [10].

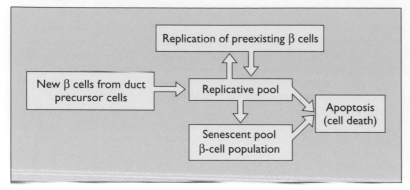

FIGURE 1-6. Mechanisms responsible for maintenance of β-cell mass. In normal development and in experimental studies, it has become apparent that the population of β cells within an adult pancreas is dynamic and responds to metabolic demand with changes in mass and function in an effort to maintain euglycemia. The mass of β cells can change by cell number or cell size. The cell size or volume can change dramatically in moving from an atrophied to a hypertrophy state. Two mechanisms add new β cells: differentiation from precursor or stem cells in the ducts (often called *neogenesis*) and replication from preexisting β cells [11]. It has been suggested that most cell types have a limited number of replications, after which the ability to respond to replication signals is lost and they are considered as senescent cells. These senescent cells can be long lived and are functional, even with functions (terminally differentiated) that are not present in younger replicative cells. Additionally, as with all cell types, β cells must have a finite lifespan and die by apoptosis [12]. The turnover of β cells implies that there are differently aged β cells at any stage of development. Adult β cells have only a low basal rate of replication, but this rate must be enough to counterbalance cell loss and to accommodate functional demand.

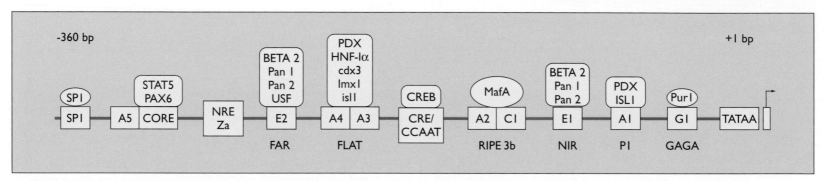

FIGURE 1-7. The promoter region of the insulin gene showing key enhancer elements and known binding transcription factors. Insulin gene expression is regulated by sequences at least 4 kb upstream from the transcription start site (represented by an *arrow* and designated as +1 bp) of the insulin gene. In adult mammals, insulin is selectively expressed in pancreatic β cells. A small (< 400 bp) region of insulin promoter that is highly conserved in various mammalian species can regulate this selective expression and contains the major glucose control elements. This region can also recapitulate glucose responsive insulin gene expression.

In the figure, the organization of the proximal portion (-360 to +1 bp) of the insulin promoter is shown. Functionally conserved enhancer elements are illustrated as *boxes*. New names for these elements are shown within the boxes, and old names are shown below each box. Above the boxes are shown the names of cloned transcription factors that can bind corresponding elements. Enhancer elements E1, A2-C1, A4-A3, and E2 have been implicated in β-cell–specific expression of the insulin gene. The cell type–specific expression is mediated by

the restricted cellular distribution of the transcription factors (such as BETA 2, MafA, and PDX-1) that bind these elements [3]. Furthermore, these elements, along with element Za, are also responsible for glucose-regulated insulin gene expression. Other enhancer elements, CRE/CCAAT and CORE, regulate insulin gene expression in response to other signals such as cAMP (cyclic adenosine 3',5'-monophosphate) by regulating cAMP response element-binding (CREB) protein and growth hormone or leptin (via signal transducer and activator of transcription [STAT] factor 5).

In addition to their role in regulating cell-specific and glucose responsive expression, insulin gene transcription factors are involved in pancreatic development and differentiation of β cells. Lack of transcription factors such as PDX-1, BETA 2, PAX6, HNF-1α, and ISL1 results in complete absence of or abnormal pancreatic development. Although humans with a mutant allele for PDX-1, BETA 2, or HNF-1α develop maturity-onset diabetes of youth, individuals with mutations in both PDX-1 alleles show pancreatic agenesis. (*Adapted from* Sander and German [3].)

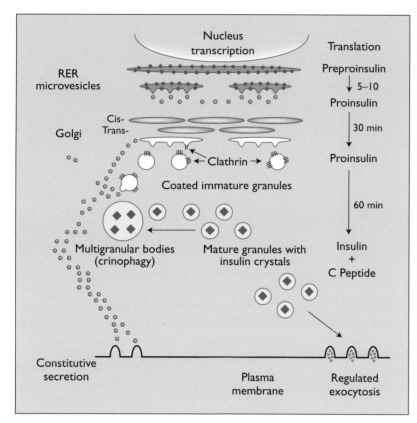

FIGURE 1-8. Pathways of insulin biosynthesis. Glucose stimulates the production of preproinsulin through effects on transcription and even stronger influences on translation. Shortly after its inception, preproinsulin is cleaved to proinsulin, which is then transported through the Golgi and packaged into clathrin-coated immature granules, where proinsulin is further processed to proinsulin-like peptides, insulin, and C peptide. Granules containing crystallized insulin can either remain in a storage compartment; be absorbed into multigranular bodies, where they are degraded by the process of crinophagy; or be secreted via the regulated pathway of secretion, the final event being exocytosis. Although the vast majority of insulin is secreted through the regulated pathway, a small amount can be released from microvesicles through the pathway of constitutive secretion [9,13,14].

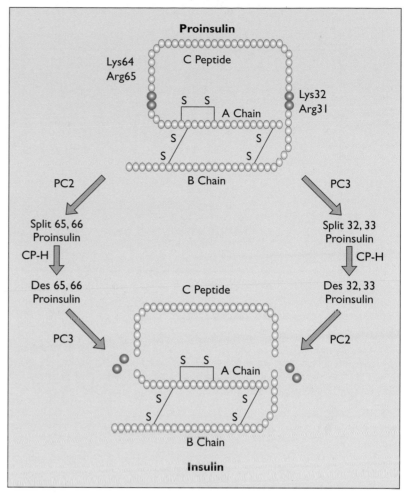

FIGURE 1-9. Proinsulin processing. Proinsulin is cleaved by endopeptidases contained in secretory granules, which act at the two dibasic sites, Arg31, Arg32 and Lys64, Arg65. PC2 also is known as type II proinsulin-processing endopeptidase, and PC3 is the type I endopeptidase. After cleavage by either PC2 or PC3, the dibasic amino acids are removed by the exopeptidase carboxypeptidase H (CP-H). Insulin and C peptide are usually released in equimolar amounts. Of the secreted insulin immunoreactivity, about 2% to 4% consists of proinsulin and proinsulin-related peptides. Because the clearance of these peptides in the circulation is considerably slower than that of insulin, they account for 10% to 40% of circulating insulin immunoreactivity. About one third of proinsulin-like immunoreactivity is accounted for by proinsulin, and most of the rest by des 32-33 split proinsulin, with only small amounts of des 65-66 split proinsulin being present. In type 2 diabetes, the ratio of proinsulin-like peptides to insulin is increased; in impaired glucose tolerance, this finding is less consistent. The increased proportion of secreted proinsulin-like peptides is thought to be caused by depletion of mature granules from the increased secretory demand by hyperglycemia, leading to the release of the incompletely processed contents of the available immature granules [13,14]. (*Adapted from* Rhodes [13].)

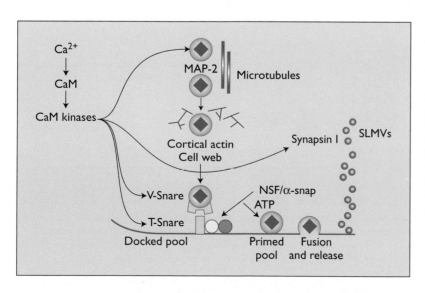

FIGURE 1-10. Distal steps of secretion. Insulin-containing secretory granules are associated with microtubules, and then move to the cell surface via further interactions with the microfilaments of the cortical actin web. Increased cytosolic calcium plays a key role in several distal steps. Initially, calcium binds to calmodulin (CaM), which can bind the CaM kinases. CaM kinase II has been localized to insulin secretory granules. These kinases can then phosphorylate proteins such as microtubule-associated protein-2 (MAP-2) and synapsin I, which may be involved in the exocytosis of synaptic-like microvesicles (SLMV). They may also regulate the key proteins involved in the docking of granules, v-SNARES (synaptobrevin [VAMP] and cellubrevin) and t-SNARES (SNAP-25 and syntaxin). The docking complex binds to α-SNAP (soluble NSF attachment protein) and NSF (N-ethyl-maleimide-sensitive fusion protein), the latter having ATPase activity, which probably allows the formation of fusion competent granules that are primed for release as the first phase of insulin secretion. (*Adapted from* Easom [15].)

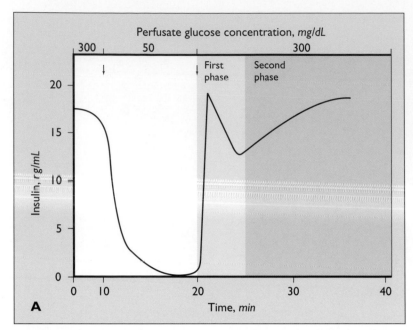

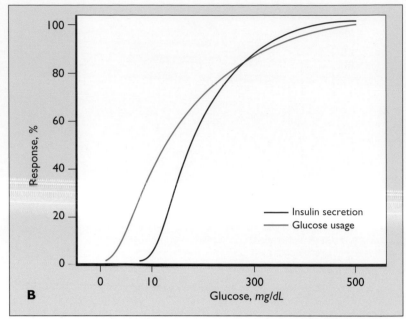

FIGURE 1-11. Glucose stimulation of insulin secretion. **A,** Insulin secretion from the isolated perfused rat pancreas. At glucose concentrations at 50 mg/dL or below, insulin secretory rates are very low. Challenge with a high concentration of glucose provokes a biphasic pattern of insulin response [16]. **B,**Comparative rates of insulin secretion and glucose utilization in isolated rat islets.

Glucose utilization was measured by the conversion of 5-tritiated glucose to tritiated H_2O [17]. The curves show the close relationship between the two except at glucose concentrations below 4 mmol. Similar relationships are found between insulin secretion and glucose oxidation as measured by conversion of labeled glucose to carbon dioxide. (Adapted from Leahy et al. [16].)

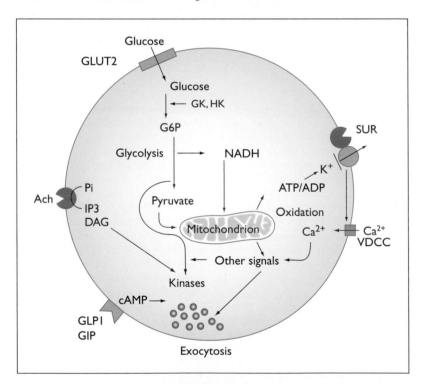

FIGURE 1-12. Mechanisms of β-cell secretion. Glucose enters the β cell through a facultative glucose transporter that allows rapid equilibration between extra- and intracellular glucose concentrations. Although glucose transporter 2 (GLUT2) is dominant in many species, glucose transporter 1 (GLUT1) may be more important in humans. Glucose is phosphorylated mainly by glucokinase (GK) rather than hexokinase (HK) [17]. Metabolism increases the ratio of adenosine triphosphate (ATP) to adenosine diphosphate (ADP), through oxidation via pyruvate and by nicotinamide adenine dinucleotide phosphate (NADP) that is brought by shuttles into mitochondria [18]. The increases in the ATP-to-ADP ratio inhibit the ATP-sensitive potassium channel, which leads to depolarization and opening of voltage-dependent calcium channels (VDCC), with a resultant major increase in cytosolic calcium, which, in turn, triggers exocytosis. Glucose-stimulated insulin secretion is caused by two mechanisms: the triggering pathway, which is potassium channel ATP dependent, and the amplifying pathway, which is potassium channel ATP independent [19]. The molecular basis of the latter pathway is unknown. Cytosolic calcium levels can also be increased by release of calcium from the endoplasmic reticulum. Insulin secretion can also be stimulated by agents such as acetylcholine (Ach) that, via muscarinic receptors, work through lipid mediators such as inositol 1,4,5-triphosphate (IP3) and diacylglycerol (DAG). Glucagon-like peptide 1 (GLP-1) and gastric inhibitory peptide (GIP) are hormones released from the gut with meals that stimulate secretion via adenylate cyclase and cyclic adenosine 3',5'-monophosphate (cAMP) [20]. Many other agents also influence insulin secretion.

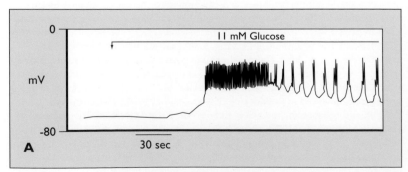

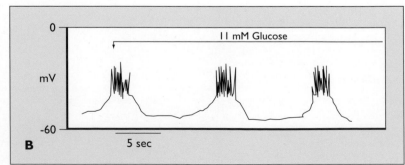

FIGURE 1-13. Glucose-induced electrical activity of the mouse β cell. **A,** The electrical activity of a mouse β cell contained in an isolated islet induced by stimulation with 11-mM glucose. When the membrane depolarizes to about -50 mV, bursting occurs, which is periodic electrical activity. Note the biphasic pattern of electrical activity, which may be related to the first phase of insulin

secretion but is shorter in duration and unlikely to be the full explanation. **B,** When depolarization reaches about -35 mV, action potentials, or spikes, occur, which are best seen in the expanded scale here. When glucose levels are very high (> 22 mM), continuous spiking activity is observed.

(Continued on next page)

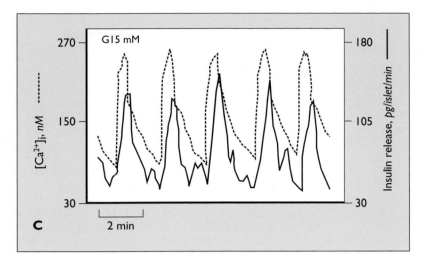

FIGURE 1-13. *(Continued)* **C,** Comparison of the oscillations of insulin release and calcium in a single pancreatic mouse islet during steady state stimulation with 15-mM glucose, suggesting a cause-and-effect relationship. Calcium was measured with fluorescence of fura-2 loaded into islets. Increased calcium spikes come mainly from entrance of extracellular calcium through L-type voltage-gated calcium channels. The depolarization is mainly caused by closure of adenosine triphosphate–regulated potassium channels [19]. (*Panels A and B adapted from* Mears and Atwater [21]; *panel C adapted from* Gilon et al. [22].)

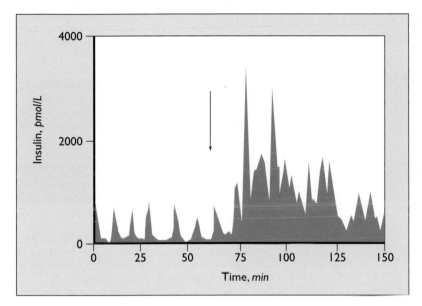

FIGURE 1-14. Pulsatile insulin secretion. Insulin is normally secreted in coordinated secretory bursts. In humans, pulses occur about every 10 minutes. In dogs, they occur somewhat more rapidly, at about 7-minute intervals in a basal state. Although the variations in peripheral insulin levels are modest, marked variations can be found in the portal vein [23]. Basal pulsation is depicted during the 60-minute period. After oral ingestion of glucose (*arrow*), which produces a glucose stimulus and an incretin effect, an increase in the amplitude of the bursts is seen, as well as an increase in frequency, with intervals decreasing from about 7 to 5 minutes. The mechanisms controlling the oscillations are uncertain. Metabolic oscillation of glycolysis must play a key role, but there may also be some kind of neural network that can coordinate communication between islets in different parts of the pancreas. (*Adapted from* Porksen et al. [23].)

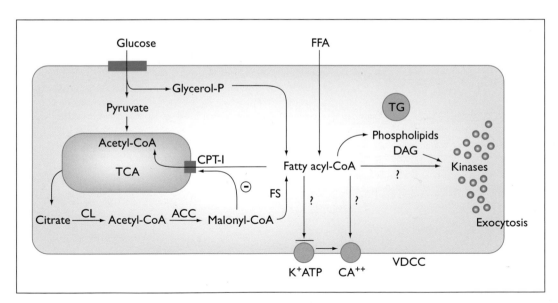

FIGURE 1-15. Fatty acid influence on β-cell function. Fat metabolism is likely to have important influences upon insulin secretion, but the mechanisms responsible for these effects are still not well understood. It appears that the modest elevations of free fatty acids (FFAs) of obesity contribute to the hyperinsulinemia of that state. Depletion of circulating FFAs during prolonged fasting when glucose levels are low and β-cell lipid stores depleted results in impairment of insulin secretion. Excessive elevations of FFAs can have an inhibitory influence on insulin secretion.

Some of glucose-stimulated insulin secretion may be mediated not only by glucose metabolism but also by fatty acid mediators. Thus, increases in glucose metabolism may produce increased cytosolic concentrations of citrate, which can be converted by citrate lyase (CL) to acetyl-CoA, which can be turned into malonyl-coenzyme A (CoA) by acetyl-CoA carboxylase (ACC). Malonyl-CoA, can inhibit carnitine palmitoyltransferase I (CPT-I), which helps control the entrance of fatty acyl-CoA into the fatty acid oxidation pathways of mitochondria. By inhibiting the entrance of fatty acyl-CoA into mitochondria, fatty acid mediators may be generated in the cytoplasm that may influence insulin secretion.

Fatty acids that enter the β cell could be converted to fatty acid mediators, which can act upon ion channels, kinases, or through other mechanisms to stimulate the exocytosis of insulin. Some of the lipid mediators include the phospholipid inositol 1,4,5-triphosphate (IP3) and diacylglycerol (DAG), which can act via protein kinase C. Alternatively, fatty acids could be stored as triglycerides (TGs) for use during times of fuel deprivation. Under some circumstances fatty acid oxidation may contribute to ATP formation and thus help close the ATP-sensitive potassium channel (K^+ ATP) resulting in depolarization and opening of the voltage-dependent calcium channels (VDCC). TCA—tricarboxylic acid cycle. (*Adapted from* McGarry and Dobbins [24] and Prentki and Corkey [25].)

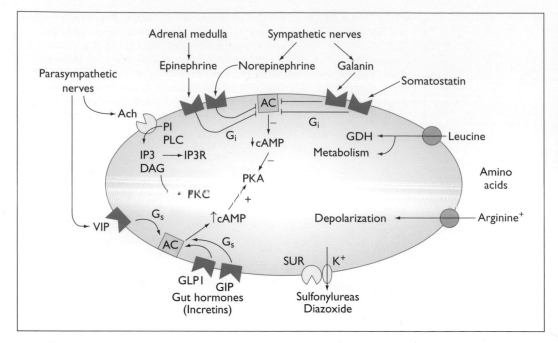

FIGURE 1-16. Effects on insulin secretion by the autonomic nervous system, gut hormones, amino acids, and drugs. The parasympathetic arm of the autonomic nervous system has a stimulatory influence upon insulin secretion exerted by acetylcholine acting mainly through phospholipase C (PLC) to generate inositol phosphate mediators and diacylglycerol (DAG). Parasympathetic stimulation also leads to release of the

peptide mediator vasoactive intestinal peptide (VIP), which enhances secretion via stimulatory G proteins (G_S) acting through adenylate cyclase (AC). The sympathetic nervous system inhibits insulin secretion, with epinephrine and norepinephrine having a negative effect on AC through inhibitory G proteins (G_i). The sympathetic peptide mediator galanin and somatostatin have inhibitory effects on insulin secretion through similar mechanisms. The gut hormones glucagon-like peptide-1 (GLP-1) and gastric inhibitory peptide (GIP) stimulate insulin secretion through cAMP (cyclic adenosine 3',5'-monophosphate) and protein kinase A (PKA). Sulfonylureas stimulate insulin secretion by acting on the sulfonylurea receptor (SUR) to close the adenosine triphosphate (ATP)-sensitive potassium channel, which causes depolarization. Diazoxide has an opposite effect, leading to hyperpolarization, which is inhibitory. Amino acids stimulate insulin secretion by several mechanisms. Arginine is positively charged, producing depolarization when transported into β cells, but this is not an important mechanism at physiologic concentrations of arginine. Leucine can influence insulin secretion by being oxidized via acetyl coenzyme A (CoA) or through a more complex metabolic effect mediated by glutamate dehydrogenase (GDH). IP3—inositol 3 phosphate; IP3R—inositol 3 phosphate receptor.

Insulin Secretion in Type 2 Diabetes

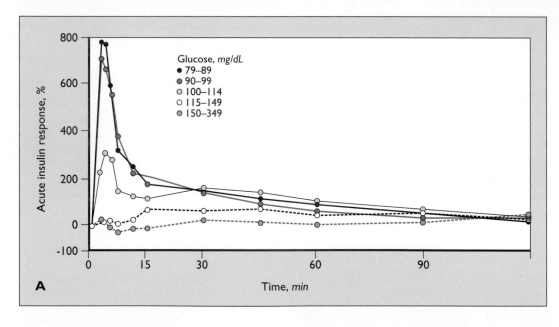

A

FIGURE 1-17. Insulin secretory characteristics in type 2 diabetes. **A,** Loss of early insulin secretory response to an intravenous (IV) glucose challenge as fasting plasma glucose increases in subjects progressing from the normal state toward type 2 diabetes [26]. It should be noted that impaired insulin responses to glucoses can even be seen before glucose levels increase to levels required for the diagnosis of impaired glucose tolerance (fasting glucose levels ≥ 110 mg/dL).

(Continued on next page)

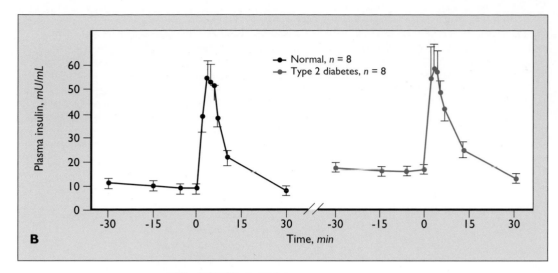

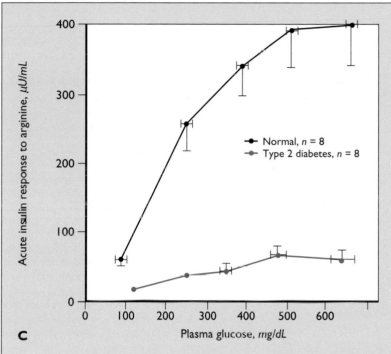

FIGURE 1-17. *(Continued)* **B,** Preservation of acute insulin secretion in response to an IV pulse of arginine in type 2 diabetes [27]. The acute insulin responses to glucose were lost in these subjects. Insulin responses are also preserved for a variety of other secretagogues, including isoproterenol, sulfonylureas, and the gut hormone glucagon-like peptide 1 (GLP-1). **C,** Loss of glucose influence on arginine-stimulated insulin secretion in type 2 diabetes [28]. The insulin secretory responses to a 350 mg/dL glucose concentration in subjects with type 2 diabetes were similar to the responses to an 80 mg/dL glucose concentration in control subjects. However, when the glucose concentrations in control subjects were increased with glucose infusions, the insulin responses far exceeded those of subjects with type 2 diabetes. Because individuals with type 2 diabetes have been found to have a β-cell mass approximately 50% of normal, the response in these subjects, which is only about 15% of control subjects, suggests that the secretory capacity for a given β-cell mass is severely impaired. (*Adapted from* Ward et al. [28].)

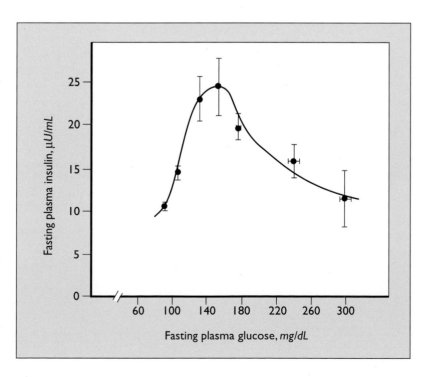

FIGURE 1-18. Inverted U-shaped curve of insulin secretion during progression from normal state to type 2 diabetes. Fasting plasma insulin levels rise as fasting glucose levels climb into the range of impaired glucose tolerance but then fall as diabetes develops and worsens. A similar pattern can be seen for plasma insulin levels obtained after an oral glucose or meal challenge. The rising insulin levels are likely to reflect a compensatory response to increasing insulin resistance, while the falling levels are indicative of β-cell failure, probably through a combination of impaired function and reduced β-cell mass. (*Adapted from* DeFronzo *et al.* [29].)

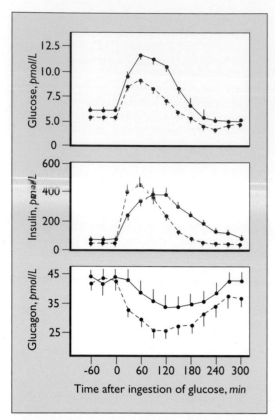

FIGURE 1-19. Insulin secretory profiles in the state of impaired glucose tolerance (IGT) (*solid line*) during an oral glucose tolerance test (OGTT). The insulin responses at 60 and 90 minutes may be higher than those found in control patients (*broken line*), which probably reflects the combined influence of higher glucose levels at these time points and insulin resistance. Importantly, the insulin responses at 30 minutes in patients with IGT are typically lower than normal, indicating the presence of a reduction in early impairment of glucagon suppression, leading to an inefficient suppression of hepatic glucose output, which contributes to the higher glucose levels found in the latter stages of OGTT. The early insulin responses found after oral glucose are higher than those seen after an intravenous glucose challenge. This is thought to be attributable to the insulinotropic effects of the gut peptides glucagon-like peptide-1 (GLP-1) and gastric inhibitory peptide (GIP) and possibly to some influence from activation of the parasympathetic nervous system. (*Adapted from* Mitrakou et al. [30].)

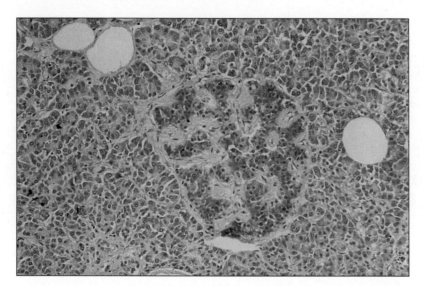

FIGURE 1-20. Amyloid deposits in islets in type 2 diabetes. In this photomicrograph of an islet, insulin-containing cells are immunostained, and amyloid deposition can be seen in the pericapillary space. The amyloid, found in a high proportion of the islets of people with type 2 diabetes, consists of β-pleated sheets of the islet amyloid polypeptide (IAPP, amylin), which consists of 37 amino acids. The sequence between positions 20 and 29 is important for the ability of this peptide to form amyloid. Production of IAPP is restricted to β cells, and its content is only approximately 1% that of insulin. Amyloid deposition adjacent to β cells is found in patients with diabetes and some insulinomas but not in the normal state nor in obesity, with its insulin resistance and high rates of insulin secretion [31]. The mechanisms responsible for its deposition are not known. It is also unclear whether this amyloid formation contributes to the pathogenesis of type 2 diabetes, but it has been shown that human IAPP aggregates have a toxic effect on islet cells.

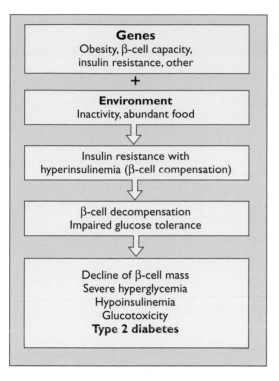

FIGURE 1-21. Pathogenesis of type 2 diabetes. This schema shows the various factors that contribute to the pathogenesis of type 2 diabetes [30]. Genes are likely to determine how well β cells can function over a lifetime. For example, most of the gene defects of maturity-onset diabetes of youth ([MODY] 1, 3, and 4) and some mutations of mitochondrial DNA lead to diabetes, which often does not become manifest until middle age. Some genes probably exist that limit the ability of β-cell mass to compensate for insulin resistance over decades and even lead to a critical reduction in β-cell mass. Everything is made worse by the challenges of Western lifestyle, with its plentiful food and lack of exercise. After hyperglycemia develops, glucose toxicity can produce further impairment of β-cell function and worsen insulin resistance. Lipotoxicity also appears to have adverse effects on the same two sites.

STAGES OF β CELL DECOMPENSATION IN DIABETES

Compensation for insulin resistance

β-cell hypertrophy

β-cell hyperplasia

Shift to the left of glucose dose-response curve

(Increased secretion per cell at given glucose level)

"Normal" or increased glucose-induced insulin secretion

Decompensation: mild hyperglycemia

Loss of glucose-induced insulin secretion

Preservation of responses to nonglucose secretagogues (arginine and others)

Normal insulin stores

Early β-cell dedifferentiation

Decreased gene expression of GLUT2, glucokinase, mGPDH, pyruvate carboxylase, VDCC, SERCA3, IP3R-II, and trascription factors (pdx-1, HNFs, Nkx 6.1, and pax-6)

Increased gene expression of LDH, hexokinase, glucose-6-phosphatase, and the transcription factor c-myc

Decompensation: severe hyperglycemia

Loss of glucose-induced insulin secretion

Impairment of responses to nonglucose secretagogues (arginine and others)

Increased ratio of secreted proinsulin to insulin

Reduced insulin stores (degranulation)

More severe β-cell dedifferentiation

Decreased gene expression of insulin, IAPP, glucokinase, Kir 6.2, SERCA2b, and transcription factor BETA 2

Increased gene expression of glucose-6-phosphatase, 12-lipoxygenase, fatty acid synthase, and the transcription factor C/EBPβ

FIGURE 1-22. Stages of β-cell decomposition in diabetes [32–36]. GLUT2—glucose transporter 2; HNF—hepatocyte nuclear factor; IAPP—islet amyloid polypeptide; IP3R-II—IP3 receptor; LDH—lactate dehydrogenase; mGPDH—mitochondrial glycerol phosphate dehydrogenase; SERCA—sarco-endoplasmic reticulum Ca²⁺-ATPase; VDCC—voltage-dependent calcium channel.

β CELL GLUCOTOXICITY AND LIPOTOXICITY

Abnormal β-cell function in diabetes: β-cell function in diabetes is abnormal, whether in type 2 diabetes, early type 1 diabetes, or with an inadequate number of transplanted islets. A variety of secondary abnormalities have been identified, most notably loss of glucose-stimulated insulin secretion (GSIS), thought to be caused by exposure of β cells to the diabetic milieu

Definition problem: Descriptive terms include the following: glucotoxicity, lipotoxicity, exhaustion, excess demand, decreased reserve, fatigue, overwork, desensitization, stress, dysfunction, and others

Glucotoxicity

Loss of GSIS is tightly tied to modest climbs in glucose levels

Reduction of GSIS can be seen with fasting plasma glucose (FPG) of 100 mg/dL

Complete loss usually when FPG is greater than 115 mg/dL

Abnormal GSIS in a diabetic state can be seen in absence of free fatty acid (FFA) increase

Lipotoxicity

FFAs are important for β-cell function, at least as a permissive factor

Increased FFAs of obesity are associated with high GSIS

Close correlation between FFAs of mild diabetes and loss of GSIS is not well established

Very high FFAs inhibit GSIS

Synergy between FFAs and hyperglycemia is not yet understood

FFAs are important for maintaining insulin secretion during a prolonged fast

FIGURE 1-23. β-cell glucotoxicity and lipotoxicity [24,25,35,36].

References

1. Edlund H: Transcribing pancreas. *Diabetes* 1998, 47:1817–1823.

2. Olbrot M, Rud J, Moss LG, Sharma A: Identification of beta-cell-specific insulin gene transcription factor RIPE3b1 as mammalian MafA. *Proc Natl Acad Sci U S A* 2002, 99:6737–6742.

3. Sander M, German MS: The β-cell transcription factors and development of the pancreas. *J Mol Med* 1997, 75:327–340.

4. Kawaguchi Y, Cooper B, Gannon M, et al.: The role of the transcriptional regulator Ptf1a in converting intestinal to pancreatic progenitors. *Nat Genet* 2002, 32:128–34.

5. Matsuoka TA, Artner I, Henderson E, et al.: The MafA transcription factor appears to be responsible for tissue-specific expression of insulin. *Proc Natl Acad Sci U S A* 2004, 101:2930–2933.

6. Bonner-Weir S, Orci L: New perspectives on the microvasculature of the islets of Langerhans in the rat. *Diabetes* 1982, 31:883–939.

7. Weir GC, Bonner-Weir S: Islets of Langerhans: the puzzle of intraislet interactions and their relevance to diabetes. *J Clin Invest* 1990, 85:983–987.

8. Prado CL, Pugh-Bernard AE, Elghazi L, et al.: Ghrelin cells replace insulin-producing beta cells in two mouse models of pancreas development. *Proc Natl Acad Sci U S A* 2004, 101:2924–2929.

9. Orci L: The insulin factory: a tour of the plant surroundings and a visit to the assembly line. *Diabetologia* 1985, 28:528–546.

10. Guest PC, Bailyes EM, Rutherford NG, Hutton JC: Insulin secretory granule biogenesis. *Biochem J* 1991, 274:73–78.

11. Bonner-Weir S, Baxter LA, Schuppin GT, Smith FE: A second pathway for regeneration of the adult exocrine and endocrine pancreas: a possible recapitulation of embryonic development. *Diabetes* 1993, 42:1715–1720.

12. Finegood DT, Scaglia L, Bonner-Weir S: (Perspective) Dynamics of β-cell mass in the growing rat pancreas: estimation with a simple mathematical model. *Diabetes* 1995, 44:249–256.

13. Rhodes CJ: Processing of the insulin molecule. In *Diabetes Mellitus: A Fundamental and Clinical Text*, edn 3. Edited by LeRoith D, Taylor SI, Olefsky JM. Philadelphia: Lippincott Williams & Wilkins; 2004:27–50.

14. Rhodes CJ, Alarcon C: What β-cell defect could lead to hyperproinsulinemia in NIDDM: some clues from recent advances made in understanding the proinsulin conversion mechanism. *Diabetes* 1994, 3:511–517.

15. Easom RA: CaM kinase II: a protein kinase with extraordinary talents germane to insulin exocytosis. *Diabetes* 1999, 48:675–684.

16. Leahy JL, Cooper HE, Deal DA, Weir GC: Chronic hyperglycemia is associated with impaired glucose influence on insulin secretion: a study in normal rats using chronic in vivo glucose infusions. *J Clin Invest* 1986, 77:908–915.

17. Meglasson MD, Matschinsky FM: New perspectives on pancreatic islet glucokinase. *Am J Physiol* 1984, 246:E1–E13.

18. Eto K, Tsubamoto Y, Terauchi Y, et al.: Role of NADH shuttle system in glucose-induced activation of mitochondrial metabolism and insulin secretion. *Science* 1999, 283:981–985.

19. Henquin JC: Triggering and amplifying pathways of regulation of insulin secretion by glucose. *Diabetes* 2000, 49:1751–1760.

20. Holst JJ, Gromada J: Role of incretin hormones in the regulation of insulin secretion in diabetic and nondiabetic humans. *Am J Physiol Endocrinol Metab* 2004, 287:E199–E206

21. Mears D, Atwater I: Electrophysiology of the pancreatic β-cell. In *Diabetes Mellitus: A Fundamental and Clinical Text*, edn 2. Edited by LeRoith D, Taylor SI, Olefsky JM. Philadelphia: Lippincott Williams & Wilkins; 2000:47–60.

22. Gilon P, Shepherd RM Henquin JC: Oscillations of secretion driven by oscillations of cytoplasmic Ca2 as evidenced in single pancreatic islets. *J Biol Chem* 1993, 268:22265–22268.

23. Porksen N, Munn S, Steers J, et al.: Effects of glucose ingestion versus infusion on pulsatile insulin secretion. *Diabetes* 1996, 45:1317–1323.

24. McGarry JD Dobbins RL: Fatty acids, lipotoxicity and insulin secretion. *Diabetologia* 1999, 42:128–138.   Prentki M, Corkey BE: Are the β-cell signaling molecules malonyl-CoA and cytosolic long-chain acyl-CoA implicated in multiple tissue defects of obesity and NIDDM? *Diabetes* 1996, 45:273–283.

26. Brunzell JD, Robertson RP, Lerner RL, et al.: Relationships between fasting plasma glucose levels and insulin secretion during intravenous glucose tolerance tests. *J Clin Endocrinol Metab* 1976, 42:222–229.

27. Ward WK, Beard JC, Halter JB, et al.: Pathophysiology of insulin secretion in non–insulin-dependent diabetes mellitus. *Diabetes Care* 1984, 7:491–502.

28. Ward WK, Bolgiano DC, McKnight B, et al.: Diminished β-cell secretory capacity in patients with noninsulin-dependent diabetes mellitus. *J Clin Invest* 1984, 74:1318–1328.

29. DeFronzo RA, Ferrannini E, Simonson DC: Fasting hyperglycemia in noninsulin-dependent diabetes mellitus: contributions of excessive hepatic glucose production and impaired tissue glucose uptake. *Metabolism* 1989, 38:387–395.

30. Mitrakou A, Kelley D, Mokan M, et al.: Role of suppression of glucose production and diminished early insulin release in impaired glucose tolerance. *N Engl J Med* 1992, 326:22–29.

31. Hull RL, Westermark GT, Westermark P, Kahn SE. Islet amyloid: a critical entity in the pathogenesis of type 2 diabetes. *J Clin Endocrinol Metab* 2004, 89:3629-3643.

32. Tokuyama Y, Sturis J, Depaoli AM, et al.: Evolution of β-cell dysfunction in the male Zucker diabetic fatty rat. *Diabetes* 1995, 44:1447–1457.

33. Jonas JC, Sharma A, Hasenkamp W, et al.: Chronic hyperglycemia triggers loss of pancreatic beta-cell differentiation in an animal model of diabetes. *J Biol Chem* 1999, 274:14112–14121.

34. Weir GC, Laybutt DR, Kaneto H, et al.: Beta-cell adaptation and decompensation during the progression of diabetes. *Diabetes* 2001, 50(suppl):S154–S159.

35. Weir GC, Bonner-Weir S: Insulin secretion in type 2 diabetes. In *Diabetes Mellitus: A Fundamental and Clinical Text*, edn 3. Edited by LeRoith D, Taylor SI, Olefsky JM. Philadelphia: Lippincott Williams & Wilkins; 2004:887–898.

36. Weir GC, Bonner-Weir S: Five stages of evolving beta cell dysfunction during progression to diabetes. *Diabetes* 2004, 53(suppl):S16–S21.

THE MECHANISMS OF INSULIN ACTION

Morris F. White and Tracey L. Fisher

2

The storage and release of energy during feeding and fasting and somatic growth are regulated by the insulin/insulin-like growth factor (IGF) signaling system. Insulin is best known for its role in the regulation of blood glucose, as it suppresses hepatic gluconeogenesis and promotes glycogen synthesis and storage in liver and muscle; triglycerides synthesis in liver and storage in adipose tissue; and amino acid storage in muscle [1]. However, the insulin signaling system has a broader role in mammalian physiology because it is shared with the IGF-1 receptor (IGFr1). During development, the insulin/IGF signaling system promotes somatic growth [2,3]; after birth, it promotes growth and survival of many tissues, including pancreatic β-cells, bone, neurons, and retina, to name a few [4–8]. Except for insulin, which can be replaced by injection as a treatment for diabetes, the complete dysfunction of essential components in the insulin/IGF signaling system is rare and invariably lethal. By contrast, a partial failure of the insulin/IGF signaling system, frequently called insulin resistance, is associated with many metabolic disorders, including dyslipidemia, hypertension, female infertility, and glucose intolerance that eventually progresses to diabetes [9].

Diabetes is an epidemic disorder that arises when insulin secretion from pancreatic β cells fails to maintain blood glucose levels in the normal range, especially when exacerbated by peripheral insulin resistance. The underlying pathophysiology of diabetes is diverse, but pancreatic β cell failure is the common theme [10]. Type 2 diabetes is the most common form, and it arises when pancreatic β-cell insulin secretion fails to compensate for peripheral insulin resistance [11]. Work over the past decade suggests that type 2 diabetes begins with skeletal muscle insulin resistance [12]; however, peripheral insulin resistance might not be enough because transgenic mice lacking muscle insulin receptors and patients with muscle insulin resistance owing to defective mRNA splicing do not ordinarily develop diabetes [13,14]. Despite incontrovertible evidence of genetic links for type 2 diabetes, diabetes is not a Mendelian disorder, so the genes responsible have been difficult to identify [15]. Consequently, linkage analysis with well-defined populations has made slow progress, although a possible role for the serine protease CAPN10 was recently revealed [16,17].

The mechanism by which insulin regulates energy metabolism and promotes cell growth has been studied extensively. Almost 50 years ago, the pioneering work of Levine and coworkers led to the hypothesis that the effect of insulin on glucose utilization was attributable to increased glucose transport across the plasma membrane. In 1971, Freychet and colleagues [18] discovered the insulin receptor, which lead to identification of its tyrosine kinase activity a decade later and, ultimately, to the discovery of the insulin receptor substrates (IRS) proteins and the mechanism of insulin action.

Insulin exerts its diverse actions by inducing tyrosine phosphorylation of its cell surface receptor, which promotes the activity of the intracellular catalytic domain that phosphorylates tyrosine residues on other intracellular proteins [19]. Autophosphorylation further activates the receptor as a tyrosine-specific protein kinase, allowing the activated receptor to phosphorylate a host of cytosolic and membrane-bound proteins. Phosphorylation of protein substrates is required to mediate insulin action. The proximal effectors of insulin action have been convincingly identified; they include IRS proteins and several others [20]. IRS proteins serve an important function as "docking" molecules, favoring the assembly of multiprotein complexes and generation of intracellular signals. Much work remains to be done to understand how these intracellular signals coordinate biologic effects.

Understanding the molecular basis of insulin action will reveal the pathophysiology of diabetes. It is firmly established that patients with type II diabetes have defects of insulin action, commonly referred to as insulin resistance. Our approach to understanding diabetes has been based on the hypothesis that common signaling pathways might mediate both peripheral insulin action and pancreatic β-cell function. When elements of these pathways fail, owing to a combination of genetic variation and epigenetic challenge, diabetes might ensue. Evidence supporting this hypothesis emerged from our work on the IRS proteins. Disruption of the gene for Irs2 in mice causes diabetes because of peripheral insulin resistance and dysregulated hepatic gluconeogenesis that is exacerbated by pancreatic β-cell failure [21]. Although all the experimental evidence is not yet available, failure of components that are regulated by the IRS2 branch of the insulin/IGF signaling pathway might be an important cause of diabetes.

Overview of Insulin Effects

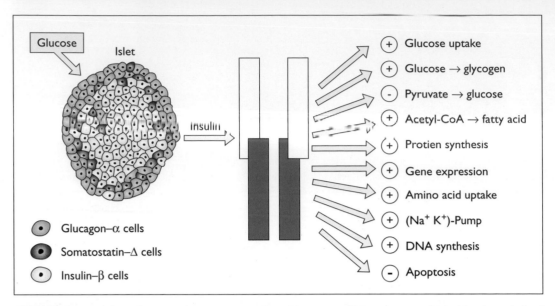

FIGURE 2-1. Insulin actions in peripheral tissues. Increases in circulating glucose levels lead to the secretion of insulin from pancreatic β cells found in the islets of Langerhans. Insulin action in the peripheral tissues requires the presence of the insulin receptor and subsequent intracellular protein phosphorylation upon hormone binding. The intracellular subunit of the receptor is a tyrosine-specific kinase that autophosphorylates and catalyzes the phosphorylation of several proteins that promote the multifaceted actions of insulin. Different tissues are known to respond differently to insulin. Although tissue sensitivity to the hormone correlates with the levels of insulin receptors expressed on the plasma membrane, it is clear that the assembly of different components of the insulin signaling pathway also confers specificity of insulin action on target cells. Insulin stimulates glucose turnover, favoring its transport across the plasma membrane, followed either by oxidative or nonoxidative disposal, the latter being associated with glycogen synthesis. Insulin-stimulated glucose transport is observed only in skeletal muscle, adipose cells, and the heart because these tissues express the insulin-dependent glucose transporter, GLUT4. In the liver and kidney, insulin inhibits gluconeogenesis because of the tissue-specific expression of hormone-sensitive metabolic enzymes involved in this process. Insulin simultaneously stimulates lipid synthesis while preventing lipolysis in adipose cells, skeletal muscle, and liver. By contrast, insulin promotes protein synthesis in almost all tissues by virtue of combined changes in gene transcription, messenger RNA translation, and amino acid uptake. Insulin also acts as a mitogen via increased DNA synthesis and prevention of programmed cell death, or apoptosis. In addition, insulin stimulates ion transport across the plasma membrane of multiple tissues. There is increasing evidence for a direct role of insulin, acting through the insulin or insulin-like growth factor (IGF) receptors, to regulate pancreatic b-cell growth, survival, and insulin release [21,22].

Insulin Receptor

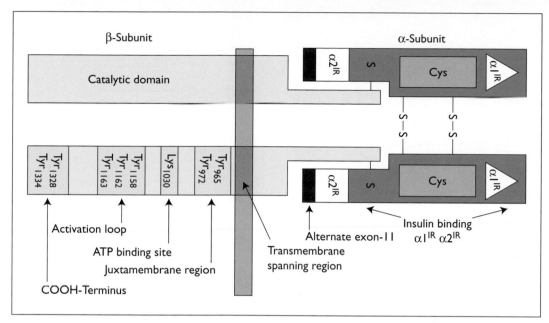

FIGURE 2-2. Insulin receptor (IR) structure. The IR is required to mediate insulin action. The product of a single copy gene located on the short arm of chromosome 19 (cytogenetic band 19p13), the insulin receptor is synthesized as a single-chain polypeptide precursor that undergoes posttranslational cleavage forming separate α and β subunits, which form heterodimers (α-β) that are exported to the plasma membrane. During maturation, the receptor is glycosylated, acylated, and forms a heterotetramer composed of two α and two β subunits (α_2-β_2). The α subunit is entirely extracellular and contains both a high- and low-affinity binding sites for insulin ($\alpha1^{IR}$-$\alpha2^{IR}$). The asymmetric insulin molecules interact with the β subunits by binding to an $\alpha1IR$ and an $\alpha2IR$ site on adjacent subunits. The β subunit spans the plasma membrane once and is linked to the α subunit through disulfide bridges and noncovalent interactions. The insulin receptor is expressed as two variably spliced isoforms, resulting from inclusion (isoform IR-A) or exclusion (isoform IR-

B) of exon-11 during messenger RNA processing. Exon-11 encodes a peptide with 12 amino acids located at the COOH-terminal end of the receptor α subunit. The resultant IR-A isoform has a lower affinity for insulin [23]. The intracellular portion of the β subunit contains a tyrosine-specific protein kinase domain. Insulin binding to the receptor extracellular domain causes a conformational modification in the intracellular domain such that the receptor undergoes autophosphorylation and can bind adenosine triphosphate (ATP). Several tyrosine residues are phosphorylated, including tyrosine 972, that promotes substrate binding and phosphorylation [20,24]. Specific phosphorylation sites in the catalytic domain (tyrosine 1158, 1162, and 1163) are essential to promote the kinase activity of the receptor toward other protein substrates [25]. The role of the COOH-terminal phosphorylation sites (tyrosine 1328 and 1334) is more controversial, with certain studies suggesting that these sites play a role in stimulating the mitogenic activity of the receptor. These identified sites both in this figure and text are numbered according to the human IR-A isoform amino acid sequence. The inclusion of exon-11, resulting in isoform IR-A, is developmentally regulated. IR-A predominates in fetal tissues and the adult central nervous system, and IR-B is preferentially expressed in adult insulin-sensitive tissues such as muscle, adipose tissue, and the liver [26,27]. Dysregulation of insulin receptor gene splicing alters fetal growth patterns and contributes to insulin resistance in adults [14,23].

Role of Insulin Receptor Substrate Proteins in Insulin Signaling

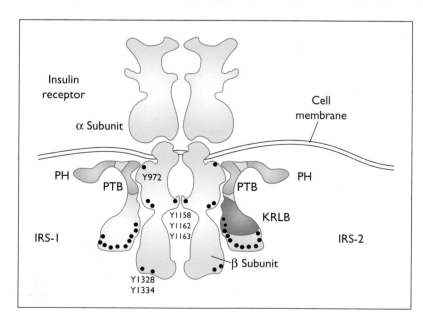

FIGURE 2-3. Model for the interaction of insulin receptors (IR) and insulin receptor substrate (IRS) molecules. The IRS proteins were identified as tyrosine-phosphorylated proteins in cells treated with insulin [28–30]. In addition to insulin, other agents such as insulin-like growth factors (IGFs) and interleukins stimulate IRS protein phosphorylation [20]. Upon activation of the IR kinase, the phosphotyrosine-binding (PTB) domain of IRS becomes closely associated with the juxtamembrane region of the insulin receptor. This interaction requires phosphorylation of tyrosine 972 in the insulin receptor. In addition, the pleckstrin homology (PH) domain of IRS may stabilize this interaction. The PH domain is located at the amino-terminal end of the IRS protein, which may promote interaction with the membrane lipid bilayer because many PH domains bind phospholipids [31]. An additional domain found only in IRS2 interacts with the catalytic activation loop of the IR. Interaction of the IRS2 kinase regulatory loop-binding (KRLB) domain with IR requires phosphorylation of tyrosine residues in the catalytic domain of the receptor (tyrosine 1158, 1162, and 1163). Because the KRLB is only present in IRS2, it may determine specificity of the interaction between the insulin receptor and its substrates [32,33]. Gene ablation experiments in mice indicate that various IRS proteins have unique functions. Mice lacking Irs1 are growth retarded and mildly insulin resistant, suggesting that Irs1 plays an important role in both insulin and IGF-I receptor function [34]. By contrast, mice lacking Irs2 develop severe insulin resistance and display impaired pancreatic β-cell development, suggesting that Irs2 is important for metabolic regulation in response to insulin [4,21]. The IRS proteins appear critical for insulin action in humans, as evidenced by polymorphisms in IRS1 and IRS2 that have been linked to obesity and insulin resistance in certain ethnic populations [35–37].

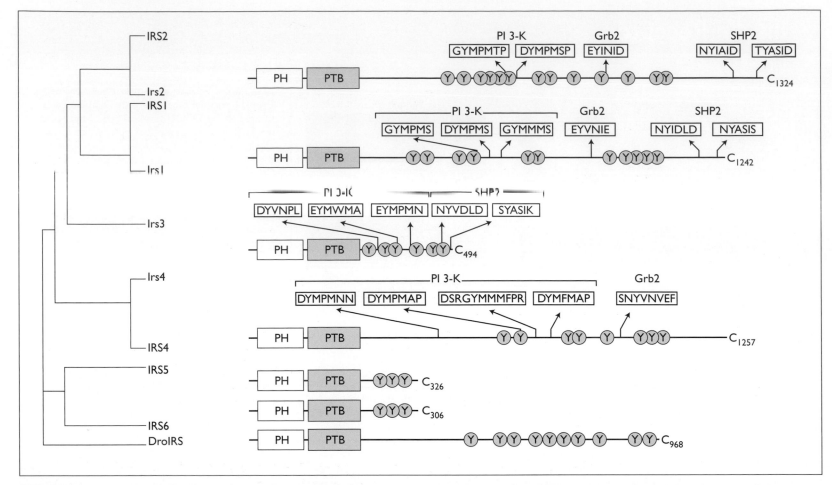

FIGURE 2-4. Structure of the insulin receptor substrate (IRS) proteins. The IRS proteins lack intrinsic catalytic activities but are composed of multiple inter-action domains and phosphorylation motifs. The various proteins that bind to IRS subsequent to receptor activation provide the molecular basis for the diversity of insulin signaling. All IRS proteins are characterized by the presence of an NH2-terminal pleckstrin homology (PH) domain adjacent to a phosphoty-rosine-binding (PTB) domain, followed by a variable length COOH-terminal tail that contains numerous tyrosine phosphorylation sites (*circled Y*). At least three IRS proteins occur in mice and humans, including IRS1 and IRS2, that are widely expressed, and IRS4, the mouse homolog of which expression is limited to the thymus, brain, kidney, and liver [38]. Rodents also express Irs3, which is largely restricted to adipose tissue and displays activity similar to Irs1; however, evidence for this short ortholog has not been found in the human genome [39,40]. Phylogenetic analysis reveals a close evolutionary relationship between IRS1/Irs1 and IRS2/Irs2 from humans/mice, which may have diverged from IRS4/Irs4. Two additional human IRS proteins, IRS5 and IRS6, were identified via

their adjacent PH and PTB domains [41]. These IRS proteins contain few tyro-sine residues in their short COOH-terminal tails, and their function remains unknown [41]. The *Drosophila melanogaster* IRS protein, Chico, is weakly related to its mammalian orthologs because it contains few conserved COOH-terminal tyrosine phosphorylation sites [42]. The PH and PTB domains of IRS proteins mediate specific interactions with the insulin and insulin-like growth factor (IGF) receptor kinases [43,44]. The PTB domain binds to phosphorylated NPXY motifs in the receptors for insulin, IGF-I, or interleukin-4; however, other recep-tors that promote IRS protein tyrosine phosphorylation do not contain NPXY-motifs [45]. Candidate PH domain binding partners include phospholipids, acidic peptides, and specific proteins such as PHIP (pleckstrin homology interacting protein) [46,47]. The p85 subunit of phosphatidylinositol 3-kinase (PI 3-K), the enzymatic activity of which is crucial in stimulating many biologic actions of insulin, is the most prominent protein shown to bind specific tyrosine phospho-rylated sites in IRS proteins [48]. Other IRS-interacting proteins include growth factor receptor binding protein 2 (GRB-2) and the tyrosine phosphatase SHP2.

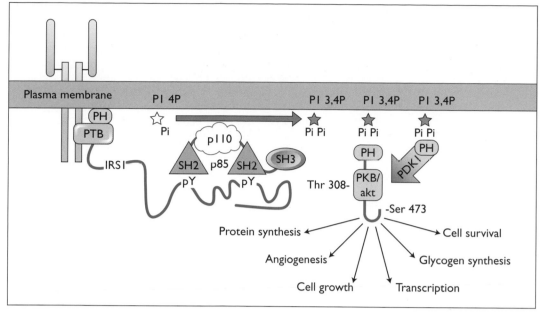

FIGURE 2-5. Tyrosine phosphorylation occurs in various amino acid sequence motifs that create binding sites for so-called SH2 (for src homology 2) motifs [49]. SH2 motifs are 50 to 100 amino acids long that bind with high affinity to phosphotyrosine residues in various intracellular signaling molecules. During insulin stimulation, tyrosine phosphorylated insulin receptor substrate (IRS) proteins bind to both SH2 domains in the regulatory subunit (p85) of phosphatidylinositol 3-kinase (PI 3-K), resulting in activation of the p110 catalytic subunit. The p110 subunit catalyzes phosphorylation of phosphatidylinositol (PI) on the D3 position of the inositol ring, leading to the generation of PI 3-phosphate from PI; PI 3,4-bisphosphate from PI 4-phosphate;

and PI 3,4,5-trisphosphate from PI 4,5-bisphosphate. Increasing evidence suggests that D3-phosphorylated inositides act as intracellular messengers, leading to activation of PI-dependent kinases, changes in intracellular trafficking, and growth stimulation [50]. Products of the PI 3-kinase interact with cytosolic serine kinases such as PDK and PKB/Akt to generate a membrane-bound signaling system that mediates various biological processes, including glycogen synthesis and glucose transport. Whereas the PH domain of Akt binds to the PI 3-phosphate, maximal enzyme activity requires PDK-mediated phosphorylation of Thr^{308} and Ser^{473} [51]. In addition to its role in metabolic regulation, Akt promotes insulin-like growth factor I–mediated inhibition of apoptosis, as well as the activation of the $p70^{S6}$ kinase with attendant protein synthesis, regulation of entry into the cell cycle, and cellular differentiation [52]. Analyses of mice carrying deletions in either *Akt1* or *Akt2* demonstrate a physiological divergence of these two isoform functions. The $Akt^{1-/-}$ mice are growth retarded but display no metabolic defects; $Akt^{2-/-}$ mice are insulin resistant, and a subset of these animals develop overt diabetes [53–55]. Recent work describes a human-dominant *AKT2* mutation found in a family that correlates with an incidence of diabetes mellitus [56]. PDK—phosphatidylinositol-dependent protein kinase; PKB—protein kinase B.

Downstream Signaling Pathways

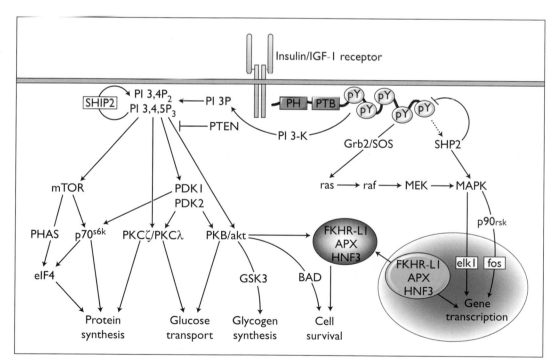

FIGURE 2-6. Insulin receptor substrate (IRS) proteins coordinate multiple downstream signaling pathways. The diversity of insulin action in different tissues is partly explained by the different outputs coupled to the pathways activated by the hormone. There are two main limbs that propagate the signal generated through the insulin receptor, including the phosphatidylinositol-3 (PI-3) kinase branch and the Ras/mitogen-activated protein kinase branch. The IRS proteins bind PI 3-kinase, Grb2/SOS, and SHP-2. The GRb2/SOS complex mediates the activation of $p21^{ras}$, thereby activating the ras—>raf—> MAPK kinase (MEK)—> microtubule-

associated protein (MAP) kinase cascade. SHP2 feeds back to inhibit IRS protein phosphorylation by directly dephosphorylating the IRS protein, but it might also transmit an independent signal to activate MAP kinase. The activated MAP kinase phosphorylates p90 ribosomal S6 kinase ($p90^{rsk}$), which itself phosphorylates the transcription factor c-fos, increasing its transcriptional activity. MAP kinase likewise phosphorylates elk1, increasing its transcriptional activity. The activation of PI 3-kinase by IRS protein recruitment results in the generation of PI 3,4P2 and PI 3,4,5P3 (antagonized by the action of PTEN or SHIP2). Together, PI 3,4P2 and PI 3,4,5P3 activate various kinases, including mammalian target of rapamycin (mTOR), atypical protein kinase C(PKC) isoforms, and phospholipid-dependent protein kinase (PDK1). PDK1 is upstream of protein kinase B (PKB), which promotes glucose transport; the atypical protein kinase C (PKC) isoforms also play a role. PKB also regulates glycogen synthase kinase 3 (GSK3), which might regulate glycogen synthesis, and a variety of regulators of cell survival; PKB-mediated BAD phosphorylation inhibits apoptosis. PKB also phosphorylates the forkhead transcription factors (such as Foxo1), which restricts their location to the cytoplasm and inhibits their transcriptional activity. GAP—guanosine triphosphatase associated protein; GLUT4—glucose transporter 4; GRB-2—growth factor receptor binding protein 2; SOS—son-of-sevenless.

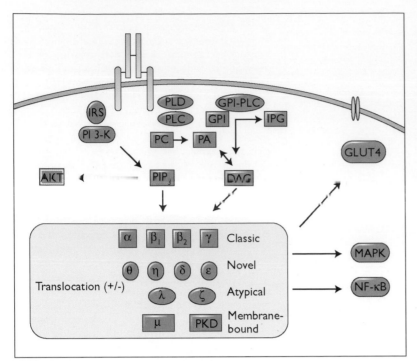

FIGURE 2-7. Members of the protein kinase C (PKC) family of serine/threonine kinases are implicated in several insulin actions. There are two subgroups of PKCs. The "classic" PKC isoforms bind calcium for activation. The atypical PKCs are activated by diacylglycerol (DAG) binding or by other phospholipids such as phosphatidylinositol 3,4,5-trisphosphate (PIP3). Insulin activates different members of this kinase family through formation of DAG and PIP3. Insulin stimulates DAG formation through phosphatidylcholine (PC) hydrolysis into DAG and phosphatidic acid (PA) or through activity of a glycosyl-phosphatidylinositol-specific phospholipase C (GPI-PLC), leading to the formation of DAG and inositol-phosphoglycan (IPG). Different isoforms of PKC have been shown to undergo translocation from the cytosol to the membrane in response to insulin stimulation in different tissues. Evidence suggests that this process may be important for the biologic activity of PKCs [57]. It is known that PKCs can directly activate the microtubule-associated protein (MAP) kinase pathway and the transcription factor nuclear factor-κB, leading to increased gene expression and protein synthesis. More recently, evidence has emerged that activation of atypical PKCs by PIP3 may be important in the process of insulin-dependent glucose transport [58].

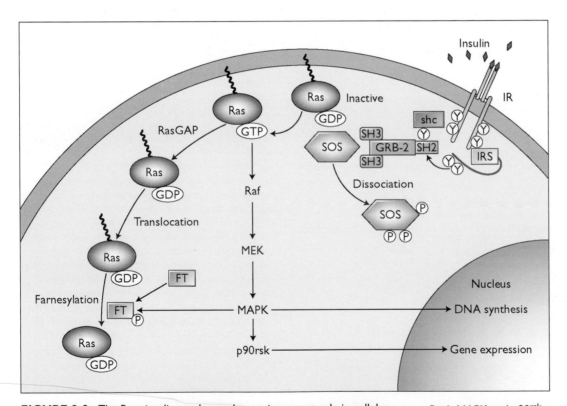

FIGURE 2-8. The Ras signaling pathway plays an important role in cellular growth and transformation [49]. Insulin activation of the Ras pathway promotes increased DNA synthesis and mitogenesis. Evidence does not exist for involvement of the Ras pathway in the metabolic actions of insulin [59]. The small G protein Ras is inactive when bound to guanosine diphosphate (GDP). Ras is active when bound to guanosine triphosphate (GTP) and anchored to the plasma membrane via a farnesylation modification [60]. Insulin promotes both GTP loading (exchange of GTP for GDP) and farnesylation of Ras. Insulin-stimulated Ras activation requires formation of a signaling complex between tyrosine phosphorylated insulin receptor substrate (IRS) or Shc (Src homology 2 [SH2]/collagen homology-containing protein) and growth factor receptor binding protein 2 (GRB-2). GRB-2 consists of one SH2 domain that binds the phosphorylated tyrosine residues (*circled Y*) in IRS or Shc, as well as two Src homology 3 (SH3) domains that recognize proline-rich motifs on the exchange factor son-of-sevenless (SOS). SOS promotes GTP loading of Ras. A Ras GTPase-activating protein (RasGAP) catalyzes the reverse reaction, forming inactive Ras-GDP. Ras-GTP activates the Raf kinase, leading to a serine/threonine kinase cascade involving subsequent phosphorylation and activation of MAPK kinase (MEK), mitogen-activated protein kinase (MAPK), and p90 ribosomal S6 kinase (p90rsk).

Both MAPK and p90rsk translocate to the nucleus upon activation to alter gene expression and promote DNA synthesis. Upon insulin stimulation, MEK also activates additional pathways that catalyze the dissociation of GRB-2 from SOS, which terminates the signal. The phosphorylation of SOS (*circled P*) is one mechanism proposed to mediate dissociation from GRB-2. Insulin also stimulates the farnesylation of Ras-GDP via an activating phosphorylation on farnesyltransferase (FT), the enzyme catalyzing this Ras modification. MAPK has been shown to mediate this FT phosphorylation, but other kinases may be involved. The FT phosphorylation in response to insulin is on a longer time course in contrast to the transient nature of insulin-stimulated Ras GTP loading. In this way, insulin is thought to prime cells for stimulation by other growth factors by increasing the pool of farnesylated Ras-GDP over time. This priming effect is specific to insulin and dependent on the presence of the insulin receptor [61]. Insulin-sensitive tissues from hyperinsulinemic animal models displayed increased farnesylated Ras [62]. Excessive maternal insulin leads to increased farnesylated Ras in fetal tissues, a condition that may contribute to the macrosomia observed in diabetic pregnancies [63]. It appears that the relative roles of IRS and shc in insulin-stimulated Ras activation via GRB-2/SOS as well as through FT phosphorylation vary in different tissues [64,65].

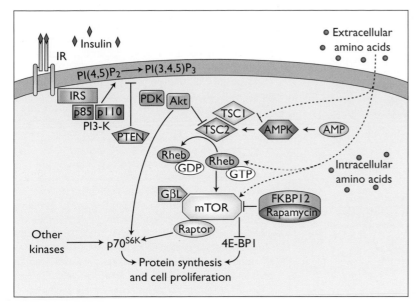

FIGURE 2-9. Insulin regulates a pathway, including the mammalian target of rapamycin (mTOR) and p70^S6 kinase (p70^S6K). Activation of these serine/threonine kinases has emerged as a major point of hormone-, growth factor– and nutrient-regulated signal integration contributing to protein synthesis and cell proliferation. Components of the mTOR and p70^S6K pathway are highly conserved from yeast to fruit flies and humans, many of which are sensitive to the availability of nutrients such as amino acids and energy sources, including glucose [53,66]. mTOR was originally isolated as the target of the immunosuppressive agent rapamycin. Once inside the cell, rapamycin binds to FKBP12 to form a complex inhibitory to downstream mTOR activity [53]. Insulin stimulates mTOR activity through insulin receptor substrates (IRS)–associated PI3-K activity leading to PI(3,4,5)P3-mediated

Akt activation, as described in Figures 2-5 and 2-6. Abundant amino acids increase mTOR and p70^S6K activity, and indicators of low energy, including adenosine monophosphate (AMP), are inhibitory. These nutritional inputs are independent of PI3-K or Akt activities and, therefore, act downstream to regulate mTOR and p70^S6K [67]. Recent work has identified signaling molecules through which Akt acts to regulate mTOR function, and these protein activities are sensitive to nutrient availability. The ubiquitously expressed Rheb (Ras homolog expressed in the brain) is a small G protein, and its guanosine triphosphate (GTP)–bound form functions to activate mTOR through an unknown mechanism [53,68]. The tuberous sclerosis gene products TSC1 and TSC2 form a negative regulatory complex in the cell, inhibiting the insulin pathway by blocking mTOR activation [69]. This occurs because of the GTPase-activating protein (GAP) activity of TSC2 toward Rheb that leads to the formation of inactive Rheb-GDP [68]. Upon insulin stimulation, Akt phosphorylates TSC2, abrogating its GAP activity, favoring Rheb-GTP and the activation of mTOR [60]. Much experimental evidence indicates that the TSC1/2 complex and Rheb are required for mTOR to sense nutritional sufficiency. Recent work demonstrates that in a low-energy phase, when AMP is high, the AMP kinase (AMPK) is activated and phosphorylates TSC2, a modification that enhances its Rheb-GAP activity [60]. Well-characterized downstream effectors of mTOR activity are p70^S6K and 4E-BP1. 4EBP-1 serves as a translational repressor until phosphorylated by mTOR and other mitogen-activated kinases. The p70^S6K occurs as two isoforms called S6K1 and S6K2. Disruption of s6k1 in mice causes glucose intolerance owing to reduced size of pancreatic islet β cells; by contrast, peripheral insulin action might be enhanced, suggesting that S6K1 contributes to feedback inhibition of insulin signaling [70]. S6K1 is activated in vivo through multi-site phosphorylation events from various kinase activities in response to insulin and other mitogens if a sufficient supply of amino acids is available or to high concentrations of amino acids alone [71]. This nutrient-stimulated activation of p70^S6K is rapamycin sensitive and apparently dependent on mTOR activation. Two mTOR-interacting proteins, raptor (regulatory associated protein of mTOR) and GβL, have been identified that may function to enhance substrate recruitment to the complex [63,72].

The Regulation of Glucose Transport and Metabolism

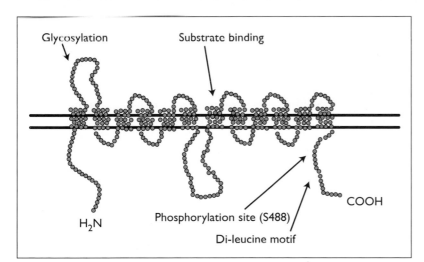

FIGURE 2-10. Glucose transporters (GLUTs). Glucose transport is mediated by a family of facilitative glucose carriers, or GLUTs. These proteins have a typical structure, including a cytoplasmic amino-terminus followed by 12 membrane-spanning domains and a cytoplasmic carboxyl-terminal tail. The proposed structure of the insulin-responsive glucose transporter GLUT4 is shown. Whereas the first exofacial loop contains glycosylation sites, the cytoplasmic carboxyl-terminal domain contains a putative phosphorylation site (serine 488) and a di-leucine motif thought to play a role in the rapid endocytosis of GLUT4. The proposed substrate-binding site is also shown [73]. There is evidence for at least 12 different members of the GLUT gene family divided into three subclasses based on sequence similarities [74]. Class I includes the well-characterized GLUT1–4 proteins. GLUT1 is ubiquitously expressed and accounts for most basal (insulin-independent) glucose uptake. GLUT2 is mainly expressed in liver and pancreatic β-cells; because of its relatively low affinity yet high capacity for glucose, it serves to provide a constant flux of glucose into these organs at physiologic plasma glucose concentrations (5 mM). In the β-cell, the uptake of glucose through GLUT2 is the first step in the detection of

circulating glucose levels. GLUT3, although broadly expressed, is most abundant in the central nervous system, where glucose concentrations are lower than in the blood stream. GLUT3 possesses a relatively high affinity for glucose and, thus, provides a mechanism for efficient glucose uptake by neurons. GLUT4 is the proto-typical insulin-responsive glucose transporter, and it is found in intracellular vesicles in insulin-responsive tissues, including skeletal muscle, adipose cells, and the heart. The class II facilitative transporters include GLUT5, GLUT7, GLUT9, and GLUT11. GLUT5 is a fructose transporter expressed mainly in the intestinal epithelial membrane, testes, and kidneys. GLUT7 protein has been detected in the intestine and can functionally transport fructose and glucose [75]. GLUT9 is expressed in human chondrocytes and may be critical for cartilage development [76,77]. The two splice variants of GLUT11 have different substrate specificities as well as nonoverlapping tissue expression patterns. The GLUT11 short form has a low affinity for glucose and is expressed in heart and skeletal muscle. The GLUT11 long form can transport fructose and is detected in the liver, lung, and brain [74]. The class III facilitative transporters include GLUT6, GLUT8, GLUT10, and GLUT12. Structurally, these proteins contain the described glycosylation sites of class I members in loop 9 as opposed to loop 1, and class III GLUTs each contain specific intracellular targeting motifs [74]. The significance of these structural differences remains unclear. GLUT6 can transport glucose and is expressed in the brain, spleen, and leukocytes [74]. Interestingly, although GLUT8 is a glucose transporter with intracellular targeting motifs similar to GLUT4 and is widely expressed in many insulin-responsive (as well as insulin-independent) tissues, evidence for GLUT8 insulin responsiveness has thus far only been detected in blastocysts [74,78]. The GLUT10 protein is highly expressed in the liver and pancreas, and the corresponding gene, SLC2A10, lies within a chromosomal location linked to type 2 diabetes [74,79]. Investigations into variants of the SLC2A10 gene and associations with type 2 diabetes in various populations are in progress [80]. The GLUT12 gene was originally cloned from a breast epithelial carcinoma cell line [81]. Evidence exists that GLUT12 may be another insulin-responsive glucose transporter. GLUT12 is also expressed in the prostate, small intestine, placenta, skeletal muscle, and adipocytes [81,82]. Recent work suggests GLUT12 expression is higher in malignant breast and prostate tissues, where it may provide increased glucose usage for the proliferation of cancerous cells [83,84].

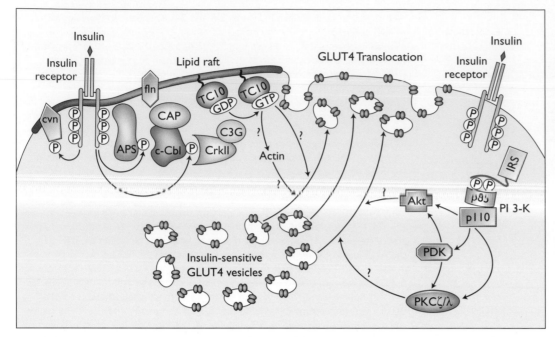

FIGURE 2-11. Insulin action on glucose transport. In tissues that are insulin responsive for glucose uptake, GLUT4 exists under basal conditions in intracellular vesicles. During insulin stimulation, GLUT4-containing vesicles move from their intracellular storage compartment and reach the cell surface through targeted exocytosis. Simultaneously, GLUT4 endocytosis is repressed, leading to an overall increase in glucose uptake [85]. The mechanism of insulin-induced redistribution of glucose transporters is referred to as *translocation*. It is not clear whether the effect of insulin to stimulate glucose uptake in muscle and fat can be entirely accounted for by the translocation hypothesis. Other factors, such as an increase in the activity of glucose transporters, may play a role. Substantial evidence exists to suggest that at least two molecularly distinct pathways mediate the effect of insulin on glucose transport. One pathway relies on phosphatidylinositol 3-kinase (PI 3-K) activation of downstream effectors, including phosphoinositide-dependent kinase (PDK), the product of the proto-oncogene Akt, and the atypical protein kinase C (aPCK) isoforms Ω and λ [86–88]. The other PI 3-K-independent pathway leads to the activation of TC10, a small G protein of the Rho family localized to lipid rafts in the plasma membrane [89]. Lipid rafts are microdomains on the cell surface that contain specific glycolipids, sphingolipids, proteins, and cholesterol that do not mix with other lipids within the plasma membrane. The insulin receptor is localized to caveolae, a specific lipid raft subset, where it phosphorylates and associates with caveolin (cvn) [89]. The localization of the insulin receptor to caveolae appears critical for the activation of the PI 3-K-independent signal leading to GLUT4 translocation in adipocytes [90]. Upon insulin stimulation, the autophosphorylated insulin receptor recruits the adapter protein APS, an adipocyte-specific insulin receptor substrate, through interaction with its SH2 domain [86]. Subsequently, the insulin receptor phosphorylates a specific tyrosine residue within APS that then binds to the SH2 domain of the c-Cbl proto-oncogene, recruiting c-Cbl for tyrosine phosphorylation by the insulin receptor [91]. In most insulin-responsive cells, c-Cbl is constitutively associated with the adapter protein CAP (c-Cbl associated protein), which binds to proline-rich sequences in c-Cbl through the CAP carboxyl-terminal SH3 domain. Recruitment of the c-Cbl-CAP proteins further stabilizes the growing caveolae-localized insulin receptor complex upon CAP binding to flotillin (fln), a hydrophobic protein found in lipid rafts. Flotillin interacts with the amino-terminal SoHo (gut peptide Sorbin homology) domain of CAP [86]. The tyrosine-phosphorylated c-Cbl recruits the CrkII adapter protein to caveolae through interaction with the CrkII SH2 domain. CrkII is constitutively bound to C3G, a guanine nucleotide-exchange factor that catalyzes the exchange of GTP for GDP in the small G protein TC10 [92]. The GTP-bound and activated TC10 results from the localization of the CrkII-C3G complex to the lipid raft microdomain, where the small G protein resides [93]. Proper localization to the lipid raft through specific posttranslational modifications of TC10 and its activation are critical for insulin-stimulated GLUT4 translocation and glucose transport [93]. The identity of TC10 downstream effectors remains unclear, but other members of the Rho small G-protein family participate in actin cytoskeleton regulation. TC10 activation may lead to cortical actin stabilization, contributing to intracellular vesicle movement and organization. The TC10 signal originating from hormone binding to insulin receptor localized within lipid rafts is necessary in parallel with the insulin stimulation of the PI 3-K pathway to activate GLUT4 translocation and glucose transport.

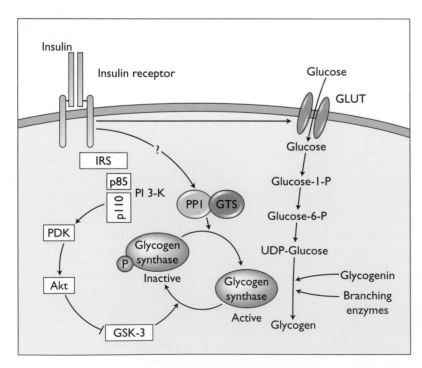

FIGURE 2-12. Insulin stimulation of glycogen synthesis. Insulin plays a key role in stimulating glycogen synthesis in many tissues. This process involves the regulation of multiple enzymatic activities. Glycogen synthase(GS) activity is regulated by phosphorylation. This crucial enzyme is inactive when phosphorylated [94]. Glycogen synthase kinase-3 (GSK-3) is an enzyme that catalyzes the phosphorylation and inactivation of glycogen synthase. GSK-3 itself is inactivated by phosphorylation. Insulin stimulates GSK-3 phosphorylation through activation of the Akt kinase (product of the Akt proto-oncogene kinase). Akt is activated in response to phosphatidylinositol 3-kinase (PI 3-K) through PI-dependent kinases 1 and 2 (PDK1 and PDK2). Akt can phosphorylate and inactivate GSK-3, thus decreasing the net rate of GS phosphorylation [95]. Additionally, insulin has been shown to increase the activity of the glycogen-bound form of the serine/threonine protein phosphatase-1 (PP1), which dephosphorylates and activates GS [96]. The exact mechanism of PP1 stimulation by insulin remains unclear [97]. Glycogen synthesis requires the assembly of a complex of proteins, including glycogenin to provide a molecular scaffold, branching enzymes, and a variety glycogen targeting subunits (GTS) that regulate PP1 localization and activity [98]. The extent to which insulin regulates GTS localization or function is currently under investigation. Insulin-stimulated glucose transport has also been shown to contribute to GS regulation [99].

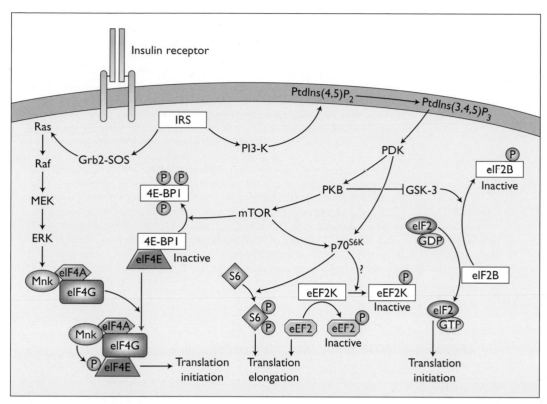

FIGURE 2-13. Regulation of protein synthesis by insulin. Insulin stimulates protein synthesis by altering the intrinsic activity or binding properties of key translation initiation and elongation factors (eIFs and eEFs, respectively) as well as critical ribosomal proteins. This occurs via phosphorylation or sequestration of repressive factors into inactive complexes. Components of the translational machinery that are targets of insulin regulation include eIF2B, eIF4E, eEF1, eEF2, and the S6 ribosomal protein [100]. The eIF2B multisubunit guanine nucleotide exchange factor for eIF2 is kept inactive via phosphorylation of the eIF2Bε subunit at Ser535 by glycogen synthase kinase-3 (GSK-3) [101]. Insulin stimulates the inhibition of GSK-3, leading to the activation of eIF2B and the formation of eIF2-GTP that can then recruit the initiator methionyl-tRNA to the ribosome [101–103]. The insulin-stimulated activation of eIF2B leads to an overall increase in translation initiation [104]. Severely diabetic rats have significantly lower eIF2B activity in muscle [105]. The eIF4F complex, including eIF4A/4G/4E and other proteins is required for cap-dependent translation initiation. The mRNA cap-binding protein, eIF4E, is inactive when bound to 4E-BP1. Insulin activates eIF4E by stimulating mammalian target of rapamycin (mTOR)-mediated phosphorylation of 4E-BP1, resulting in a dissociation of this complex [106]. The release of eIF4E allows for binding to eIF4G, the scaffold protein for the eIF4F complex. Transgenic mice carrying a genetic *4E-BP1* deletion have increased insulin sensitivity and dramatically decreased white adipose tissue depots [107]. Mnk, an insulin-stimulated kinase activated through the Ras/ERK cascade, also resides in the eIF4F complex, where it phosphorylates eIF4E at Ser209 [108,109]. Phosphorylation of eIF4E increases the binding affinity of the factor for mRNA caps. Formation of the active cap-binding complex leads to increased translation initiation. Insulin also stimulates translation elongation by phosphorylation of eEF1 by an undetermined mechanism. Insulin-stimulated phosphorylation of the ribosomal S6 protein by p70S6K may promote elongation of specific mRNAs corresponding to components of the translational machinery [72]. An elongation factor critical for ribosomal translocation along the mRNA, eEF2, is inactive when phosphorylated at Thr56 by the eEF2kinase (eEF2K) [110,111]. Insulin stimulates the dephosphorylation of eEF2 via a rapamycin sensitive route potentially involving the phosphorylation and inactivation of eEF2K by p70S6K [110]. In vitro, p70S6K phosphorylates eEF2K at Ser366, a modification that greatly reduces the activity of the kinase [110]. Activation of the atypical protein kinase C-zeta (PKCΩ) is also required for insulin-stimulated protein synthesis although its downstream effectors remain undetermined [112]. Nutrient availability impacts many of the aforementioned insulin-stimulated changes in protein synthesis [67,113]. Some reactions require additional signals from amino acids or energy sources such as glucose that indicate sufficient nutritional resources exist to support protein synthesis. At other steps of translation, initiation, and elongation, nutrient availability is permissive but not absolutely required. One point of convergence between nutritional and insulin signals occurs at the level of mTOR activity regulation [67,72,114].

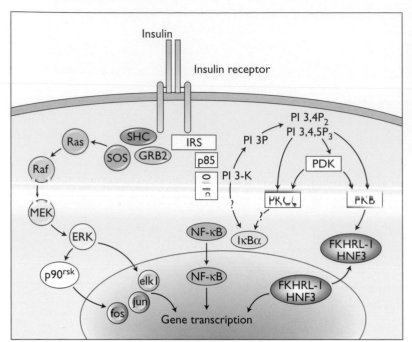

FIGURE 2-14. Regulation of gene expression by insulin. Insulin affects target gene expression in a variety of cells and organs. Both the phosphatidylinositol 3-kinase (PI3-K) and the Ras/extracellular-regulated kinase (ERK) signaling pathways have been shown to mediate insulin action on gene transcription in different tissues. The Ras/ERK pathway activates p90[rsk] whereby individually ERK and p90[rsk] translocate into the nucleus and phosphorylate transcription factors, including elk1 and fos. These phosphorylation events increase transcriptional activity mediated by such factors. The PI3-K pathway activates protein kinase B (PKB) through PI-dependent protein kinase (PDK). Active PKB phosphorylates members of the FKHR transcriptional enhancer family, including FKHR-L1 and HNF3, which, under basal conditions, are localized to the nucleus. Phosphorylation of these FKHR factors leads to their nuclear exclusion and cytoplasmic retention, effectively inhibiting specific gene transcription [115]. Insulin also affects the inhibitory complex dissociation of IκB from nuclear factor κB. Nuclear factor κB is then free to enter the nucleus and activate target gene transcription. The insulin stimulation of NFκB has been shown to be sensitive to inhibitors of PI3-K, implicating the involvement of the PI3-K pathway [116]. Activation of atypical protein kinase C (PKC), such as PKCΩ, may also contribute to activation of nuclear factor κB. The regulation of nuclear factor κB by insulin remains unclear.

Insulin Resistance

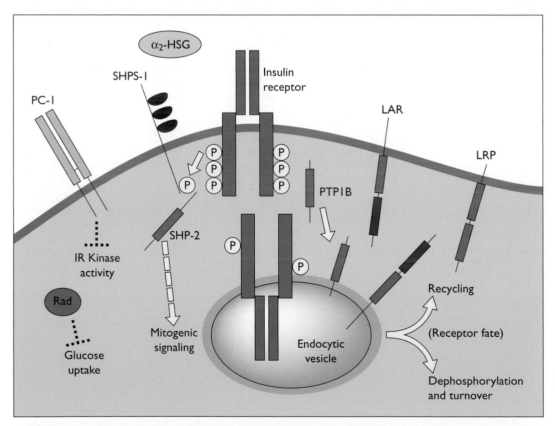

phatases include leukocyte antigen related (LAR) and leukocyte receptor protein (LRP) as well as protein tyrosine phosphatase 1B ([PTP1B] cytosolic). These phosphatases may also alter insulin signaling by targeting insulin receptor substrates for dephosphorylation. Transgenic mouse studies show that overexpression of LAR in muscle results in whole-body insulin resistance [123]. PTP1B knockout mice are resistant to obesity and demonstrate increased insulin sensitivity [124,125].

A variety of other molecules affect insulin action. The membrane glycoprotein PC-1 has been proposed to exert a negative effect on insulin receptor function by dampening its kinase activity [126]. Studies indicate a correlation between PC-1 expression and insulin resistance in patients with type II diabetes [127]. Another inhibitor of the insulin receptor kinase is the serum glycoprotein a2–Heremans Schmid glycoprotein. This 63-kDa protein has been reported to inhibit insulin-induced receptor autophosphorylation and phosphorylation of insulin receptor substrate-1 and the insulin receptor substrate Shc, with an associated decrease of the mitogenic actions of insulin. No effect of a2-HSG has been reported on the metabolic functions of insulin [128]. Rad (ras-like protein associated with diabetes) was originally identified by subtractive hybridization as a gene overexpressed in patients with diabetes. Although subsequent studies have failed to confirm this association, it is interesting that overexpression of Rad in transfected cells impairs insulin-dependent glucose uptake [129]. The transmembrane glycoprotein SHP substrate (SHPS)-1 is phosphorylated and forms a complex with SHP-2, a non-receptor PTP, in response to insulin. This complex appears to enhance extracellular-regulated kinase (ERK) activity in response to insulin [130].

FIGURE 2-15. Modulators of insulin action. Multiple signals converge on the insulin receptor to modulate its function. Protein tyrosine phosphatases (PTPs) appear to play an important role in deactivating the insulin receptor, providing a mechanism for regulating the insulin response. The endocytic step that occurs after insulin binding, with internalization of the ligand/receptor complex into clathrin-coated vesicles, may be another point for receptor dephosphorylation. The endosome has been identified as a major site of tyrosine phosphatase activity toward the insulin receptor [117]. Many studies of obese, insulin-resistant humans and rodents demonstrate alterations in the expression or activity of PTPs in insulin-responsive tissues [118–122]. The two major classes of tyrosine phosphatases are the receptor type (membrane bound) and the nonreceptor type (cytosolic). Tyrosine phosphatases identified as insulin receptor phos-

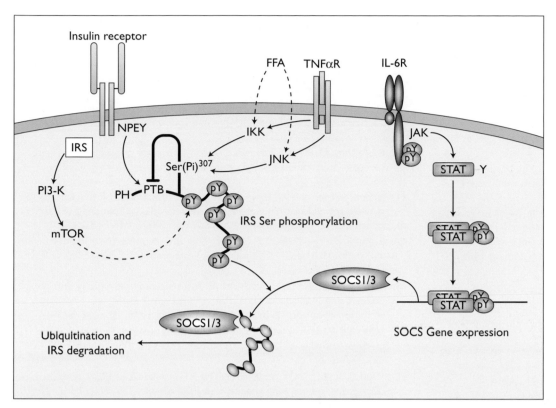

FIGURE 2-16. Insulin resistance as a product of altered insulin receptor substrate (IRS) function. Both increased IRS serine/threonine (Ser/Thr) phosphorylation and decreased IRS protein levels have been observed in insulin resistant as well as diabetic humans [131,132]. Recent work reveals potential molecular mechanisms for insulin signal termination caused by IRS ser/thr phosphorylation, including disruption of interaction with upstream receptors, disruption of interaction with downstream effectors, and targeted degradation of the protein. Many insulin-resistant stimuli, including inflammatory cytokines such as tumor necrosis factor-α and interleukin-6 (IL-6), excess free fatty acids (FFAs) attributable to obesity and hyperlipidemia as well as hyperinsulinemia, lead to ser/thr phosphorylation of IRS proteins [131,132]. One identified serine phosphorylation site on IRS1, Ser307, is located near the phosphotyrosine-binding (PTB) domain, a region that interacts with the activated insulin receptor. Phosphorylation of IRS1 Ser307 correlates with a decrease in overall IRS1 phosphotyrosine content [133]. The c-Jun kinase (JNK), a proto-type stress-induced ser/thr kinase that is stimulated by many agonists during acute or chronic inflammation, can target IRS1 Ser307 [133]. Phosphorylation of Ser307 by JNK has been shown to abrogate the interaction of IRS1 with the insulin receptor [134]. JNK activity is also elevated in obesity and stimulated by FFAs [135]. JNK is a candidate for physiological IRS1 ser/thr kinase because Jnk[-/-] mice have

increased insulin sensitivity and are resistant to weight gain on high-fat diets [136]. Genetically obese mice, ob/ob, have reduced weight gain when carrying a Jnk1 gene deletion [136]. Other kinases, including IKK-β and mammalian target of rapamycin (mTOR), have been shown to phosphorylate Ser307 as well as other sites on IRS1 [137]. Insulin-stimulated phosphorylation of IRS1 at Ser307 does not involve JNK and is sensitive to rapamycin, implying mTOR involvement [137]. Other identified Ser/Thr phosphorylation sites on IRS1 are located in the COOH-terminal tail near tyrosine residues critical for interaction of downstream effectors such as the p85 subunit of phosphatidylinositol 3-kinase (PI3-K). Additionally, recent work reveals a mechanism leading to IRS1/2 protein degradation through suppressor of cytokine signaling (SOCS) association [138]. The expression of SOCS proteins is induced by cytokines such as IL-6 through stimulation of Janus kinases (JAKs) and activating phosphorylation of the signal transducer and activator of transcription (STAT) transcription factors. SOCS binding to IRS1/2 leads to ubiquitinylation of the IRS proteins and targets them for proteasome-mediated degradation [138]. Indeed, SOCS1-/- mice are hypersensitive to insulin action [139]. A model for proteasome-mediated degradation of IRS proteins involves phosphorylation of specific Ser/Thr residues contributing to recognition of IRS by SOCS proteins, thus promoting ubiquitinylation and degradation.

References

1. DeFronzo RA, Ferrannini E: Regulation of intermediary metabolism during fasting and feeding. In *Endocrinology*. edn 4. Edited by DeGroot LJ, Jameson JL. Philadelphia: WB Saunders; 2001:737–755.

2. Baker J, Liu JP, Robertson EJ, Efstratiadis A: Role of insulin-like growth factors in embryonic and postnatal growth. *Cell* 1993, 75:73–82.

3. Liu JP, Baker J, Perkins JA, *et al.*: Mice carrying null mutations of the genes encoding insulin-like growth factor I (Igf-1) and type I IGF receptor (Igf1r). *Cell* 1993, 75:59–72.

4. Withers DJ, Burks DJ, Towery HH, *et al.*: Irs-2 coordinates Igf-1 receptor-mediated beta-cell development and peripheral insulin signalling. *Nat Genet* 1999 23:32–40.

5. Lupu F, Terwilliger JD, Lee K, *et al.*: Roles of growth hormone and insulin-like growth factor I in mouse postnatal growth. *Dev Biol* 2001 229:141–162.

6. Dudek H, Datta SR, Franke TF, *et al.*: Regulation of neuronal survival by the serine-threonine protein kinase Akt. *Science* 1997, 275:661–665.

7. Hellstrom A, Perruzzi C, Ju M, *et al.*: Low IGF-I suppresses VEGF-survival signaling in retinal endothelial cells: direct correlation with clinical retinopathy of prematurity. *Proc Natl Acad Sci U S A* 2001, 98:5804–5408.

8. Pete G, Fuller CR, Oldham JM, *et al.*: Postnatal growth responses to insulin-like growth factor I in insulin receptor substrate-1-deficient mice. *Endocrinology* 1999, 140:5478–5487.

9. Reaven GM: Banting Lecture 1988. Role of insulin resistance in human disease. 1988 [classical article]. *Nutrition* 1997, 13:65.

10. Halban PA, Kahn SE, Lernmark A, Rhodes CJ: Gene and cell-replacement therapy in the treatment of type I diabetes: how high must the standards be set? *Diabetes* 2001, 50:2181–2191.

11. DeFronzo RA: Pathogenesis of type 2 diabetes: metabolic and molecular implications for identifying diabetes genes. *Diabetes Rev* 1997, 5:177–269.

12. Cline GW, Rothman DL, Magnusson I, *et al.*: 13C-nuclear magnetic resonance spectroscopy studies of hepatic glucose metabolism in normal subjects and subjects with insulin-dependent diabetes mellitus. *J Clin Invest* 1994, 94:2369–2376.

13. Bruning JC, Michael MD, Winnay JN, et al.: A muscle-specific insulin receptor knockout exhibits features of the metabolic syndrome of NIDDM without altering glucose tolerance. Mol Cell 1998, 2:559–569.

14. Savkur RS, Philips AV, Cooper TA: Aberrant regulation of insulin receptor alternative splicing is associated with insulin resistance in myotonic dystrophy. Nat Genet 2001 29:40–47.

15. Burghes AH, Vaessin HE, de La CA: Genetics. The land between Mendelian and multifactorial inheritance. Science 2001, 293:2213–2214.

16. Sreenan SK, Zhou YP, Otani K, et al.: Calpains play a role in insulin secretion and action. Diabetes 2001, 50:2013–2020.

17. Horikawa Y, Oda N, Cox NJ, et al.: Genetic variation in the gene encoding calpain-10 is associated with type 2 diabetes mellitus. Nat Genet 2000, 26:163–175.

18. Freychet P, Roth J, Neville DM Jr: Insulin receptors in the liver: specific binding of [125I] insulin to the plasma membrane and its relation to insulin bioactivity. Proc Natl Acad Sci U S A 1971, 68:1833–1837.

19. White MF, Kahn CR: The insulin signaling system. J Biol Chem 1994, 269:1–4.

20. Yenush L, White MF: The IRS-signaling system during insulin and cytokine action. Bio Essays 1997, 19:491–500.

21. Withers DJ, Gutierrez JS, Towery H, et al.: Disruption of IRS-2 causes type 2 diabetes in mice. Nature 1998, 391:900–904.

22. Kulkarni RN, Bruning JC, Winnay JN, et al.: Tissue-specific knockout of the insulin receptor in pancreatic b cells creates an insulin secretory defect similar to that in Type 2 diabetes. Cell 1999, 96:329–339.

23. Frasca F, Pandini G, Scalia P, et al.: Insulin receptor isoform A, a newly recognized, high-affinity insulin-like growth factor II receptor in fetal and cancer cells. Mol Cell Biol 1999, 19:3278–3288.

24. White MF, Livingston JN, Backer JM, et al.: Mutation of the insulin receptor at tyrosine 960 inhibits signal transmission but does not affect its tyrosine kinase activity. Cell 1988, 54:641–649.

25. White MF, Shoelson SE, Keutmann H, Kahn CR: A cascade of tyrosine autophosphorylation in the b-subunit activates the insulin receptor. J Biol Chem 1988, 263:2969–2980.

26. Moller DE, Yokota A, Caro JF, Flier JS: Tissue-specific expression of two alternatively spliced insulin receptor mRNAs in man. Mol Endocrinol 1989, 3:1263–1269.

27. Mosthaf L, Grako K, Dull TJ, Coussens L, et al.: Functionally distinct insulin receptors generated by tissue-specific alternative splicing. EMBO J 1990, 9:2409–2413.

28. White MF, Maron R, Kahn CR: Insulin rapidly stimulates tyrosine phosphorylation of a Mr 185,000 protein in intact cells. Nature 1985, 318:183–186.

29. Sun XJ, Rothenberg PL, Kahn CR, et al.: The structure of the insulin receptor substrate IRS-1 defines a unique signal transduction protein. Nature 1991, 352:73–77.

30. Sun XJ, Wang LM, Zhang Y, et al.: Role of IRS-2 in insulin and cytokine signalling. Nature 1995, 377:173–177.

31. Itoh T, Takenawa T: Phosphoinositide-binding domains: Functional units for temporal and spatial regulation of intracellular signalling. Cell Signal 2002, 14:733–743.

32. Sawka-Verhelle D, Tartare-Deckert S, White MF, Van Obberghen E: Insulin receptor substrate-2 binds to the insulin receptor through its phopshotyrosine-binding domain and through a newly identified domain comprising amino acids 591–786. J Biol Chem 1996, 271:5980–5983.

33. He W, Craparo A, Zhu Y, et al.: Interaction of insulin receptor substrate-2 (IRS-2) with the insulin and insulin-like growth factor I receptors. Evidence for two distinct phosphotyrosine-dependent interaction domains within IRS-2. J Biol Chem 1996, 271:11641–11645.

34. Tamemoto H, Kadowaki T, Tobe K, et al.: Insulin resistance and growth retardation in mice lacking insulin receptor substrate-1. Nature 1994, 372:182–186.

35. Sesti G, Federici M, Hribal ML, et al.: Defects of the insulin receptor substrate (IRS) system in human metabolic disorders. FASEB J 2001, 15:2099–2111.

36. Stefan N, Kovacs P, Stumvoll M, et al.: Metabolic effects of the Gly1057Asp polymorphism in IRS-2 and interactions with obesity. Diabetes 2003, 52:1544–1550.

37. Le Fur S, Le Stunff C, Bougneres P: Increased insulin resistance in obese children who have both 972 IRS-1 and 1057 IRS-2 polymorphisms. Diabetes 2002, 51(suppl 3):S304–S307.

38. Fantin VR, Lavan BE, Wang Q, et al.: Cloning, tissue expression, and chromosomal location of the mouse insulin receptor substrate 4 gene. Endocrinology 1999, 140:1329–1337.

39. Smith-Hall J, Pons S, Patti ME, et al.: The 60-kDa insulin receptor substrate functions like an IRS-protein (pp60IRS3) in adipose cells. Biochemistry 1997, 36:8304–8310.

40. Bjornholm M, He AR, Attersand A, et al.: Absence of functional insulin receptor substrate-3 (IRS-3) gene in humans. Diabetologia 2002, 45:1697–1702.

41. Jellema A, Mensink RP, Kromhout D, et al.: Metabolic risk markers in an overweight and normal weight population with oversampling of carriers of the IRS-1 972Arg-variant. Atherosclerosis 2003, 171:75–81.

42. Bohni R, Riesgo-Escovar J, Oldham S, et al.: Autonomous control of cell and organ size by CHICO, a Drosophila homolog of vertebrate IRS1-4. Cell 1999, 97:865–875.

43. Yenush L, Zanella C, Uchida T, et al.: The pleckstrin homology and phosphotyrosine binding domains of insulin receptor substrate 1 mediate inhibition of apoptosis by insulin. Mol Cell Biol 1998, 18:6784–6794.

44. Burks DJ, Pons S, Towery H, et al.: Heterologous PH domains do not mediate coupling of IRS-1 to the insulin receptor. J Biol Chem 1997, 272:27716–27721.

45. Wolf G, Trub T, Ottinger E, et al.: The PTB domains of IRS-1 and Shc have distinct but overlapping specificities. J Biol Chem 1995, 270:27407–27410.

46. Burks DJ, Wang J, Towery H, et al.: IRS pleckstrin homology domains bind to acidic motifs in proteins. J Biol Chem 1998, 273:31061–31067.

47. Farhang-Fallah J, Yin X, Trentin G, et al.: Cloning and characterization of PHIP, a novel insulin receptor substrate-1 pleckstrin homology domain interacting protein. J Biol Chem 2000, 275:40492–40497.

48. Shepherd PR, Withers DJ, Siddle K: Phosphoinositide 3-kinase: the key switch mechanism in insulin signalling. Biochem J 1998, 333(pt 3):471–490.

49. Pawson T, Scott JD: Signaling through scaffold, anchoring, and adaptor proteins. Science 1997, 278:2075–2080.

50. Toker A, Cantley LC: Signalling through the lipid products of phosphoinosite-3-OH kinase. Nature 1997, 387:673–676.

51. Cross DAE, Alessi DR, Cohen P, et al.: Inhibition of glycogen synthase kinase-3 by insulin mediated protein kinase B. Nature 1996, 378:785–787.

52. Brazil DP, Hemmings BA: Ten years of protein kinase B signalling: a hard Akt to follow. Trends Biochem Sci 2001, 26:657–664.

53. Cho H, Thorvaldsen JL, Chu Q, et al.: Akt1/PKBalpha is required for normal growth but dispensable for maintenance of glucose homeostasis in mice. J Biol Chem 2001, 276:38349–38352.

54. Cho H, Mu J, Kim JK, et al.: Insulin resistance and a diabetes mellitus-like syndrome in mice lacking the protein kinase Akt2 (PKB beta). Science 2001, 292:1728–1731.

55. Garofalo RS, Orena SJ, Rafidi K, et al.: Severe diabetes, age-dependent loss of adipose tissue, and mild growth deficiency in mice lacking Akt2/PKB beta. J Clin Invest 2003, 112:197–208.

56. George S, Rochford JJ, Wolfrum C, et al.: A family with severe insulin resistance and diabetes due to a mutation in AKT2. Science 2004, 304:1325–1328.

57. Farese RV. Insulin-sensitive phospholipid signaling systems and glucose transport. Update II. Exp Biol Med (Maywood) 2001 Apr, 226:283–295.

58. Standaert ML, Bandyopadhyay G, Kanoh Y, et al.: Insulin and PIP3 activate PKC-zeta by mechanisms that are both dependent and independent of phosphorylation of activation loop (T410) and autophosphorylation (T560) sites. Biochemistry 2001, 40:249–255.

59. Ceresa BP, Pessin JE: Insulin regulation of the Ras activation/inactivation cycle. Mol Cell Biochem 1998, 182:23–29.

60. Goalstone ML, Draznin B: What does insulin do to Ras? Cell Signal 1998, 10:297–301.

61. Goalstone ML, Leitner JW, Wall K, et al.: Effect of insulin on farnesyltransferase. Specificity of insulin action and potentiation of nuclear effects of insulin-like growth factor-1, epidermal growth factor, and platelet-derived growth factor. J Biol Chem 1998, 273:23892–23896.

62. Goalstone ML, Wall K, Leitner JW, et al.: Increased amounts of farnesy-lated p21Ras in tissues of hyperinsulinaemic animals. Diabetologia 1999, 42:310–316.

63. Stephens E, Thureen PJ, Goalstone ML, et al.: Fetal hyperinsulinemia increases farnesylation of p21 Ras in fetal tissues. Am J Physiol Endocrinol Metab 2001, 281:E217–E223.

64. Rui L, Archer SF, Argetsinger LS, Carter-Su C: Platelet-derived growth factor and lysophosphatidic acid inhibit growth hormone binding and signaling via a protein kinase C-dependent pathway. J Biol Chem 2000, 275:2885–2892.

65. Goalstone ML, Leitner JW, Berhanu P, et al.: Insulin signals to prenyltrans-ferases via the Shc branch of intracellular signaling. J Biol Chem 2001, 276:12805–12812.

66. Long X, Muller F, Avruch J: TOR action in mammalian cells and in Caenorhabditis elegans. Curr Top Microbiol Immunol 2004, 279:115–138.

67. Stefan N, Fritsche A, Machicao F, et al.: The Gly1057Asp polymorphism in IRS-2 interacts with obesity to affect beta cell function. Diabetologia 2004, 47:2248.

68. Garami A, Zwartkruis FJ, Nobukuni T, et al.: Insulin activation of Rheb, a mediator of mTOR/S6K/4E-BP signaling, is inhibited by TSC1 and 2. Mol Cell 2003, 11:1457–1466.

69. Harrington LS, Findlay GM, Grgay A, et al.: The TSC1-2 tumor supressor controls insulin-PI3K signaling via regulation of IRS proteins. J Cell Biol 2004, 166:213–223.

70. Pende M, Kozma SC, Jaquet M, et al.: Hypoinsulinaemia, glucose intoler-ance and diminished beta-cell size in S6K1-deficient mice. Nature 2000, 408:994–997.

71. Isotani S, Hara K, Tokunaga C, et al.: Immunopurified mammalian target of rapamycin phosphorylates and activates p70 S6 kinase alpha in vitro. J Biol Chem 1999, 274:34493–34498.

72. Begum N, Sandu OA, Ito M, et al.: Active Rho kinase (ROK-alpha) asso-ciates with insulin receptor substrate-1 and inhibits insulin signaling in vascular smooth muscle cells. J Biol Chem 2002, 277:6214–6222.

73. Czech MP: Molecular actions of Insulin on glucose transport. Annu Rev Nutr 1995, 15:441–471.

74. Wood IS, Trayhurn P: Glucose transporters (GLUT and SGLT): expanded families of sugar transport proteins. Br J Nutr 2003, 89:3–9.

75. Li Q, Manolescu A, Ritzel M, et al.: Cloning and functional characteriza-tion of the human GLUT7 isoform SLC2A7 from the small intestine. Am J Physiol Gastrointest Liver Physiol 2004, 287:G236–G242.

76. Mobasheri A, Neama G, Bell S, et al.: Human articular chondrocytes express three facilitative glucose transporter isoforms: GLUT1, GLUT3 and GLUT9. Cell Biol Int 2002, 26:297–300.

77. Richardson S, Neama G, Phillips T, et al.: Molecular characterization and partial cDNA cloning of facilitative glucose transporters expressed in human articular chondrocytes, stimulation of 2-deoxyglucose uptake by IGF-I and elevated MMP-2 secretion by glucose deprivation. Osteoarthritis Cartilage 2003, 11:92–101.

78. Carayannopoulos MO, Chi MM, Cui Y, et al.: GLUT8 is a glucose trans-porter responsible for insulin-stimulated glucose uptake in the blasto-cyst. Proc Natl Acad Sci U S A 2000, 97:7313–7318.

79. McVie-Wylie AJ, Lamson DR, Chen YT: Molecular cloning of a novel member of the GLUT family of transporters, SLC2a10 (GLUT10), local-ized on chromosome 20q13.1: a candidate gene for NIDDM suscepti-bility. Genomics 2001, 72:113–117.

80. Andersen G, Rose CS, Hamid YH, et al.: Genetic variation of the GLUT10 glucose transporter (SLC2A10) and relationships to type 2 diabetes and intermediary traits. Diabetes 2003, 52:2445–2448.

81. Rogers S, Macheda ML, Docherty SE, et al.: Identification of a novel glucose transporter-like protein-GLUT-12. Am J Physiol Endocrinol Metab 2002, 282:E733–E738.

82. Gude NM, Stevenson JL, Rogers S, et al.: GLUT12 expression in human placenta in first trimester and term. Placenta 2003, 24:566–570.

83. Rogers S, Docherty SE, Slavin JL, et al.: Differential expression of GLUT12 in breast cancer and normal breast tissue. Cancer Lett. 2003, 193:225–233.

84. Chandler JD, Williams ED, Slavin JL, et al.: Expression and localization of GLUT1 and GLUT12 in prostate carcinoma. Cancer 2003, 97:2035–2042.

85. Pessin JE, Thurmond DC, Elmendorf JS, et al.: Molecular basis of insulin-stimulated GLUT4 vesicle trafficking. Location! Location! Location! J Biol Chem 1999, 274:2593–2596.

86. Khan AH, Pessin JE: Insulin regulation of glucose uptake: a complex inter-play of intracellular signalling pathways. Diabetologia 2002, 45:1475–1483.

87. Farese RV: Function and dysfunction of aPKC isoforms for glucose trans-port in insulin-sensitive and insulin-resistant states. Am J Physiol Endocrinol Metab 2002, 283:E1–E11.

88. Bandyopadhyay G, Standaert ML, Sajan MP, et al.: Protein kinase C-lambda knockout in embryonic stem cells and adipocytes impairs insulin-stimu-lated glucose transport. Mol Endocrinol 2004, 18:373–383.

89. Saltiel AR, Pessin JE: Insulin signaling in microdomains of the plasma membrane. Traffic 2003, 4:711–716.

90. Cohen AW, Razani B, Wang XB, et al.: Caveolin-1-deficient mice show insulin resistance and defective insulin receptor protein expression in adipose tissue. Am J Physiol Cell Physiol 2003, 285:C222–C235.

91. Liu J, Kimura A, Baumann CA, Saltiel AR: APS facilitates c-Cbl tyrosine phosphorylation and GLUT4 translocation in response to insulin in 3T3-L1 adipocytes. Mol Cell Biol 2002, 22:3599–3609.

92. Chiang SH, Baumann CA, Kanzaki M, et al.: Insulin-stimulated GLUT4 translocation requires the CAP-dependent activation of TC10. Nature 2001, 19:410:944–948.

93. Watson RT, Shigematsu S, Chiang SH, et al.: Lipid raft microdomain compartmentalization of TC10 is required for insulin signaling and GLUT4 translocation. J Cell Biol 2001, 154:829–840.

94. Roach PJ: Control of glycogen synthase by hierarchal protein phosphory-lation. FASEB J 1990, 4:2961–2968.

95. Cross DA, Alessi DR, Cohen P, et al.: Inhibition of glycogen synthase kinase-3 by insulin mediated by protein kinase B. Nature 1995, 378:785–789.

96. Haystead TAJ, Sim AT, Carling D, et al.: Effects of the tumour promoter okadaic acid on intracellular protein phosphorylation and metabolism. Nature 1989, 337:78–81.

97. Brady MJ, Saltiel AR: The role of protein phosphatase-1 in insulin action. Recent Prog Horm Res 2001, 56:157–173.

98. Newgard CB, Brady MJ, O'Doherty RM, Saltiel AR: Organizing glucose disposal: emerging roles of the glycogen targeting subunits of protein phosphatase-1. Diabetes 2000, 49:1967–1977.

99. Brady MJ, Kartha PM, Aysola AA, Saltiel AR: The role of glucose metabo-lites in the activation and translocation of glycogen synthase by insulin in 3T3-L1 adipocytes. J Biol Chem 1999, 274:27497–27504.

100. Rhoads RE: Signal transduction pathways that regulate eukaryotic protein synthesis. J Biol Chem 1999, 274:30337–30340.

101. Hartley D, Cooper GM: Role of mTOR in the degradation of IRS-1: regulation of PP2A activity. J Cell Biochem 2002, 85:304–314.

102. Plas DR, Thompson CB: Akt activation promotes degradation of tuberin and FOXO3a via the proteasome. J Biol Chem 2003, 278:12361–12366.

103. Kim JK, Fillmore JJ, Chen Y, et al.: Tissue-specific overexpression of lipoprotein lipase causes tissue-specific insulin resistance. Proc Natl Acad Sci U S A 2001, 98:7522–7527.

104. Proud CG, Denton RM: Molecular mechanisms for the control of trans-lation by insulin. Biochem J 1997, 328(pt 2):329–341.

105. Jaeschke A, Hartkamp J, Saitoh M, et al.: Tuberous sclerosis complex tumor suppressor-mediated S6 kinase inhibition by phosphatidylinosi-tide-3-OH kinase is mTOR independent. J Cell Biol 2002, 159:217–224.

106. Brunn GJ, Hudson CC, Sekulic A, et al.: Phosphorylation of the transla-tional repressor PHAS-I by the mammalian target of rapamycin. Science 1997, 277:99–101.

107. Tsukiyama-Kohara K, Poulin F, Kohara M, et al.: Adipose tissue reduction in mice lacking the translational inhibitor 4E-BP1. Nat Med 2001, 7:1128–1132.

108. Waskiewicz AJ, Johnson JC, Penn B, et al.: Phosphorylation of the cap-binding protein eukaryotic translation initiation factor 4E by protein kinase Mnk1 in vivo. Mol Cell Biol 1999, 19:1871–1880.

109. Minich WB, Balasta ML, Goss DJ, Rhoads RE: Chromatographic resolution of in vivo phosphorylated and nonphorphorylated eukaryotic translation initiation factor eIF-4E: increased cap affinity of the phosphorylated form. *Proc Natl Acad Sci U S A* 1994, 91:7668–7672.

110. Proud CG, Wang X, Patel JV, et al.: Interplay between insulin and nutrients in the regulation of translation factors. *Biochem Soc Trans* 2001, 29(pt 4):541–547.

111. Redpath NT, Price NT, Severinov KV, Proud CG: Regulation of elongation factor-2 by multisite phosphorylation. *Eur J Biochem* 1993, 213:689–699.

112. Mendez R, Kollmorgen G, White MF, Rhoads RE: Requirement of protein kinase C zeta for stimulation of protein synthesis by insulin. *Mol Cell Biol* 1997, 17:5184–5192.

113. White MF, Sun XJ, Pierce JH, inventors; Joslin Diabetes Center I, assignee: DNA encoding an insulin receptor substrate. MA patent 5,858,701. 1999 Jan 12.

114. Lu Z, Hu X, Li Y, et al.: Human papillomavirus 16 E6 oncoprotein interferences with insulin signaling pathway by binding to tuberin. *J Biol Chem* 2004, 279:35664–35670.

115. Kilberg MS, Handlogten ME, Christensen HN: Characteristics of an amino acid transport system in rat liver for glutamine, asparagine, histidine, and closely related analogs. *J Biol Chem* 1980, 255:4011–4019.

116. Pandey SK, He HJ, Chesley A, et al.: Wortmannin-sensitive pathway is required for insulin-stimulated phosphorylation of inhibitor kappaBalpha. *Endocrinology* 2002, 143:375–385.

117. Di Guglielmo GM, Drake PG, Baass PC, et al.: Insulin receptor internalization and signalling. *Mol Cell Biochem* 1998, 182:59–63.

118. Ahmad F, Azevedo JL, Cortright R, et al.: Alterations in skeletal muscle protein-tyrosine phosphatase activity and expression in insulin-resistant human obesity and diabetes. *J Clin Invest* 1997, 100:449–458.

119. Ahmad F, Considine RV, Bauer TL, et al.: Improved sensitivity to insulin in obese subjects following weight loss is accompanied by reduced protein-tyrosine phosphatases in adipose tissue. *Metabolism* 1997, 46:1140–1145.

120. Ahmad F, Goldstein BJ: Increased abundance of specific skeletal muscle protein-tyrosine phosphatases in a genetic model of insulin-resistant obesity and diabetes mellitus. *Metabolism* 1995, 44:1175–1184.

121. Ahmad F, Considine RV, Goldstein BJ: Increased abundance of the receptor-type protein-tyrosine phosphatase LAR accounts for the elevated insulin receptor dephosphorylating activity in adipose tissue of obese human subjects. *J Clin Invest* 1995, 95:2806–2812.

122. McGuire MC, Fields RM, Nyomba BL, et al.: Abnormal regulation of protein tyrosine phosphatase activities in skeletal muscle of insulin-resistant humans. *Diabetes* 1991, 40:939–942.

123. Zabolotny JM, Kim YB, Peroni OD, et al.: Overexpression of the LAR (leukocyte antigen-related) protein-tyrosine phosphatase in muscle causes insulin resistance. *Proc Natl Acad Sci U S A* 2001, 98:5187–5192.

124. Elchebly M, Payette P, Michaliszyn E, et al.: Increased insulin sensitivity and obesity resistance in mice lacking the protein tyrosine phosphatase-1B gene [see comments]. *Science* 1999, 283:1544–1548.

125. Klaman LD, Boss O, Peroni OD, et al.: Increased energy expenditure, decreased adiposity, and tissue-specific insulin sensitivity in protein-tyrosine phosphatase 1B-deficient mice. *Mol Cell Biol* 2000, 20:5479–5489.

126. Goldfine ID, Maddux BA, Youngren JF, et al.: Membrane glycoprotein PC-1 and insulin resistance. *Mol Cell Biochem* 1998, 182:177–184.

127. Frittitta L, Ercolino T, Bozzali M, et al.: A cluster of three single nucleotide polymorphisms in the 3'- untranslated region of human glycoprotein PC-1 gene stabilizes PC-1 mRNA and is associated with increased PC-1 protein content and insulin resistance-related abnormalities. *Diabetes* 2001, 50:1952–1955.

128. Srinivas PR, Deutsch DD, Mathews ST, et al.: Recombinant human alpha 2-HS glycoprotein inhibits insulin-stimulated mitogenic pathway without affecting metabolic signalling in Chinese hamster ovary cells overexpressing the human insulin receptor. *Cell Signal* 1996, 8:567–573.

129. Moyers JS, Bilan PJ, Reynet C, Kahn CR: Overexpression of Rad inhibits glucose uptake in cultured muscle and fat cells. *J Biol Chem* 1996, 271:23111–23116.

130. Takada T, Matozaki T, Takeda H, et al.: Roles of the complex formation of SHPS-1 with SHP-2 in insulin- stimulated mitogen-activated protein kinase activation. *J Biol Chem* 1998, 273:9234–9242.

131. Johnston AM, Pirola L, Van Obberghen E: Molecular mechanisms of insulin receptor substrate protein-mediated modulation of insulin signalling. *Growth Regul* 2003, 546:32–36.

132. Pirola L, Johnston AM, Van Obberghen E: Modulators of insulin action and their role in insulin resistance. *Int J Obes Relat Metab Disord* 2003, 27(suppl 3):S61–S64.

133. Aguirre V, Uchida T, Yenush L, et al.: The c-Jun NH(2)-terminal kinase promotes insulin resistance during association with insulin receptor substrate-1 and phosphorylation of Ser(307). *J Biol Chem* 2000, 275:9047–9054.

134. Aguirre V, Werner ED, Giraud J, et al.: Phosphorylation of Ser[307] in insulin receptor substrate-1 blocks interactions with the insulin receptor and inhibits insulin action. *J Biol Chem* 2002, 277:1531–1537.

135. Marchand-Brustel Y, Gual P, Gremeaux T, et al.: Fatty acid-induced insulin resistance: role of insulin receptor substrate 1 serine phosphorylation in the retroregulation of insulin signalling. *Biochem Soc Trans* 2003, 31(pt 6):1152–1156.

136. Hirosumi J, Tuncman G, Chang L, Gorgun, et al.: A central role for JNK in obesity and insulin resistance. *Nature* 2002, 420:333–336.

137. Rui L, Aguirre V, Kim JK, Shulman et al.: Insulin/IGF-1 and TNF-alpha stimulate phosphorylation of IRS-1 at inhibitory Ser[307] via distinct pathways. *J Clin Invest* 2001, 107:181–189.

138. Rui L, Yuan M, Frantz D, et al.: SOCS-1 and SOCS-3 block insulin signaling by ubiquitin-mediated degradation of IRS1 and IRS2. *J Biol Chem* 2002, 277:42394–42398.

139. Kawazoe Y, Naka T, Fujimoto M, et al.: Signal transducer and activator of transcription (STAT)-induced STAT inhibitor 1 (SSI-1)/suppressor of cytokine signaling 1 (SOCS1) inhibits insulin signal transduction pathway through modulating insulin receptor substrate 1 (IRS-1) phosphorylation. *J Exp Med* 2001, 193:263–269.

INSULIN RESISTANCE

Ele Ferrannini

3

At the whole-body level, hormone response is the compounded result of secretory rate and cellular sensitivity. For many hormones, action is modulated through hormonal feedback (*eg,* corticotropin-releasing hormone [CRH] and adrenocorticotropic hormone [ACTH] for cortisol, gonadotrophin-releasing hormone and gonadotrophins for sex steroids). With this design, sensitivity is provided by the specific hormone receptors on target tissues as well as on the companion gland of the feedback loop. In the case of insulin, there is no major pituitary or hypothalamic relay; target tissues control secretion directly by determining the level of positive and negative stimuli. Thus, the circulating concentrations of substrates (mostly glucose, but also amino acids, free fatty acids [FFA], and ketone bodies), which result from insulin action on intermediary metabolism in different tissues, feed signals back to the β cell. Sensitivity gating is provided by insulin receptors on target tissues (and on the β cell itself). Possibly as a consequence of the peculiar system design, insulin resistance is a relatively common phenomenon in physiology as well as pathophysiology.

Insulin exerts multiple actions on many cell types, but the primary servoregulated signal for insulin release is the plasma glucose concentration. According to this construct, insulin resistance is a reduced sensitivity of glucose uptake to insulin stimulation sensed by the β cell through elevated plasma glucose levels. Consequently, insulin resistance is defined as defective glucose disposal in the face of raised glucose and insulin concentrations.

Insulin sensitivity is set not only by the number and affinity of the insulin receptors but also by the functional state of the intracellular signaling pathways that transduce insulin binding to the various effectors (*eg,* glucose transport, phosphorylation and oxidation, glycogen synthesis, lipolysis, and ion exchange). Therefore, a massive reduction in the number of insulin receptors (or the presence of high titers of circulating anti-insulin or anti–insulin-receptor autoantibodies) is associated with a form of insulin resistance that is generalized and extreme (*ie,* all pathways are involved). These are, however, rare cases. More commonly, cellular resistance of the glucose pathway is caused by a malfunction of the signal transduction machinery. The various insulin effectors are, at least in part, independent of one another. As a consequence, cellular insulin resistance can be of any degree and usually is incomplete, or pathway specific. In addition, resistance in the glucose pathway reinforces the insulin signal to other pathways (*eg,* protein turnover) via stimulation of β cell activity. To the extent that they have preserved their sensitivity, other pathways are overly stimulated by the compensatory hyperinsulinemia. The pathophysiologic implication of this phenomenon is that, in insulin-resistant states, any abnormality that is found to be associated with defective glucose metabolism (*eg,* dyslipidemia, higher blood pressure, platelet hypercoagulation, or prothrombotic changes) theoretically can be the result of either the insulin resistance itself or the chronic effects of the attendant hyperinsulinemia. This is the origin of the insulin resistance syndrome.

Definition and Measurement

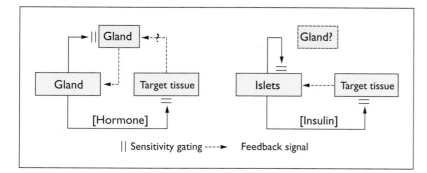

FIGURE 3-1. General organization of an endocrine system and peculiarity of the insulin system. For many protein and non-protein hormones, action is modulated by at least one, often two, hierarchical hormonal feedback paths (eg, corticotropin-releasing hormone and adrenocorticotropic hormone for cortisol, gonadotrophin-releasing hormone and gonadotrophins for sex steroids). Sensitivity is provided by the circulating hormone concentrations ([hormone]) acting upon specific hormone receptors located on target tissues as well as on the companion gland of the feedback loop. In the case of insulin, there is no major pituitary or hypothalamic relay; target tissues control secretion directly by determining the level of positive and negative stimuli. Thus, the circulating concentrations of substrates (mostly glucose, but also amino acids, free fatty acids, and ketone bodies), which result from insulin action on intermediary metabolism in different tissues, feed signals back to the β cell. Sensitivity gating is provided by insulin receptors on target tissues; some degree of autoregulation is given by insulin receptors on the β cell itself.

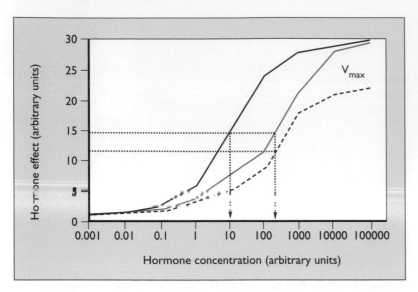

FIGURE 3-2. Shape and parameters of the dose-response curve for a hormone. In general, the relationship between concentration and action of a hormone is sigmoidal (*black line*): the response is sluggish in the low concentration range, then rises in an approximately linear manner, and then tapers off to saturation. Mathematically, this kind of dose-response relationship can be approximated by a Michaelis-Menten equation, in which the maximal effect is termed V_{max}, the hormone concentration at which the effect is half-maximal is termed K_m, and sensitivity is expressed by the ratio V_{max}/K_m. The figure exemplifies two types of abnormal response: reduced sensitivity, characterized by a 20-fold increase in K_m (*blue line*), and the same reduction in sensitivity coupled with an impaired maximal response (*dotted line*).

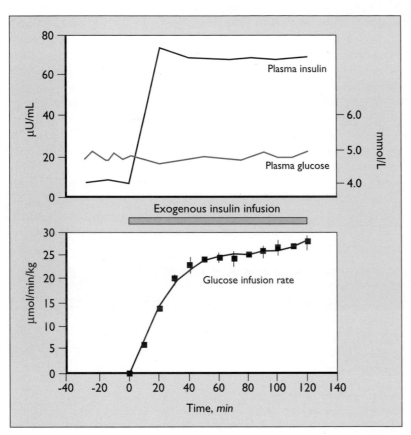

FIGURE 3-3. Euglycemic hyperinsulinemic insulin clamping. Euglycemic hyper-insulinemic insulin clamping is regarded as the gold standard for the measurement of insulin sensitivity in vivo [1,2]. Exogenous insulin is infused in a primed-constant format to raise plasma insulin concentrations to any desired level (in this figure, the postprandial range). As peripherally infused insulin is cleared rapidly from the plasma (at the rate of 0.6 to 1.4 L/min in nonobese healthy subjects [3]), a stable hyperinsulinemic plateau is reached within 20 minutes. Exogenous glucose is infused simultaneously to prevent insulin-induced hypoglycemia; the glucose infusion rate is adjusted every 5 to 10 minutes under the guidance of on-line plasma glucose measurements. During the second hour of a 2-hour clamp study, endogenous glucose release generally is suppressed, and the glucose infusion rate equals the total amount of glucose taken up by all tissues in the body. The *black squares* in the *lower panel* of the figure represent mean (± standard error of the mean [SEM]) values of whole-body insulin-mediated glucose uptake (normalized for body weight) in 30 nondiabetic patients of a range of ages and body weights.

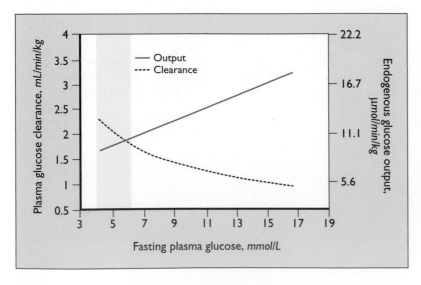

FIGURE 3-4. Glucose turnover in the fasting state. The use of a glucose isotope, either stable or radioactively labeled, allows one to measure the rate at which glucose is produced endogenously and cleared from the plasma in the fasting state. Following a prolonged primed-constant intravenous infusion, the tracer reaches isotopic equilibrium (*ie,* constant specific activity) throughout the body glucose space. Under these circumstances, the ratio of the tracer infusion rate to its steady-state plasma concentration measures whole-body glucose clearance (expressed in mL/min/kg of body weight). Endogenous glucose output (mostly from the liver) then is calculated as the product of glucose clearance by the fasting plasma glucose concentration and expressed in μmol/min per kg of body weight. The graph shows how glucose clearance and endogenous glucose output vary across a range of fasting plasma glucose concentrations, encompassing the normal (*shaded area*) and diabetic state. Whereas glucose clearance is reduced already for minor degrees of fasting hyperglycemia (< 7 mmol/L), endogenous glucose output increases in approximate proportion to the severity of hyper-glycemia [4].

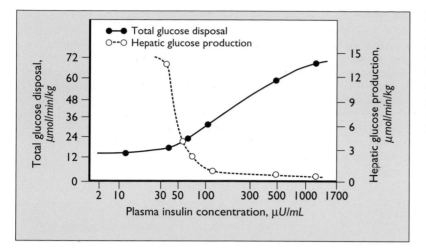

FIGURE 3-5. Insulin dose-response curves for stimulation of whole-body glucose uptake and inhibition of endogenous glucose production in healthy subjects. Curves were constructed by combining the insulin clamp technique at five insulin levels encompassing the physiologic and pharmacologic concentration range with tracer glucose infusion. The effect of insulin on endogenous (hepatic) glucose release is already maximal at plasma insulin concentrations that are submaximal for stimulation of glucose uptake [5]. Thus, under physiologic conditions, the earliest and most effective action of insulin to limit postprandial hyperglycemia is to suppress release of endogenous glucose into the systemic circulation.

Insulin Action

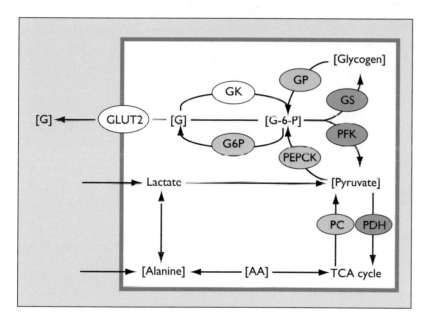

FIGURE 3-6. Hepatic glucose production. Simplified scheme of the main intracellular pathways of glucose production in the liver, glycogenolysis and gluconeogenesis (*thick lines*). *Shaded ovals* indicate key insulin-sensitive enzymes in the pathway. Substrate concentrations are in brackets; insulin-sensitive enzymes are inscribed in circles, shaded to indicate stimulatory action or gray to indicate inhibitory action. Whereas glycogen breakdown directly increases the intracellular concentrations of glucose-6-phosphate (G-6-P), uptake of lactate, alanine, and other gluconeogenic amino acids provides 3-carbon precursors for de novo G-6-P synthesis. G—free glucose; GP—glycogen phosphorylase; GS—glycogen synthase; G6P—glucose-6-phosphatase; GK—glucokinase; PFK—phosphofructokinase; PEPCK—phosphoenolpyruvate-carboxykinase; PC—pyruvate carboxylase; PDH—pyruvate dehydrogenase; AA—amino acids; GLUT2—isoform 2 (non–insulin-sensitive) of the glucose transporter; TCA—tricarboxylic acid cycle.

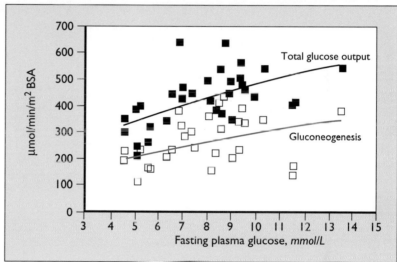

FIGURE 3-7. Contribution of gluconeogenesis to fasting plasma glucose concentration. Total endogenous glucose output (measured by the tracer dilution technique) and gluconeogenesis (determined by the deuterated water technique [6]) were simultaneously measured in fasting nondiabetic subjects and patients with type 2 diabetes mellitus. As expected (*see* Fig. 3-4), endogenous glucose output (*filled squares, solid line*) is related directly to the degree of hyperglycemia over a range of fasting plasma glucose concentrations. Gluconeogenesis (*empty squares, blue line*) makes up roughly one half of total glucose output in nondiabetic subjects, and is increased in diabetic patients, thereby contributing substantially to their fasting hyperglycemia [7]. BSA—body surface area.

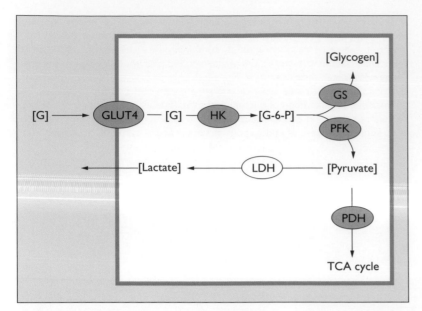

FIGURE 3-8. Peripheral glucose disposal. Simplified scheme of glycogen synthesis and glucose oxidation, the main pathways of intracellular glucose disposition in insulin target tissues. *Shaded ovals* indicate key insulin-sensitive enzymes in the pathway. G—free glucose; G-6-P—glucose-6-phosphate; GLUT4—isoform 4 (insulin-sensitive) of the glucose transporter; HK—hexokinase II; GS—glycogen synthase; PFK—phosphofructokinase; PDH—pyruvate dehydrogenase; LDH—lactic dehydrogenase; TCA—tricarboxylic acid cycle.

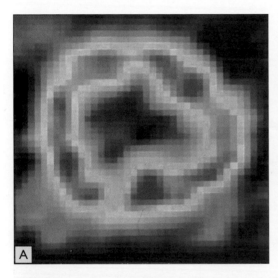

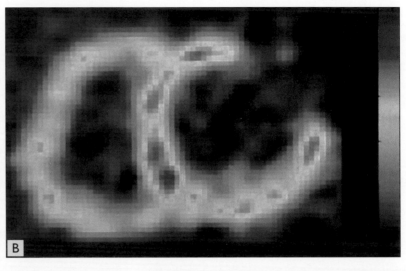

FIGURE 3-9. (See Color Plate) Insulin action in the heart. Myocardial muscle is insulin-sensitive. Whereas free fatty acids (FFA) represent the dominant fuel for cardiac muscle in the fasting state, an increase in circulating insulin concentrations inhibits lipolysis, thereby restraining FFA availability and promoting glucose uptake. By using ^{18}F-deoxyglucose (FDG), an analog of glucose (which is transported and phosphorylated in the same manner as D-glucose but not further metabolized) labeled with a short-lived radioactive isotope of fluorine (^{18}F), positron-emitting tomography (PET) detects a signal that is proportional to the rate of myocardial glucose uptake. The figure shows FDG images of human heart muscle during a euglycemic insulin clamp study like the one illustrated in Figure 3-3. The colors (with red being the most intense) indicate regions with different rates of glucose utilization. **A,** The left ventricle of a normal patient. **B,** The ventricular walls of a patient who suffered from an anterior myocardial infarction 6 months before the PET study. A "cold" area of missing glucose uptake is clearly visible at the upper right corner (the anterior wall of the left ventricle). Also evident is a diffuse decrease in insulin-mediated glucose uptake (insulin resistance) throughout the left ventricular wall, involving myocardial regions distant from the infarcted area and normally perfused (perfusion scan not shown) [8].

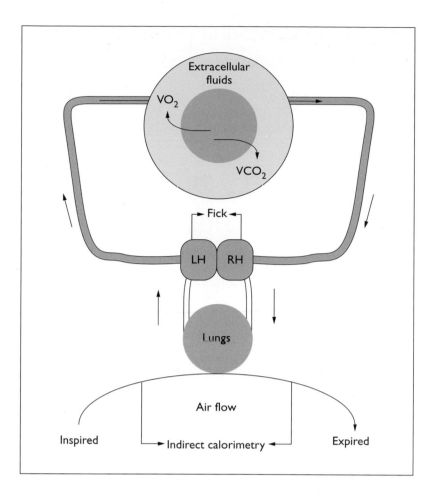

FIGURE 3-10. Measuring intracellular glucose disposition and energy expenditure in vivo via indirect calorimetry. The schematic illustrates the correspondence between indirect calorimetry (in which oxygen consumption = [O_2 in expired air - O_2 in inspired air] $\times$ air flow; carbon dioxide production = [CO_2 in expired air - CO_2 in inspired air] $\times$ air flow) and the Fick principle (by which oxygen consumption = (arterial blood O_2 - central venous blood O_2) $\times$ cardiac output; carbon dioxide production = (arterial blood CO_2 - venous blood CO_2) $\times$ cardiac output). With the use of calorimetric equations, net rates of oxidation of lipids and carbohydrates and of energy expenditure can be quantified at the whole-body as well as the organ level starting from gas-exchange data. LH—left heart; RH—right heart; VO$_2$—oxygen consumption; VCO$_2$—carbon dioxide production.

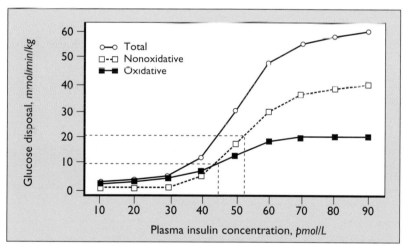

FIGURE 3-11. Dose-response curve for action of insulin on glucose oxidation and nonoxidative glucose disposal in the healthy subject. Indirect calorimetry can be combined with the insulin clamp technique to estimate glucose oxidation at various plasma insulin plateaus. Nonoxidative glucose disposal, consisting primarily of glycogen synthesis, is then obtained as the difference between total glucose uptake and net glucose oxidation. The figure presents data from healthy subjects studied over a range of plasma insulin levels; the dotted lines identify the K_m values for oxidative glucose disposal and glycogen synthesis. Glucose oxidation has a high sensitivity and low capacity; glycogen synthesis has lower sensitivity but higher capacity. Thus, under physiologic conditions, mild hyperinsulinemia stimulates glucose oxidation, whereas stronger insulinization promotes glucose storage into glycogen. Clamp studies combined with regional calorimetry have demonstrated that skeletal muscle is the insulin target tissue responsible for most (50% to 70%) insulin-mediated glucose uptake and storage in vivo [9].

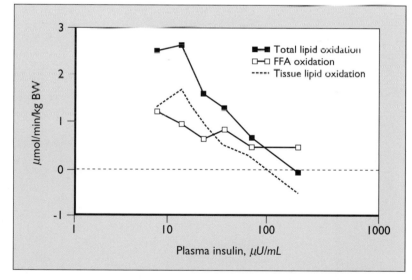

FIGURE 3-12. Dose-response curves for insulin action on lipid metabolism. Indirect calorimetry also yields estimates for total net lipid oxidation. The oxidation of circulating free fatty acid (FFA) can be measured by collecting labeled CO_2 in the expired air during the constant infusion of carbon-labeled palmitate. Tissue lipid oxidation is then defined as the difference between total lipid and FFA oxidation. In the clamp studies in normal subjects summarized in the figure, low insulin doses effectively inhibited both total lipid and FFA oxidation; high physiologic insulin doses (or chronic hyperinsulinemia) did not affect FFA oxidation any further, but caused net lipid synthesis (ie, negative values of lipid oxidation). BW—body weight. (Data from Groop et al. [10].)

Insulin Resistance

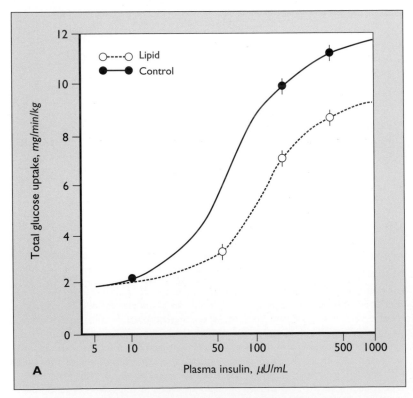

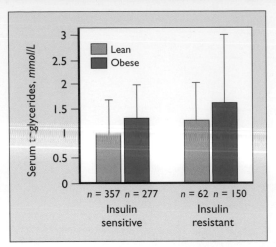

FIGURE 3-13. Relation between free fatty acid (FFA) concentrations and insulin sensitivity. In each of 450 nondiabetic subjects, plasma FFA concentrations measured in the fasting state and again at the end of a euglycemic insulin clamp (*see* Fig. 3-3) are plotted against the individual level of insulin sensitivity. The distance between the two regression lines measures the suppressive effect of insulin on lipolysis (*ie,* inhibition of tissue hormone-sensitive lipase). Lipolysis is resistant to insulin inhibition (in the fasting state as well as during insulinization) in subjects who are resistant to the effect of insulin on glucose uptake [11]. Thus, insulin sensitivity in lipolysis and glucose pathways is a coupled phenomenon. FFM—fat-free mass.

FIGURE 3-14. Insulin sensitivity and serum triglycerides. If the effect of insulin on lipolysis is deficient, both the peripheral tissues and the liver are exposed to an excess of circulating free fatty acids (FFA). In peripheral tissues, FFA impede insulin-mediated glucose uptake (by substrate competition, according to Randle [12]); in the liver, FFA are incorporated into triglycerides at an increased rate. In accordance with the latter observation, serum triglyceride concentrations are higher in insulin-resistant individuals (*ie,* subjects in the lowest quartile of the distribution of insulin sensitivity) than in more insulin-sensitive subjects, whether they are obese or lean. The figure plots median and interquartile range for four groups: insulin-sensitive lean subjects; insulin-sensitive obese subjects; insulin-resistant lean subjects; and insulin-resistant obese subjects. (*Data from* the European Group for the Study of Insulin Resistance database [11]).

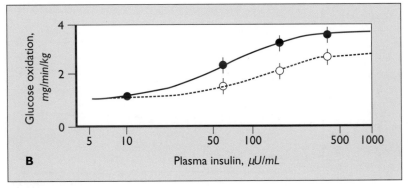

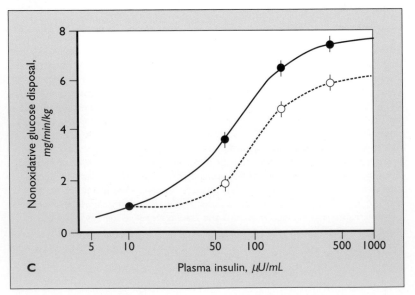

FIGURE 3-15. Experimental proof of substrate competition. Dose-response curves for total glucose uptake (**A**) and its main components, glucose oxidation (**B**), and nonoxidative glucose disposal (**C**) (equivalent to glycogen synthesis), in healthy volunteers under control conditions (*solid lines*), and during the simultaneous infusion of Intralipid (KabiVitrum, Franklin, OH), a triglyceride emulsion (*dotted lines*). Provision of exogenous fatty substrates acutely impairs total glucose uptake and its main components (glucose oxidation and glycogen synthesis), as predicated by substrate competition.

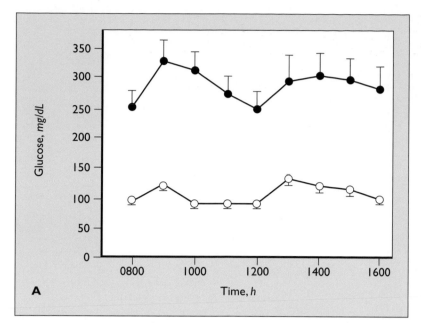

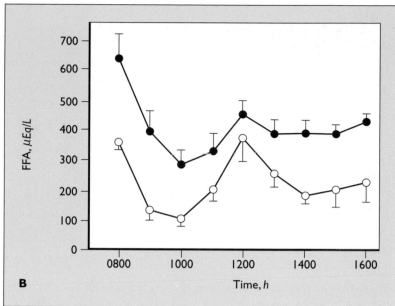

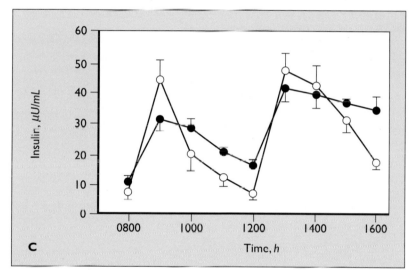

FIGURE 3-16. Day-long metabolic profile in type 2 diabetes. Plasma glucose (**A**), free fatty acids (FFA) (**B**), and insulin (**C**) concentrations in response to breakfast and lunch were measured in nondiabetic patients (*open circles*) and in type 2 diabetic patients (*closed circles*). Whereas average insulin levels were comparable in the two groups, plasma glucose and FFA were markedly elevated in the diabetic patients [12]. Thus, patients with type 2 diabetes are resistant to insulin action on glucose disposal (*ie*, higher plasma glucose concentrations) as well as lipolysis (*ic*, higher plasma FFA levels) throughout the day. Consequently, insulin target tissues are exposed to chronically elevated FFA and may become laden with triglyceride deposits. (*Adapted from* Golay *et al.* [13].)

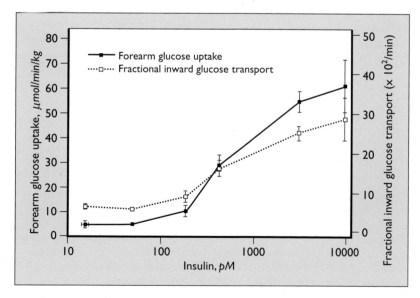

FIGURE 3-17. Glucose transport in vivo. In the human forearm, glucose transport can be measured under in vivo conditions by a triple-tracer method [14]. By this technique, the washout curves of three intra-arterially injected tracers (mannitol, to trace extracellular kinetics; 3-ortho-methylglucose, to trace glucose transport; and labeled glucose, to monitor intracellular glucose metabolism) are measured in a deep forearm vein that drains mostly muscle tissue. A compartmental model then is used on these data to calculate fractional inward glucose transport across the plasma membrane of skeletal muscle. The dose-response curve for glucose transport in the human forearm tissues was measured in healthy subjects by the triple tracer technique during graded hyperinsulinemia created by the insulin clamp technique. The graph also shows the parallelism between inward glucose transport and total glucose uptake in forearm tissues.

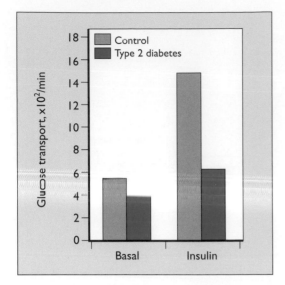

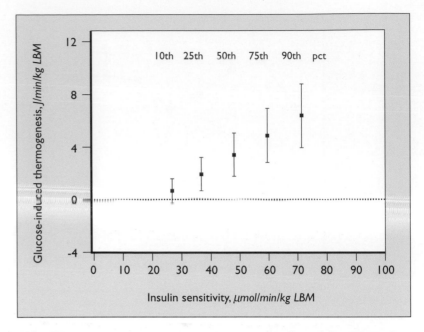

FIGURE 3-18. Defective glucose transport in type 2 diabetes. Inward glucose transport was measured by the triple-tracer technique in the basal state (overnight fast) and during euglycemic hyperinsulinemia in matched groups of patients with type 2 diabetes and nondiabetic controls. Diabetes is associated with a marked defect in the ability of insulin to stimulate glucose transport in skeletal muscle tissues [15].

FIGURE 3-19. Insulin resistance and thermogenesis. One of the actions of insulin in vivo is to stimulate energy expenditure (*ie*, thermogenesis). Glucose-induced thermogenesis (GIT) is the change in energy expenditure observed during euglycemic hyperinsulinemia, as measured by indirect calorimetry during an insulin clamp in this case. The figure shows point estimates (± Standard error of the mean [SEM]) of GIT at different percentiles (pct) of insulin sensitivity in 322 nondiabetic subjects after statistical adjustment by gender, age, and body mass index. Insulin-resistant subjects show a defect in glucose-induced thermogenesis that is proportional to the degree of insulin resistance [16]. LBM—lean body mass.

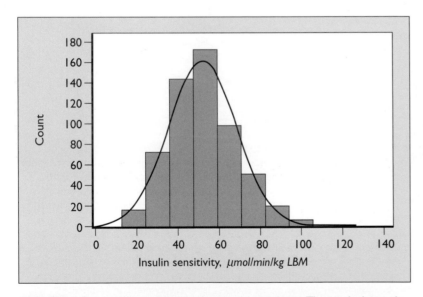

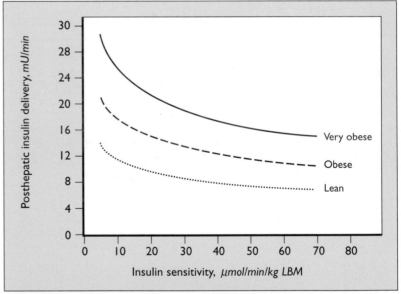

FIGURE 3-20. Insulin sensitivity in the general population. The graph shows the frequency distribution plot of insulin sensitivity (as measured by the euglycemic insulin clamp) in a cohort of 580 nondiabetic, nonobese (body mass index ≤ 25 kg/m²) white patients of both genders. The distribution is significantly different from the normal distribution. The graft is skewed to the left as a result of an excess of insulin-resistant individuals (*data from* the European Group for the Study of Insulin Resistance [17]). There is, however, no evidence to suggest a bimodal or multimodal distribution of this trait. In general terms, this distribution is compatible with a model in which genetic drive is influenced by powerful environmental factors. LBM—lean body mass.

FIGURE 3-21. Relation between insulin sensitivity and insulin secretion. In a cohort of 1200 nondiabetic white patients of both genders, the relationship between insulin sensitivity (by the insulin clamp technique) and insulin secretion (estimated from the clamping data as the posthepatic insulin delivery rate) is highly curvilinear (hyperbolic), such that in insulin-resistant individuals small changes in insulin sensitivity are associated with large (compensatory) changes in insulin secretion. The plot also shows the impact of obesity as an independent factor that greatly amplifies insulin secretion at any given level of insulin resistance. Thus, any degree of insulin hypersecretion (and, therefore, of hyperinsulinemia) can be described as the sum of a component that is secondary (compensatory) to insulin resistance and a part that is primary. The primary component is particularly common in obese individuals. (*Data from* Ferrannini *et al.* [18].)

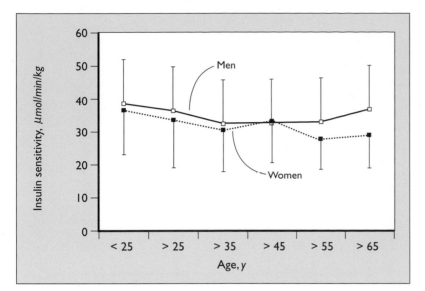

FIGURE 3-22. Impact of age on insulin sensitivity. In nondiabetic, otherwise healthy patients, aging has a marginal effect on insulin resistance [15]. Thus, the aging population tends to be insulin resistant because it is enriched with individuals with impaired glucose tolerance, essential hypertension, or obesity rather than as a result of senescence itself.

Insulin Resistance Syndrome

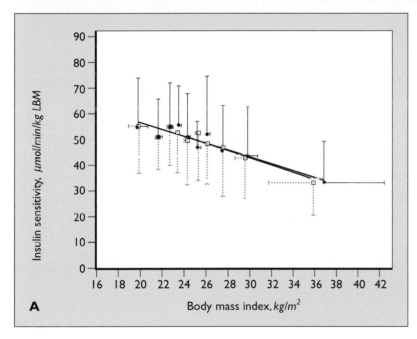

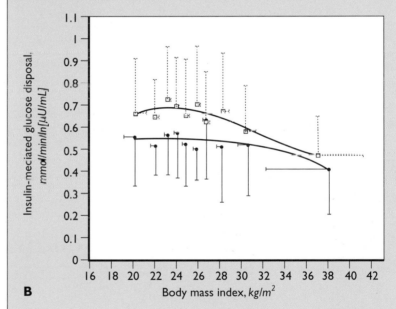

FIGURE 3-23. Insulin resistance and obesity. The dependence of insulin sensitivity on obesity (expressed as the body mass index [BMI]) is expressed in two ways in this figure. When total insulin-mediated glucose uptake is normalized by lean body mass (LBM) (**A**), insulin sensitivity declines linearly with body mass equally in men (*dotted lines*) and women (*solid bars*). However, when insulin-mediated glucose disposal is expressed in absolute terms (**B**) (in mmol/min, corrected for the steady-state plasma insulin concentration

achieved during the clamp), the negative impact of obesity is seen only in very obese individuals (BMI > 32 kg/m²). Thus, in the obese person, each unit mass of lean tissue (mostly skeletal muscle) is resistant to the action of insulin in direct proportion to the excess body fat. However, the expanded body mass of the moderately obese person compensates for the reduced insulin sensitivity and contributes to the maintenance of glucose tolerance [18].

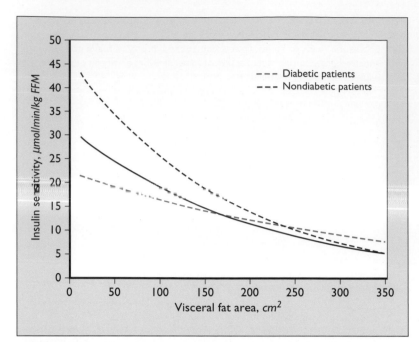

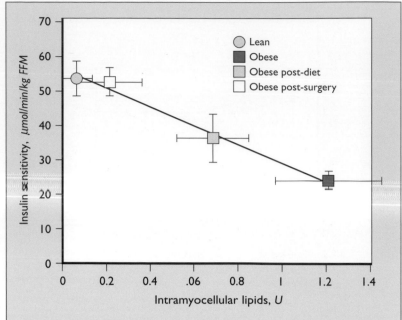

FIGURE 3-24. Fat as a determinant of insulin action. Adipose mass is not the sole link between obesity and insulin resistance. Excessive deposition of fat in the abdominal visceral area and within skeletal muscle cells is a potent determinant of insulin action. This graph shows the reciprocal association between insulin sensitivity (on the euglycemic insulin clamp) and intra-abdominal fat accumulation (measured as the visceral fat area by MRI) in adult humans. The *solid line* is the predicted relationship after adjustment by gender, age, and body mass index in 70 patients ($P < 0.001$). The *dotted lines* are the separate relationships in nondiabetic patients and diabetic patients. Note that the impact of visceral fat accumulation on insulin sensitivity is stronger in nondiabetic, insulin-sensitive subjects than in insulin-resistant diabetic patients ($P < 0.02$). FFM—fat-free mass.

FIGURE 3-25. Reciprocal association between insulin sensitivity and intramyocellular lipid accumulation (estimated by histochemistry on biopsy specimens of vastus lateralis muscle) in lean patients, morbidly obese patients, and morbidly obese patients after weight reduction by hypocaloric diet or surgery (biliopancreatic diversion). FFM—fat-free mass. (*Adapted from* Greco *et al.* [19].)

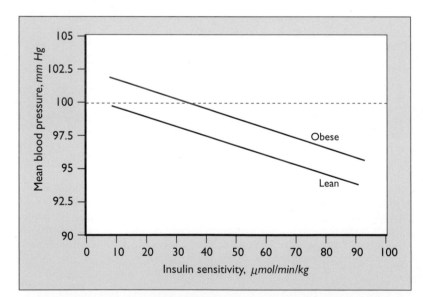

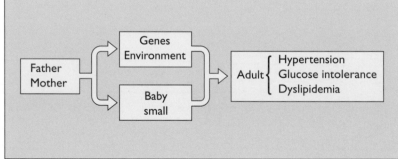

FIGURE 3-27. Insulin resistance and intrauterine development. Low birthweight has been found to be associated with the emergence in adulthood of hypertension, impaired glucose tolerance, and dyslipidemia, all states of impaired insulin action. Therefore, in addition to genes and environmental factors, insulin sensitivity may be modulated by changes that occur during intrauterine development. Thus, intrauterine growth retardation, possibly caused by maternal insulin resistance, may exert negative effects on the development of β cells, insulin sensing in target tissues, and the vasculature.

FIGURE 3-26. Insulin resistance and blood pressure. Patients with essential hypertension are, as a group, insulin resistant. This is not a special feature of essential hypertension, however, but the extension of a physiologic link to the disease domain. In fact, insulin resistance is associated with higher blood pressure levels in the normotensive population. The graph shows the significant inverse relationship between mean blood pressure and insulin sensitivity (as measured by the clamping technique) in 450 nondiabetic subjects in the European Group for the Study of Insulin Resistance cohort. The regression lines are adjusted by gender and age, and are drawn across the observed range of insulin sensitivity. The lower line (*lean*) is the predicted dependence in a subject with a body mass index of 25 kg/m², whereas the upper line (*obese*) is the function for an individual with a body mass index of 35 kg/m². The dotted line is an arbitrary threshold for clinical hypertension. Obesity and insulin resistance work together to raise arterial blood pressure [20].

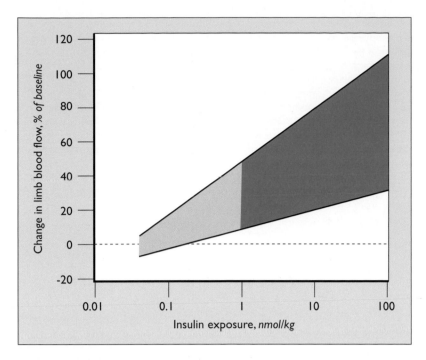

FIGURE 3-28. Hemodynamic actions of insulin: I. Insulin induces dilatation of peripheral (forearm, leg, or calf) vasculature as a function of exposure (dose of insulin × length of exposure, expressed as total nmol/kg of body weight). The lightly shaded area represents the physiologic insulin exposure, over which the average vasodilatory response is in the range 15% to 30%. This represents a compilation of a number of published studies. (*Adapted from* Yki-Järvinen and Utriainen [21]).

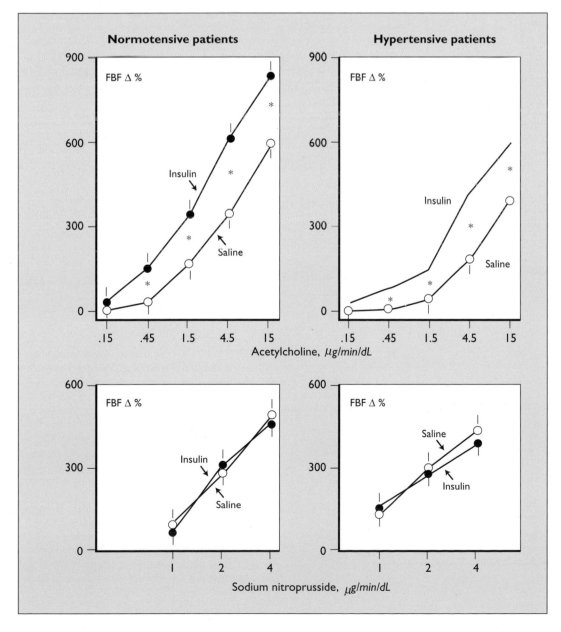

FIGURE 3-29. Hemodynamic actions of insulin: II. When infused locally (*ie,* through the brachial artery) at physiologic doses, insulin potentiates acetylcholine-induced (*top*), but not nitroprusside-induced (*bottom*), vasodilatation in humans [22], both in normotensive patients (*left*) and in patients with essential hypertension (*right*). These data suggest that insulin vasodilatation is an endothelium-dependent phenomenon. In addition, the potentiating effect of insulin was similar in healthy patients and hypertensive patients (who were resistant to the effect of insulin on glucose uptake), suggesting that the actions of insulin on the vasculature and glucose metabolism are largely independent of each other. *Asterisks* indicate mean values that are significantly different between insulin and saline infusion. FBF—forearm blood flow.

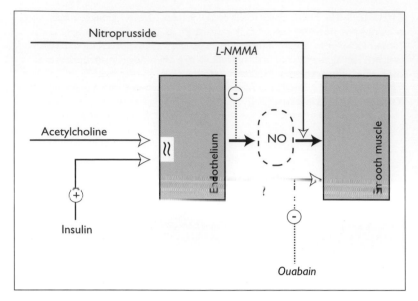

FIGURE 3-30. Hemodynamic actions of insulin: III. Insulin receptors are present on endothelial as well as on smooth muscle cells; thus, both types of cells are potential targets for insulin action. Insulin-induced vasodilatation [23] and insulin potentiation of acetylcholine-induced vasodilatation can both be blocked by L-monomethyl-arginine (L-NMMA), a competitive inhibitor of nitric oxide (NO) synthase [22], indicating that a likely mechanism for this effect of insulin is NO release from the endothelium. Direct provision of NO with nitroprusside bypasses the endothelial step. Furthermore, both insulin-induced vasodilatation [24] and insulin potentiation of acetylcholine-induced vasodilatation [22] can be blocked by ouabain, an inhibitor of sodium-potassium ATPase, suggesting that cell membrane hyperpolarization is an alternative mechanism for this action of insulin. Insulin-induced hyperpolarization can be exerted directly on the smooth muscle cell or involve the release of an unidentified hyperpolarizing factor from the endothelium.

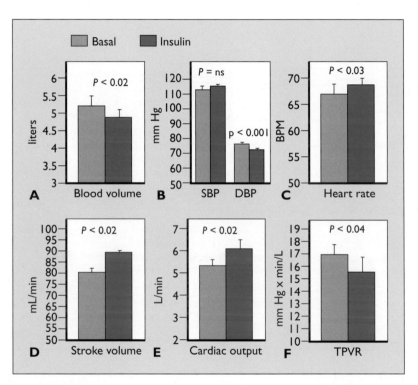

FIGURE 3-31. Hemodynamic actions of insulin: IV. Vasodilatation is not the only vascular action of insulin. Following physiologic hyperinsulinemia established by insulin clamping, blood volume is reduced (**A**); diastolic blood pressure (DBP) falls slightly, whereas systolic blood pressure (SBP) increases somewhat (**B**); heart rate goes up (**C**); stroke volume and cardiac output increase (**D** and **E**); and total peripheral vascular resistances (TPVR) decrease (**F**). This hemodynamic picture is compatible with a direct effect of insulin to reduce vascular resistance (vasodilatation) and a simultaneous effect of insulin to stimulate adrenergic activity (enhanced cardiac contractility). BPM—beats per minute.

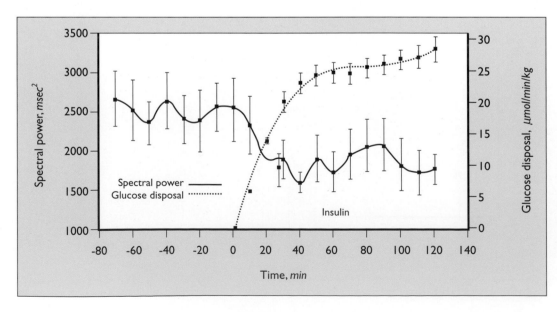

FIGURE 3-32. Hemodynamic actions of insulin: V. Spectral analysis of heart rate variability provides information on the autonomic nervous control of cardiac function. Total spectral power reflects parasympathetic and adrenergic inputs related to baroreflex control of heart rate; these inputs are mediated through the central nervous system. During a standard euglycemic insulin clamp, insulin causes a prompt and marked decline in total spectral power, which is temporally and quantitatively unrelated to insulin stimulation of glucose disposal [25]. This effect is partially independent of changes in heart rate, and therefore reflects direct desensitization of the autonomic neural reflex arch. In addition, the effect is more marked on the parasympathetic component of the autonomic arch (parasympathetic withdrawal), thereby giving rise to relative sympathetic dominance.

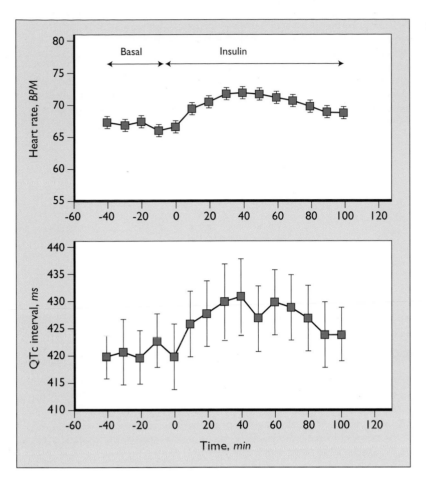

FIGURE 3-33. Electrophysiologic action of insulin. Insulin acutely hyperpolarizes plasma membranes, possibly through its stimulatory effect on ATP-dependent sodium-potassium exchange. The graph shows the changes in heart rate and corrected QT (QTc) interval on the electrocardiogram during a euglycemic insulin clamp in healthy volunteers. Despite a tachycardic effect (*top*), insulin causes a prolongation of the QTc interval (*bottom*), indicating a prolongation of the repolarization phase. In chronically hyperinsulinemic individuals, this action of insulin may sensitize the heart to arrhythmias, particularly in at-risk individuals. BPM—beats per minute. (*Adapted from* Gastaldelli et al. [26].)

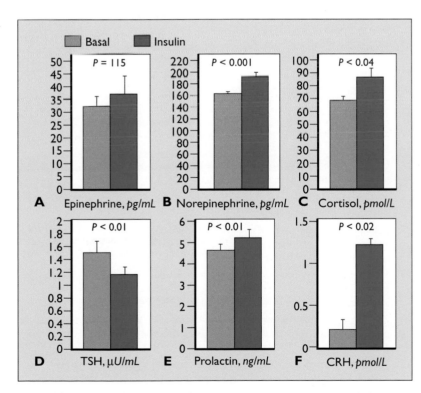

FIGURE 3-34. Insulin action and the central nervous system. Physiologic euglycemic hyperinsulinemia is associated with a rise in the circulating levels of norepinephrine (**A** and **B**), cortisol (**C**), prolactin (**E**), and corticotropin-releasing hormone (CRH) (**F**), and a decrease in thyroid-stimulating hormone (TSH) (**D**) [25]. This pattern of hormonal responses is compatible with a moderate stress reaction orchestrated by CRH. Thus, the hemodynamic, autonomic nervous, and hormonal responses to peripheral hyperinsulinemia coherently indicate that insulin acts in the central nervous system, most probably following transport from the plasma across the blood-brain barrier [27].

NATIVE AND EXPERIMENTAL INSULIN RESISTANCE

Physiologic	Nonendocrine
Puberty	Essential hypertension
Pregnancy	Chronic uremia
Bed rest	Liver cirrhosis
Contraceptives	Rheumatoid arthritis
High-fat diet	Acanthosis nigricans
Metabolic	Chronic heart failure
Type 2 diabetes	Myotonic dystrophia
Uncontrolled type 1 diabetes	Trauma, burns, sepsis
Diabetic ketoacidosis	Surgery
Obesity	Neoplastic cachexia
Severe malnutrition	Experimental
Hyperuricemia	Short-term hyperglycemia
Insulin-induced hypoglycemia	Short-term hypoglycemia
Excessive alcohol consumption	Short-term hyperinsulinemia
Endocrine	Short-term hypoinsulinemia
Thyrotoxicosis	Fat infusion
Hypothyroidism	Amino acid infusion
Cushing syndrome	Infusion of counterregulatory hormones
Pheochromocytoma	
Acromegaly	Acidosis

FIGURE 3-35. Native and experimental insulin resistance. This table lists conditions that have been found to be associated with insulin resistance or under which insulin resistance can be produced experimentally.

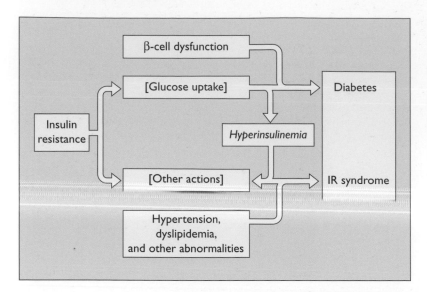

FIGURE 3-36. Insulin action and the insulin resistance syndrome: a working hypothesis. Insulin resistance (IR) in the glucose pathway combines with β-cell dysfunction to produce the hyperglycemia of diabetes. Insulin resistance also induces compensatory hyperinsulinemia. Insulin pathways other than glucose metabolism (lipids, blood pressure, endothelial function, autonomic nervous system) may themselves be resistant or, if normally sensitive, be overly stimulated by the hyperinsulinemia. The signs and symptoms of the IR syndrome develop from these pathways.

References

1. DeFronzo RA, Tobin J, Andres R: Glucose clamp technique: a method for quantifying insulin secretion and resistance. *Am J Physiol* 1979, 237:E214–E223.

2. Ferrannini E, Mari A: How to measure insulin sensitivity. *J Hypertens* 1998, 16:895–906.

3. Iozzo P, Beck-Nielsen H, Laakso M, et al.: Independent influence of age on basal insulin secretion in nondiabetic humans. *J Clin Endocrinol Metab* 1999, 84:863–868.

4. DeFronzo RA, Simonson D, Ferrannini E: Hepatic and peripheral insulin resistance: a common feature of insulin-independent and insulin-dependent diabetes. *Diabetologia* 1982, 23:313–320.

5. DeFronzo RA, Ferrannini E, Hendler R, et al.: Regulation of splanchnic and peripheral glucose uptake by insulin and hyperglycemia in man. *Diabetes* 1983, 32:35–45.

6. Landau BR, Wahren J, Chandramouli V, et al.: Use of 2H2O for estimating rates of gluconeogenesis. Application to the fasted state. *J Clin Invest* 1995, 95:172–178.

7. Gastaldelli A, Baldi S, Pettiti M, et al.: Influence of obesity and type 2 diabetes on gluconeogenesis and glucose output in hormones. *Diabetes* 2000, 49:1367–1373.

8. Paternostro G, Camici PG, Lammerstma AA, et al.: Cardiac and skeletal muscle insulin resistance in patients with coronary artery disease: a study with positron-emitting tomography. *J Clin Invest* 1996, 98:2094–2099.

9. Kelley DE, Mokan M, Simoneau JA, Mandarino LJ: Interaction between glucose and free fatty acid metabolism in human skeletal muscle. *J Clin Invest* 1993, 92:91–98.

10. Groop LC, Saloranta C, Schenk M, et al.: The role of free fatty acid metabolism in the pathogenesis of insulin resistance in obesity and non–insulin-dependent diabetes mellitus. *J Clin Endocrinol Metab* 1991, 72:96–102.

11. Ferrannini E, Camastra S, Coppack SW, et al.: Insulin action and non-esterified fatty acids. *Proc Nutr Soc* 1997, 56:753–761.

12. Randle PJ, Garland PB, Hales CN, Newsholme EA: The glucose fatty acid cycle: its role in insulin sensitivity and the metabolic disturbances of diabetes mellitus. *Lancet* 1963, 1:785–789.

13. Golay A, Swilocky AL, Chen YD, Reaven GM: Relationship between plasma free fatty acid concentration, endogenous glucose production, and fasting hyperglycemia in normal and non–insulin-dependent diabetic individuals. *Metabolism* 1987, 36:692–696.

14. Bonadonna RC, Saccomani MP, Seely L, et al.: Glucose transport in human skeletal muscle: the in vivo response to insulin. *Diabetes* 1993, 42:191–198.

15. Bonadonna RC, Del Prato S, Cobelli C, et al.: Transmembrane glucose transport in skeletal muscle of patients with non–insulin-dependent diabetes. *J Clin Invest* 1993, 92:486–492.

16. Camastra S, Bonora E, Del Prato S, et al.: Effect of obesity and insulin resistance on resting and glucose-induced thermogenesis in man. EGIR (European Group for the Study of Insulin Resistance). *Int J Obes Relat Metab Disord* 1999, 23(12):1307–1313.

17. Ferrannini E, Vichi S, Beck-Nielsen H, et al.: Insulin action and age. *Diabetes* 1996, 45:947–953.

18. Ferrannini E, Natali A, Bell P, et al.: Insulin resistance and hypersecretion in obesity. *J Clin Invest* 1997, 100:1166–1173.

19. Greco AV, Mingrone G, Giancaterini A, et al.: Insulin resistance in morbid obesity: reversal with intramyocellular fat depletion. *Diabetes* 2002, 51(1):144–151.

20. Ferrannini E, Natali A, Capaldo B, et al.: Insulin resistance, hyperinsulinemia, and blood pressure. Role of age and obesity. *Hypertension* 1997, 30:1144–1149.

21. Yki-Järvinen H, Utriainen T: Insulin-induced vasodilatation: physiology or pharmacology? *Diabetologia* 1998, 41:369–379.

22. Taddei S, Virdis A, Mattei P, et al.: Effect of insulin on acetylcholine-induced vasodilation in normotensive subjects and patients with essential hypertension. *Circulation* 1995, 92:2911–2920.

23. Steinberg HO, Brechtel G, Johson A, et al.: Insulin-mediated skeletal muscle vasodilatation is nitric oxide dependent. A novel action of insulin to increase nitric oxide release. *J Clin Invest* 1994, 94:1172–1179.

24. Tack CJ, Lutterman JA, Vervoot G, et al.: Activation of the sodium-potassium pump contributes to insulin-induced vasodilatation in humans. *Hypertension* 1996, 28:426–432.

25. Muscelli E, Emdin M, Natali A, et al.: Autonomic and hemodynamic responses to insulin in lean and obese humans. *J Clin Endocrinol Metab* 1998, 83:2084–2090.

26. Gastaldelli A, Emdin M, Conforti F, et al.: Insulin prolongs the QTc interval in humans. *Am J Physiol Regul Integr Comp Physiol* 2000, 279(6):R2022–R2025.

27. Schwartz MW, Figlewicz DP, Baskin DB, et al.: Insulin in the brain: a hormonal regulator of energy balance. *Endocr Rev* 1992, 13:81–113.

CONSEQUENCES OF INSULIN DEFICIENCY

Abbas E. Kitabchi and Mary Beth Murphy

Diabetes [Mellitus] is a remarkable disorder, and not one very common to man...The disease is chronic in its character, and is slowly engendered, though the patient does not survive long when it is completely established, for the marasmus produced is rapid, and death speedy. Life too is odious and painful, the thirst is ungovernable, and the copious potations are more than equaled by the profuse urinary discharge; for more urine flows away, and it is impossible to put any restraint to the patient's drinking or making water. For if he stop for a very brief period, and leave off drinking, the mouth becomes parched, the body dry; the bowels seem on fire, he is wretched and uneasy, and soon dies, tormented with burning thirst.

Aretaeus of Cappodocia (ea. 120 A.D.–200 AD) [1]

Diabetes mellitus (type 1 or type 2) is the result of an absolute or relative insulin-deficient state that, if not corrected, gives rise to the acute metabolic decompensation of hyperglycemic crises so poignantly described above by Aretaeus of Cappodocia more than 1800 years ago. The two major hyperglycemic crises are diabetic ketoacidosis (DKA) and hyperglycemic hyperosmolar state (HHS). These two syndromes are the hallmark of insulin-deficient states. These crises continue to be important causes of mortality and morbidity among patients with diabetes. The annual incidence of DKA hospital admissions ranges from 4.6 to 8 episodes per 1000 patients with diabetes. It is estimated that DKA accounts for 4% to 9% of all hospital admissions for patients diagnosed with diabetes, whereas this figure for HHS is less than 1% [2,3].

Diabetic ketoacidosis is a proinflammatory state resulting in production of reactive oxygen species indicating oxidative stress [4,5]. Recently, it has been demonstrated that serum levels of inflammatory cytokines (interleukin [IL]-1β, IL-6, IL-8, and tumor necrosis factor-α), growth hormone, cortisol (*see* Fig. 4-12) as well as markers of cardiovascular risk factors, plasminogen activator inhibitor-1, C-reactive protein, and lipid peroxidation markers (thiobarbituric acid) and free fatty acids (*see* Fig. 4-13) are elevated in acute DKA [6]. These parameters return to normal at resolution of hyperglycemia with insulin therapy, thus demonstrating a robust anti-inflammatory effect of insulin in response to the general alarm reaction associated with the hyperglycemic ketotic state [6].

T-lymphocytes, which are usually insulin-insensitive, on activation with antigens, become insulin-sensitive and develop de novo growth factor receptors for insulin, insulin growth facor-1 and IL-2 [7]. Because DKA is a proinflammatory state, T-lymphocytes may be activated in vivo and, therefore, there may be in situ development of de novo growth factor receptors. In a recent study, T-lymphocytes (CD4+ and CD8+) were evaluated in eight patients with DKA by measuring insulin growth factor, insulin, and IL-2 receptors by flow cytometry on admission and after treatment with insulin and resolution of DKA (*see* Fig. 4-24). This study demonstrates in situ emergence of these growth factor receptors (insulin, insulin growth factor-1, and IL-2), as well as elevated levels of oxidative stress including dichloroflourescein- and thiobarbituric acid–reacting material on admission and at resolution of DKA with insulin therapy, compared with matched control subjects [8].

The most common precipitating causes for these hyperglycemic emergencies are a) infection, b) undertreatment or omission of insulin, c) previously undiagnosed diabetes, and d) presence of comorbid conditions [9]. In addition, contributing factors for the development of HHS include decreased intake of fluid and electrolytes and excessive use of such drugs as glucocorticoids, diuretics, β-blockers, as well as the use of immunosuppressive agents and diazoxide [9]. Although DKA is most frequently seen in type 1 diabetes and HHS is often associated with type 2 diabetes, each of these conditions can be seen in both types because DKA and HHS have common underlying causes, *ie*, ineffective insulin concentration, dehydration, and increased counterregulatory (stress) hormones, but at different levels. DKA can also occur in young, obese, previously undiagnosed blacks who demonstrate the characteristics of type 2 diabetes [10].

It is important to note that some patients may present with an overlapping metabolic picture of both DKA and HHS. The incidence of combined HHS and DKA in some series has been noted to be as high as 30% [11]. Hyperglycemic hyperosmolar state and DKA can also occur in relatively pure form. Generally, in DKA, the insulin deficiency is absolute whereas in HHS, the insulin may be insufficient relative to the excessive levels of stress hormones (cortisol, glucagon, catecholamines, and growth hormone).

With better understanding of the pathogenesis of insulin-deficient states, the use of more physiologic doses of insulin, and frequent monitoring of such patients in the hospital, the mortality rate has been reduced to less than 5% for DKA and 15% for HHS [3,9,12,13]. Indications for hospitalization include loss of greater than 5% body weight during the crisis, respiration rate faster than 35 per minute, intractable elevation of blood glucose, changes in mental status, uncontrolled fever, and unresolved nausea and vomiting [9]. Poor prognostic signs for DKA and HHS include advanced age, lower degree of consciousness, and lower blood pressure. The cost of these crises, in one study, was estimated to be about $13,000 per episode [14]. The annual hospital cost for patients in hyperglycemic crisis may exceed billions of dollars per year [14]. Prevention of these metabolic emergencies, therefore, poses an important medical and social challenge. Preventive procedures should include extensive educational programs which review steps to be taken during sick days for patients with diabetes, including frequent monitoring of blood glucose and urine ketones. The use of a liquid diet, containing salt and carbohydrates, close contact with health care providers, and, above all, the use of short-acting insulin are important precautionary measures for prevention of recurrence of these crises. Injection of short-acting insulin should not be stopped during sick days in patients with diabetes. In addition to educational endeavors, improved access to a health care delivery system and the availability of affordable medication in less affluent segments of society are some of the most effective methods for prevention of such crises.

Structure of the Islets of Langerhans

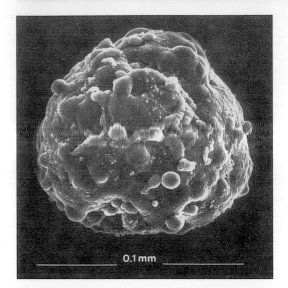

FIGURE 4-1. Surface topography of the periphery of the islet cell (× 900). (*From* Orci [15]; with permission.)

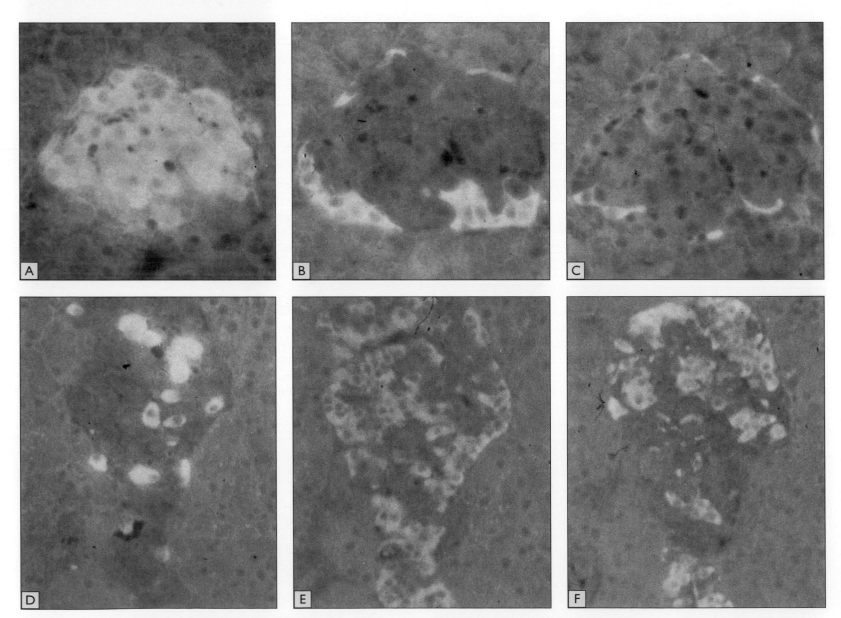

FIGURE 4-2. (See Color Plate) Consecutive serial sections of islets of Langerhans processed for indirect immunofluorescence. **A—C,** The location of insulin-, glucagon-, and somatostatin-containing cells, respectively, in the islet of a control rat. **D—F,** The profound perturbation of this normal distribution in the islet of a rat rendered experimentally diabetic for 17 months after a single intravenous injection of streptozotocin, 45 mg/kg. Note that the number of insulin-containing cells is strikingly reduced while that of glucagon- and somatostatin-containing cells is greatly increased. (*From* Orci *et al.* [16]; with permission.)

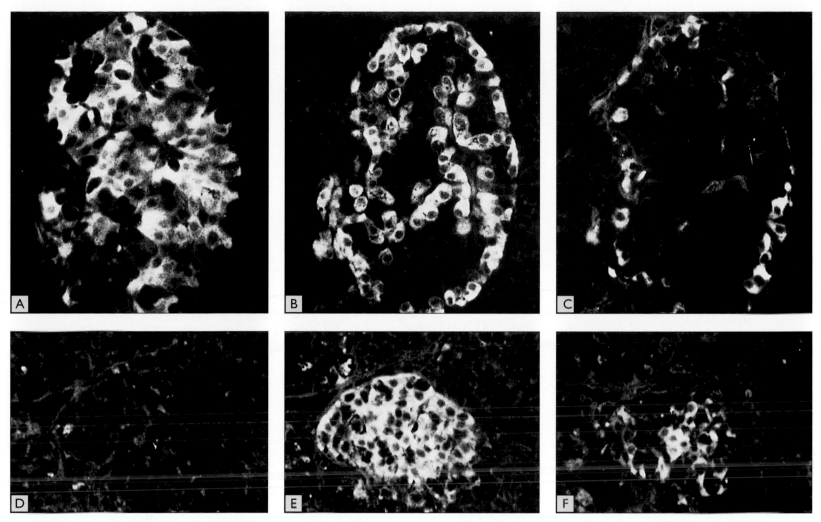

FIGURE 4-3. Distribution of β-, α-, and Δ-cells on serial sections of an islet from an adult, nondiabetic subject. The indirect immunofluorescent technique demonstrates insulin (**A**), glucagon (**B**), and somatostatin (**C**). **D—F**, Serial sections of the islet of Langerhans in a patient with type I diabetes treated with the indirect immunofluorescent technique against insulin, glucagon, and somatostatin, respectively. The only detectable immunofluorescent cells within the islet are the numerous glucagon- and somatostatin-containing cells (× 200). (*From* Orci *et al.* [16]; with permission.)

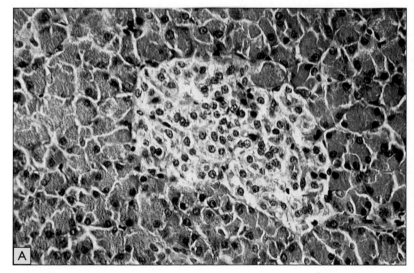 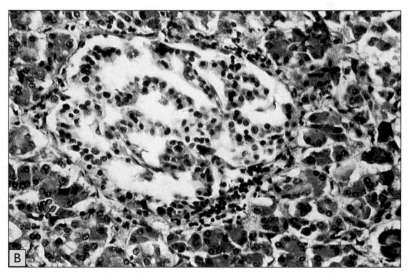

FIGURE 4-4. (See Color Plate) Islet cell necrosis and lymphocyte infiltration. **A**, Pancreatic islet section from normal, nondiabetic control patient. **B**, Pancreatic islet section from patient with type I diabetes. Lymphocytic infiltration can be seen throughout the pancreatic islets with residual islet cells.

(*Continued on next page*)

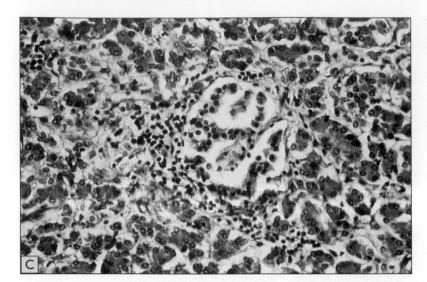

FIGURE 4-4. (See Color Plate) (*Continued*) **C**, Pancreatic islet section from patient with type 1 diabetes showing lymphocytic infiltration in the pancreatic islets, particularly the peripheral islets. (*Courtesy of* J.W. Yoon.)

Definition and Criteria for Insulin-deficient State

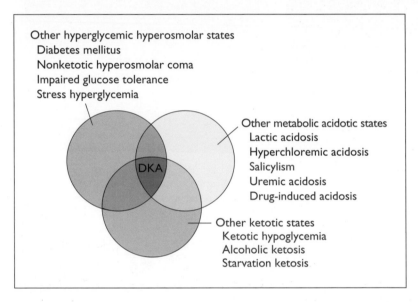

FIGURE 4-5. Other conditions in which the components of the diagnostic triad for diabetic ketoacidosis (DKA) (hyperglycemia, ketosis, and acidosis) may be found. (*Adapted from* Kitabchi and Wall [17].)

Other hyperglycemic hyperosmolar states
  Diabetes mellitus
  Nonketotic hyperosmolar coma
  Impaired glucose tolerance
  Stress hyperglycemia

Other metabolic acidotic states
  Lactic acidosis
  Hyperchloremic acidosis
  Salicylism
  Uremic acidosis
  Drug-induced acidosis

Other ketotic states
  Ketotic hypoglycemia
  Alcoholic ketosis
  Starvation ketosis

FIGURE 4-6. Diagnostic criteria and typical total body deficits of water and electrolytes in diabetic ketoacidosis (DKA) and hyperglycemic hyperosmolar syndrome (HHS). (*Adapted from* Kitabchi et al. [9].)

DIAGNOSTIC CRITERIA AND TYPICAL TOTAL BODY DEFICITS OF WATER AND ELECTROLYTES IN DIABETIC KETOACIDOSIS AND HYPERGLYCEMIC HYPEROSMOLAR SYNDROME

Diagnostic criteria and classification	DKA			HHS
	Mild	Moderate	Severe	
Plasma glucose, *mg/dL*	> 250	> 250	> 250	> 600
Arterial pH	7.25–7.30	7.00 to < 7.24	< 7.00	> 7.30
Serum bicarbonate, *mEq/L*	15–18	10 to < 15	< 10	> 15
Urine ketone*	Positive	Positive	Positive	Small
Serum ketone*	Positive	Positive	Positive	Small
Effective serum osmolality[†]	Variable	Variable	Variable	> 320 mOsm/kg
Anion gap[‡]	> 10	> 12	> 12	Variable
Mental status	Alert	Alert/drowsy	Stupor/coma	Stupor/coma
Typical deficits				
Total water, *L*	6			9
Water, *mL/kg*	100			100–200
Na+, *mEq/kq*	7–10			5–13
Cl-, *mEq/kg*	3–5			5–15
K+, *mEq/kg*	3–5			4–6
PO4, *mmol/kg*	5–7			3–7
Mg++, *mEq/kg*	1–2			1–2
Ca++, *mEq/kg*	1–2			1–2

*Nitroprusside reaction method.

[†]Calculation: Effective serum osmolality 2[measured Na+ (mEq/L + glucose (mg/dL)/18].[‡]Calculation: Anion gap $[(Na^+ + K^+)(mEq/L)]$ $[(Cl + HCO3^-) (mEq/L)]$.

LABORATORY EVALUATION OF METABOLIC CAUSES OF ACIDOSIS AND COMA

Factor Studied	Starvation of High Fat Intake	DKA	Lactic Acidosis	Uremic Acidosis	Alcoholic Ketosis (Starvation)	Salicylate Intoxication	Methanol or Ethylene Glycol Intoxication	Hyperosmolar Coma	Hypoglycemic Coma	Rhabdomyolysis
pH	Normal	↓	↓	Mild ↓	↓ ↑	↓ ↑*	↓	Normal	Normal	Mild ↓ may be ↓ ↓
Plasma glucose	Normal	↑	Normal	Normal	↓ or normal	Normal or ↓	Normal	↑ ↑ >500 mg/dL	↓ ↓<30 mg/dL	Normal
Glycosuria	Negative	++	Negative	Negative	Negative	Negative[†]	Negative	++	Negative	Negative
Total plasma ketones[†]	Slight ↑	↑ ↑	Normal	Normal	Slight to moderate ↑	Normal	Normal	Normal or slight ↑	Normal	Normal
Anion gap	Slight ↑	↑	↑	Slight ↑	↑	↑	↑	Normal	Normal	↑ ↑
Osmolality	Normal	↑	Normal	↑ or	Normal	Normal	↑ ↑	↑ ↑>330 mOsm/kg	Normal	Normal or slight ↑
Uric acid	Mild (starvation)	↑	Normal	Normal ↑ ↑	Normal	Normal	Normal	Normal	Normal	↑
Miscellaneous		May give false-positive for ethylene glycol[§]	Serum lactate >7 mM	BUN >200 mg/dL		Serum salicylate +	Serum levels positive			Myoglobinuria, hemoglobinuria

*Acetest and Ketostix measure acetoacetic acid only. Thus, misleading low values may be obtained because the majority of "ketone bodies" are β-hydroxybutyrate.
[†]Respiratory alkalosis/metabolic acidosis.
[‡]May get false-positive or false-negative urinary glucose caused by the presence of salicylate or its metabolites.
[§]Bjellerup P, et al. Clin Toxicology 1994; 32:85–86.

FIGURE 4-7. Laboratory evaluation of metabolic causes of acidosis and coma. DKA—diabetic ketoacidosis. (*Adapted from* Morris and Kitabchi [18].)

Pathophysiology of Insulin-deficient State

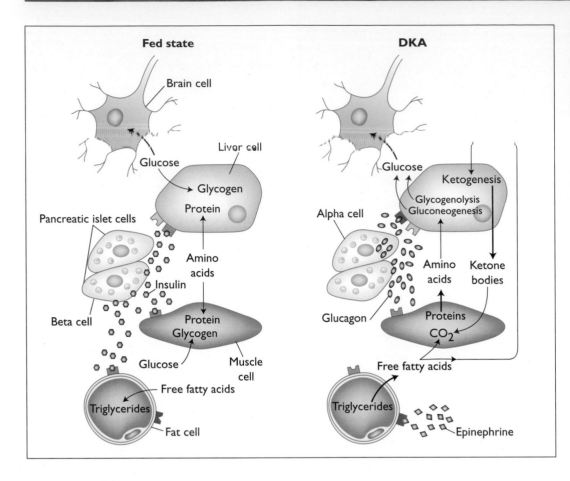

FIGURE 4-8. Mechanisms of glucose regulation. Glucose supply to the brain can be maintained for days and even weeks when the body has been deprived of caloric intake. In the fed state (*left*), assimilation of metabolic fuels and substrates is promoted by insulin in tissues sensitive to the hormone. In diabetic ketoacidosis (DKA) (*right*), counterregulatory hormones (notably glucagon and epinephrine) reverse these processes, promoting glycogenolysis and creating substrates for ketogenesis and gluconeogenesis [19–22]. Denial of glucose to insulin-sensitive tissues preserves it for the brain. Insulin receptor depicted as a *dark-notched square*; glucagons receptor depicted as a *light-notched square*. (*Adapted from* Kitabchi and Rumbak [22].)

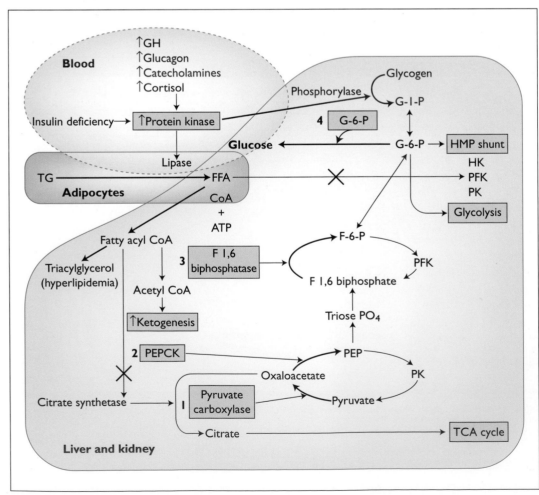

FIGURE 4-9. Proposed biochemical changes that occur during diabetic ketoacidosis. These alterations lead to increased gluconeogenesis, lipolysis, ketogenesis, and decreased glycolysis. *Note*: Lipolysis occurs mainly in adipose tissue. Other events occur primarily in the liver (except some gluconeogenesis in the kidney) [23]. *Thick arrows* indicate stimulated pathways in diabetic ketoacidosis, which consists of rate-limiting enzymes of gluconeogenesis, whereas *thin arrows* indicate inhibitory pathway in glycolysis. The tricarboxylic acid (TCA) cycle is inhibited by fatty and acyl coenzyme A (CoA)-induced inhibition of citrate synthesis, a rate-limiting enzyme in the TCA cycle. ATP—adenosine triphosphate; FFA—free fatty acids; F-6-P—fructose-6-phosphate; GH—growth hormone; G-1-P—glucose-1-phosphate; G-6-P—glucose-6-phosphotase; HK—hexokinase; HMP—hexose monophosphate; PC—pyruvate carboxylase; PEP—phosphoenolpyruvate; PEPCK— phosphoenolpyruvate carboxykinase; PFK—phosphofructokinase; PK—pyruvate kinase; TG—triglycerides; X—indicates an inhibitor effect of the compound on the particular enzyme system. (*Adapted from* Kitabchi et al. [13].)

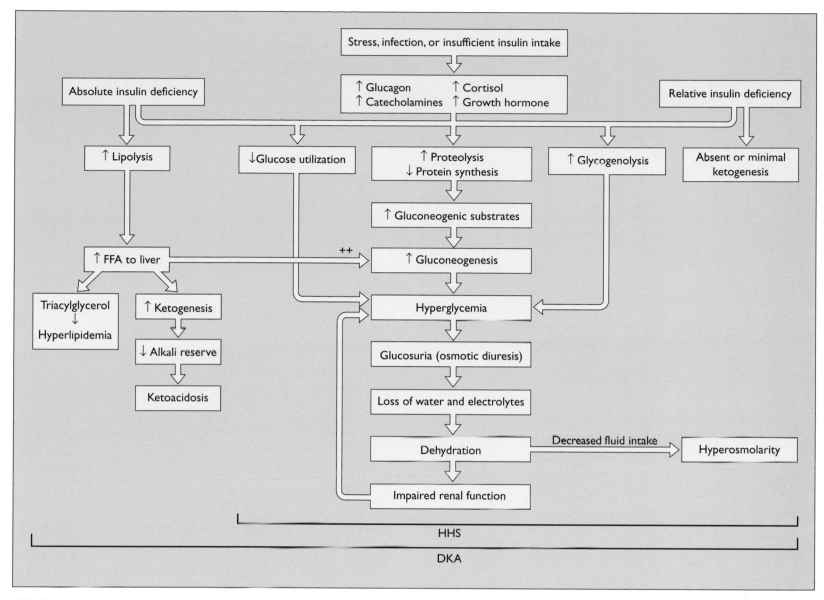

FIGURE 4-10. Pathogenesis of diabetic ketoacidosis (DKA) and hyperglycemic hyperosmolar syndrome (HHS). Alteration of fat, protein, and carbohydrate metabolism leads to metabolic changes toward catabolic states and symptoms of polyuria, polydipsia, polyphagia, osmotic diuresis, severe dehydration, and, if not treated, coma and death. The hallmark of these events is the insulin-deficient state and increased counterregulatory hormones. In HHS, in addition to the relative insulin deficiency and greater dehydration, there is also a greater amount of hyperglycemia (secondary to lower intake of fluid) than in DKA. Although the mechanism for the lack of a significant amount of ketosis and acidemia in HHS (as compared with DKA) is not entirely clear, in one study the level of C-peptide (as an indication of pancreatic insulin reserve) was shown to be five- to tenfold lower in DKA than in HHS [24]. This has been offered as a partial explanation for the lack of ketonemia in HHS. Since the required amount of insulin for its antilipolytic action is about five- to tenfold lower than for the glucose transport action [25], it follows that the larger amount of residual insulin (C-peptide) in HHS is sufficient to prevent lipolysis (thus no ketogenesis in HHS). This amount of insulin is not enough to promote glucose transport and its metabolism, thus the resultant hyperglycemia is noted in HHS without severe ketonemia. (*Adapted from* Kitabchi *et al.* [9].)

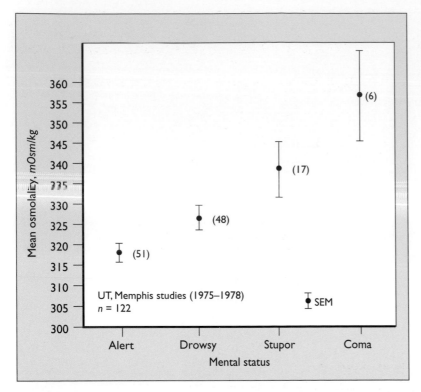

FIGURE 4-11. Calculated serum osmolality in 122 patients with diabetic ketoacidosis with relation to mental status. About one third of patients with hyperglycemic crises may present with altered mental status [11]. This can be correlated to serum osmolality but needs to be differentiated from various clinical conditions associated with altered mental status or coma (see Fig. 4-7), which may be present in diabetic patients. (*Adapted from* Kitabchi and Fisher [11].)

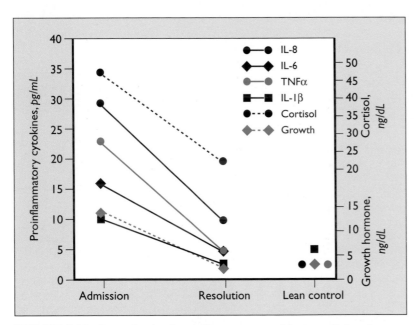

FIGURE 4-12. Serum levels of proinflammatory cytokines, cortisol, and growth hormone in lean patients with diabetic ketoacidosis on admission and after resolution of diabetic ketoacidosis with insulin therapy [6].

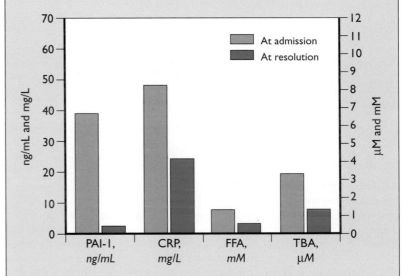

FIGURE 4-13. Serum levels of cardiovascular risk factors (plasminogen activator inhibitor-1 and C-reactive protein), free fatty acids, and lipid peroxidation (thiobarbituric acid) in lean diabetic ketoacidosis patients on admission and after resolution of diabetic ketoacidosis with insulin therapy [6].

Treatment of Acute Diabetic Complications

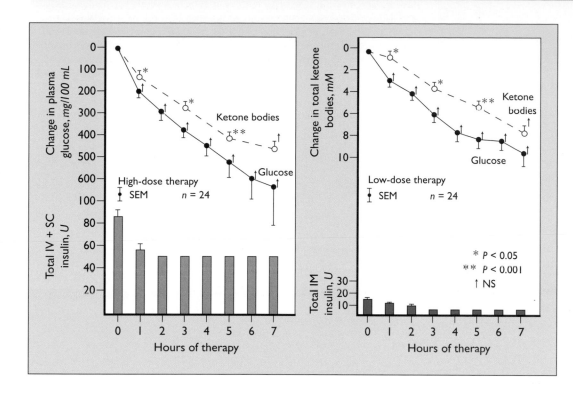

FIGURE 4-14. Efficacy of low-dose versus conventional therapy of insulin for treatment of diabetic ketoacidosis. Treatment of hyperglycemic crises has undergone numerous modifications since the discovery of insulin. In the early decades after the discovery of insulin, low-dose therapy was the norm due to the limited availability of insulin, but in subsequent decades, doses of insulin were modified from physiologic to pharmacologic and even suprapharmacologic doses until the mid-1970s. The initial observation of Alberti et al. [26] demonstrated the effectiveness of low-dose insulin and gave impetus to the first prospective randomized study, which is summarized here [27]. This study confirms the similarity of the responses to low-dose and high-dose insulin in diabetic ketoacidosis without the disadvantages of greater hypoglycemia and hypokalemia associated with high-dose insulin therapy. IV—intravenous; IM—intramuscular; SC—subcutaneous; NS—not significant. (*Adapted from* Kitabchi *et al.* [27].)

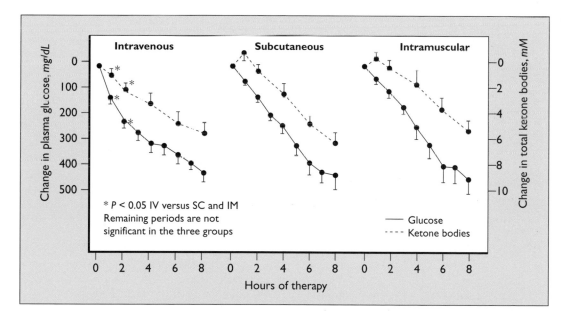

FIGURE 4-15. Comparison of the effects of randomized intravenous (IV), subcutaneous (SC), and intramuscular (IM) low-dose insulin regimens on changes in plasma glucose and total ketone bodies in patients with diabetic ketoacidosis (15 patients in each group). The low-dose insulin therapy was effective in lowering blood glucose in diabetic ketoacidosis therapy by any route of administration. (*Adapted from* Fisher *et al.* [28].)

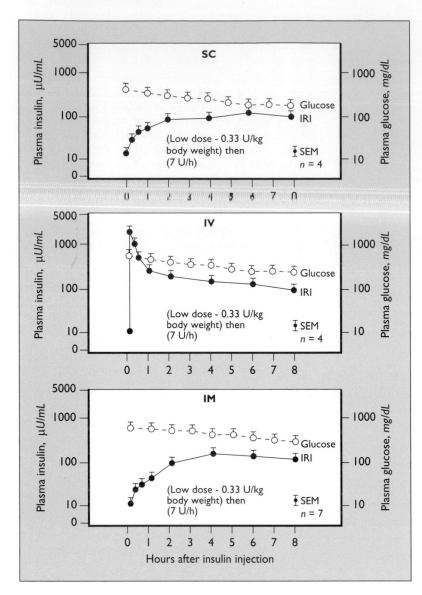

FIGURE 4-16. Comparison of the effect of low-dose insulin regimen (7 U/h) administered by subcutaneous (SC), intravenous (IV), and intramuscular (IM) injections on plasma immunoreactive insulin (IRI) levels (*closed circles*) and plasma glucose decrements (*open circles*) in three groups of diabetic ketoacidosis patients who had not previously been treated with insulin. In these patients, IV insulin caused serum insulin to rise immediately to supraphysiologic levels, whereas SC and IM injections of the same amount of insulin resulted in lower serum insulin concentrations, which reached near physiologic concentrations (postprandially) only after 2 to 3 hours. This low level of insulin may be the reason for the slow clearance of ketone bodies noted in Figure 4-13 for the IM and SC routes as compared to the IV route of the same amount of insulin injection (7 U/h). (*Adapted from* Kitabchi *et al.* [29].)

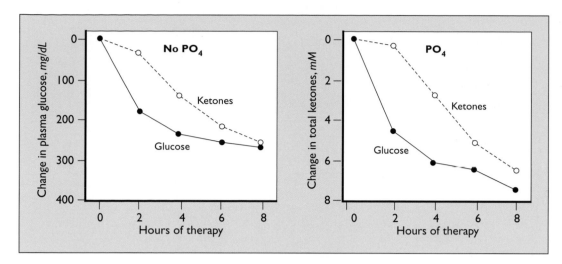

FIGURE 4-17. Use of phosphate in diabetic ketoacidosis. Another controversial issue in the management of diabetic ketoacidosis (DKA) prompted study on the use of phosphate (PO_4) replacement in DKA. This study shows that phosphate therapy does not affect the clinical and biochemical outcomes (plasma glucose and ketone bodies) of low-dose insulin therapy. However, the use of phosphate in DKA was associated with a certain degree of hypocalcemia. (*Adapted from* Fisher and Kitabchi [30].)

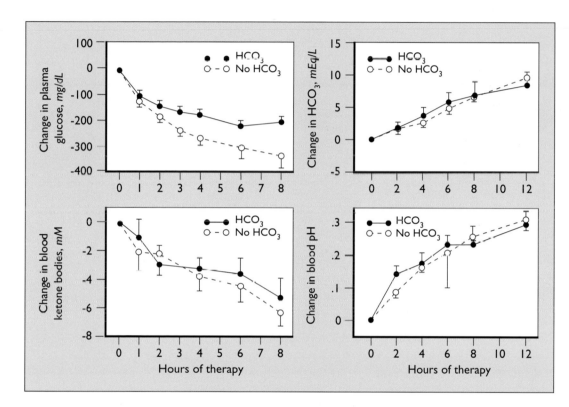

FIGURE 4-18. The role of bicarbonate therapy in the treatment of diabetic ketoacidosis [31]. This prospective randomized study shows the effect of bicarbonate (HCO_3) therapy on various recovery parameters of diabetic ketoacidosis (DKA), indicating that bicarbonate did not alter outcomes of DKA therapy on hours of recovery from hyperglycemia, acidosis, or hypocapnia [32]. There is, therefore, very little reason for the use of bicarbonate therapy in DKA, particularly when the pH level is greater than 7.0 [31]. [*Adapted from* Morris *et al.* [32].)

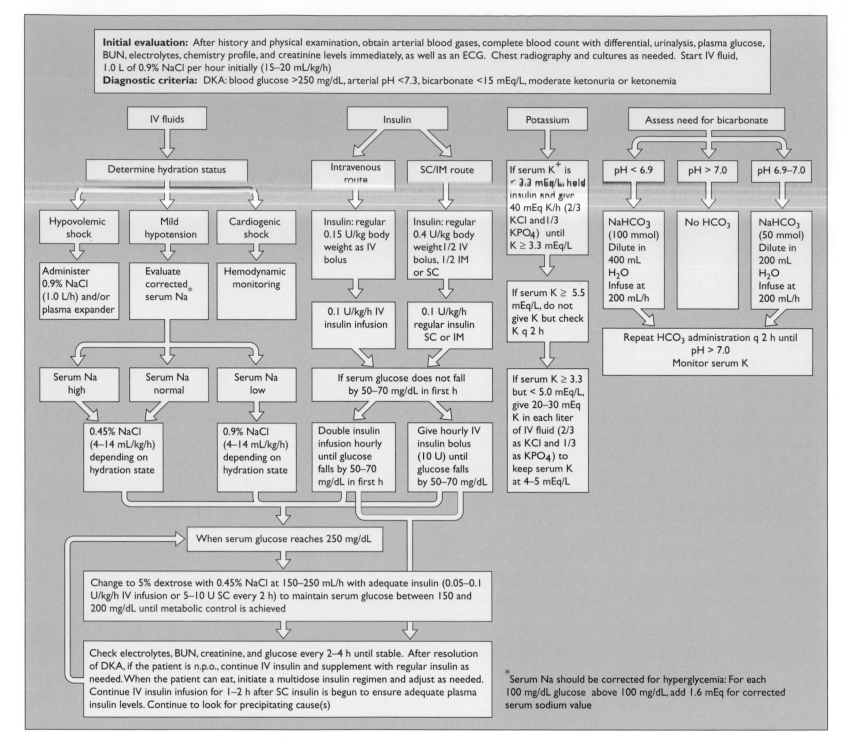

Initial evaluation: After history and physical examination, obtain arterial blood gases, complete blood count with differential, urinalysis, plasma glucose, BUN, electrolytes, chemistry profile, and creatinine levels immediately, as well as an ECG. Chest radiography and cultures as needed. Start IV fluid, 1.0 L of 0.9% NaCl per hour initially (15–20 mL/kg/h)

Diagnostic criteria: DKA: blood glucose >250 mg/dL, arterial pH <7.3, bicarbonate <15 mEq/L, moderate ketonuria or ketonemia

IV fluids

Determine hydration status

Hypovolemic shock → Administer 0.9% NaCl (1.0 L/h) and/or plasma expander

Mild hypotension → Evaluate corrected* serum Na

Cardiogenic shock → Hemodynamic monitoring

Serum Na high
Serum Na normal
Serum Na low

0.45% NaCl (4–14 mL/kg/h) depending on hydration state

0.9% NaCl (4–14 mL/kg/h) depending on hydration state

Insulin

Intravenous route

Insulin: regular 0.15 U/kg body weight as IV bolus → 0.1 U/kg/h IV insulin infusion

SC/IM route

Insulin: regular 0.4 U/kg body weight 1/2 IV bolus, 1/2 IM or SC → 0.1 U/kg/h regular insulin SC or IM

If serum glucose does not fall by 50–70 mg/dL in first h

Double insulin infusion hourly until glucose falls by 50–70 mg/dL in first h

Give hourly IV insulin bolus (10 U) until glucose falls by 50–70 mg/dL

Potassium

If serum K^+ is < 3.3 mEq/L, hold insulin and give 40 mEq K/h (2/3 KCl and 1/3 KPO_4) until K ≥ 3.3 mEq/L

If serum K ≥ 5.5 mEq/L, do not give K but check K q 2 h

If serum K ≥ 3.3 but < 5.0 mEq/L, give 20–30 mEq K in each liter of IV fluid (2/3 as KCl and 1/3 as KPO_4) to keep serum K at 4–5 mEq/L

Assess need for bicarbonate

pH < 6.9 → NaHCO₃ (100 mmol) Dilute in 400 mL H_2O Infuse at 200 mL/h

pH > 7.0 → No HCO₃

pH 6.9–7.0 → NaHCO₃ (50 mmol) Dilute in 200 mL H_2O Infuse at 200 mL/h

Repeat HCO₃ administration q 2 h until pH > 7.0 Monitor serum K

When serum glucose reaches 250 mg/dL

Change to 5% dextrose with 0.45% NaCl at 150–250 mL/h with adequate insulin (0.05–0.1 U/kg/h IV infusion or 5–10 U SC every 2 h) to maintain serum glucose between 150 and 200 mg/dL until metabolic control is achieved

Check electrolytes, BUN, creatinine, and glucose every 2–4 h until stable. After resolution of DKA, if the patient is n.p.o., continue IV insulin and supplement with regular insulin as needed. When the patient can eat, initiate a multidose insulin regimen and adjust as needed. Continue IV insulin infusion for 1–2 h after SC insulin is begun to ensure adequate plasma insulin levels. Continue to look for precipitating cause(s)

*Serum Na should be corrected for hyperglycemia: For each 100 mg/dL glucose above 100 mg/dL, add 1.6 mEq for corrected serum sodium value

FIGURE 4-19. Protocol for the therapeutic management of patients with diabetic ketoacidosis (DKA). Important interventions include the use of insulin, adequate hydration, and frequent monitoring of patients [9,11,18].

BUN—blood urea nitrogen; ECG—electrocardiogram; IM—intramuscular; IV—intravenous; n.p.o.—nothing by mouth; SC—subcutaneous. (*Adapted from* Kitabchi *et al.* [33].)

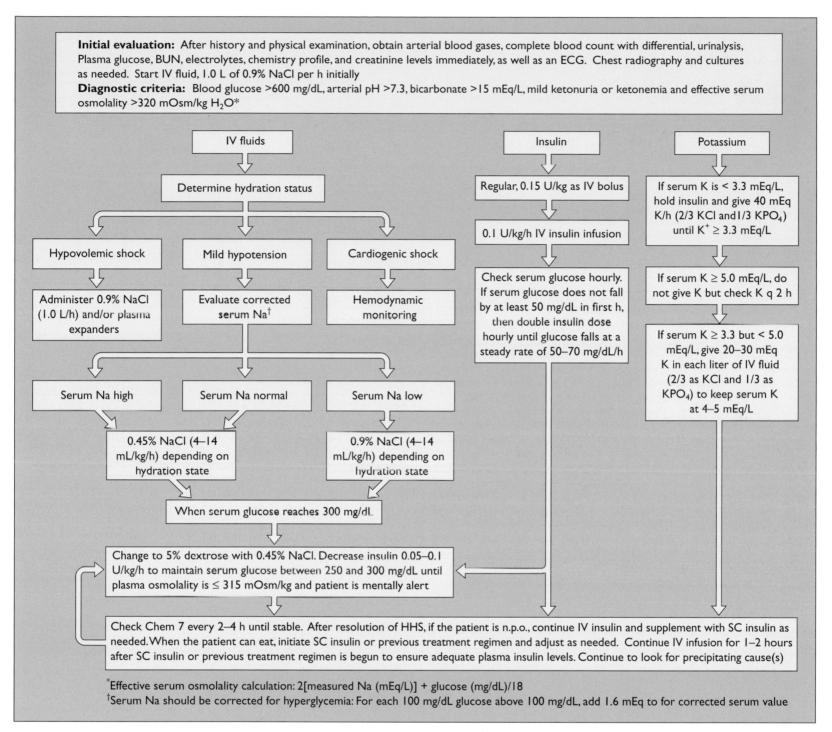

Initial evaluation: After history and physical examination, obtain arterial blood gases, complete blood count with differential, urinalysis, Plasma glucose, BUN, electrolytes, chemistry profile, and creatinine levels immediately, as well as an ECG. Chest radiography and cultures as needed. Start IV fluid, 1.0 L of 0.9% NaCl per h initially
Diagnostic criteria: Blood glucose >600 mg/dL, arterial pH >7.3, bicarbonate >15 mEq/L, mild ketonuria or ketonemia and effective serum osmolality >320 mOsm/kg H$_2$O*

IV fluids

Insulin

Potassium

Determine hydration status

Regular, 0.15 U/kg as IV bolus

If serum K is < 3.3 mEq/L, hold insulin and give 40 mEq K/h (2/3 KCl and 1/3 KPO$_4$) until K$^+$ ≥ 3.3 mEq/L

Hypovolemic shock

Mild hypotension

Cardiogenic shock

0.1 U/kg/h IV insulin infusion

Administer 0.9% NaCl (1.0 L/h) and/or plasma expanders

Evaluate corrected serum Na†

Hemodynamic monitoring

Check serum glucose hourly. If serum glucose does not fall by at least 50 mg/dL in first h, then double insulin dose hourly until glucose falls at a steady rate of 50–70 mg/dL/h

If serum K ≥ 5.0 mEq/L, do not give K but check K q 2 h

Serum Na high

Serum Na normal

Serum Na low

If serum K ≥ 3.3 but < 5.0 mEq/L, give 20–30 mEq K in each liter of IV fluid (2/3 as KCl and 1/3 as KPO$_4$) to keep serum K at 4–5 mEq/L

0.45% NaCl (4–14 mL/kg/h) depending on hydration state

0.9% NaCl (4–14 mL/kg/h) depending on hydration state

When serum glucose reaches 300 mg/dL

Change to 5% dextrose with 0.45% NaCl. Decrease insulin 0.05–0.1 U/kg/h to maintain serum glucose between 250 and 300 mg/dL until plasma osmolality is ≤ 315 mOsm/kg and patient is mentally alert

Check Chem 7 every 2–4 h until stable. After resolution of HHS, if the patient is n.p.o., continue IV insulin and supplement with SC insulin as needed. When the patient can eat, initiate SC insulin or previous treatment regimen and adjust as needed. Continue IV infusion for 1–2 hours after SC insulin or previous treatment regimen is begun to ensure adequate plasma insulin levels. Continue to look for precipitating cause(s)

*Effective serum osmolality calculation: 2[measured Na (mEq/L)] + glucose (mg/dL)/18
†Serum Na should be corrected for hyperglycemia: For each 100 mg/dL glucose above 100 mg/dL, add 1.6 mEq to for corrected serum value

FIGURE 4-20. Protocol for the therapeutic management of patients with hyperglycemic hyperosmolar syndrome (HHS). These patients may require a greater amount of hydration as well as a slower rate of glucose decrement. Chem 7—electrolytes, blood urea nitrogen (BUN), creatinine; ECG—electrocardiogram; IV—intravenous; n.p.o.—nothing by mouth; SC—subcutaneous. (*Adapted from* Kitabchi *et al.* [33].)

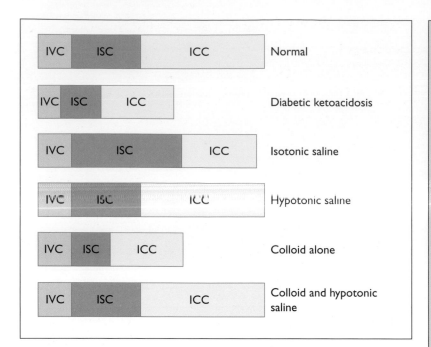

FIGURE 4-21. Use of hypotonic versus isotonic saline and plasma expanders. This figure demonstrates the effect of these solutions in various cellular compartments. The diagram depicts the decreased intravascular (IVC), interstitial (ISC), and intracellular (ICC) compartments present in patients with diabetic ketoacidosis (DKA), as compared with control patients. Subsequent panels show the effects of fluid resuscitation of DKA with different solutions. Isotonic solutions replete only IVC and ISC compartments, whereas hypotonic solutions replete all compartments. However, larger volumes of hypotonic solutions are required to produce equivalent increases in IVC. Colloid alone is restricted to the IVC; therefore, combined use of colloid plus hypotonic solution can lead to a rapid increase in IVC, followed by more gradual replacement of the other compartments. It is also important to remember that hydration in DKA and hyperglycemic hyperosmolar syndrome dilutes concentrations of the stress hormones and thus makes peripheral tissues more sensitive to lower doses of insulin [34]. (*Adapted from* Hillman [35].)

Suggested DKA/HHS Flowsheet

Weight:
0°_____
24°_____

	Date													
	Mental status*													
	Temperature													
	Pulse													
	Respiration/depth†													
	Blood pressure													
	Serum glucose, *mg/dL*													
	Serum "ketones"													
	Urine "ketones"													
Electrolytes	Serum Na^+, *mEq/L*													
Electrolytes	Serum K^+, *mEq/L*													
Electrolytes	Serum Cl^-, *mEq/L*													
Electrolytes	Serum HCO_3^-, *mEq/L*													
Electrolytes	Serum BUN, *mg/dL*													
Electrolytes	Effective osmolality 2 [measured Na mEq/L]+ glucose mg/dL/18													
Electrolytes	Anion gap													
ABG	pH venous (V) arterial (A)													
ABG	pO_2													
ABG	pCO_2													
ABG	O^2 SAT													
Insulin	Units past h													
Insulin	Route													
Intake Fluid/Metabolites	0.45% NaCl (mL) past h													
Intake Fluid/Metabolites	0.9% NaCl (mL) past h													
Intake Fluid/Metabolites	5% dextrose (mL) past h													
Intake Fluid/Metabolites	KCl (mEq) past h													
Intake Fluid/Metabolites	PO_4 (mmol) past h													
Intake Fluid/Metabolites	Other													
Output	Urine, mL													
Output	Other													

*A–Alert D–Drowsy S–Stuporous C–Comatose
†D–Deep S–Shallow N–Normal

FIGURE 4-22. Flow sheet to document serial changes in laboratory/clinical values and supplementary measures during recovery from diabetic ketoacidosis (DKA). ABG—arterial blood gases; BUN—blood urea nitrogen; HHS—hyperglycemic hyperosmolar syndrome; SAT—saturation. (*Adapted from* Kitabchi *et al.* [13].)

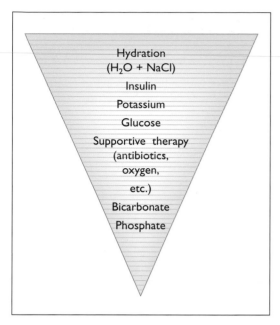

FIGURE 4-23. Treatment of hyperglycemic crisis. This figure summarizes the importance of documentation of various modalities of therapy and responses to treatment of hyperglycemic crises. The importance of frequent monitoring of patients by health care providers cannot be overemphasized. Precipitating causes of these crises must be sought while the patient is being managed, and the patient should be referred to an educational program, as discussed earlier, for prevention of future recurrence of such events. (*Adapted from* Kitabchi *et al.* [36]).

GROWTH FACTOR RECEPTORS EXPRESSION ON T-LYMPHOCYTES IN EIGHT DIABETIC KETOACIDOSIS PATIENTS

Receptor	DKA Admission		DKA Resolution	
	CD4, %	CD8, %	CD4, %	CD8, %
CD69	68 ± 6	74 ± 9	46 ± 5	49 ± 6
Insulin (IR)	18 ± 6	24 ± 7	39 ± 7	41 ± 7
IGF-1 (IGFR)	23 ± 5	29 ± 8	48 ± 6	52 ± 5
IL-2 (IL2R)	39 ± 4	43 ± 5	62 ± 6	64 ± 6

Markers of oxidative stress		
	DKA Admission	DKA Resolution
DCF (µM)	8.7 ± 0.8	3.4 ± 0.6
TBA (µM) [as malonaldehyde]	3.9 ± 0.4	1.7 ± 0.3

FIGURE 4-24. Growth factor receptor expression on T-lymphocytes and markers of oxidative stress in eight patients with diabetic ketoacidosis (DKA) [7]. DCF—dichlorofluorescein; IGF—insulin growth factor; IGFR—insulin growth factor receptor; IL-2—interleukin-2; IL2R—interleukin-2 receptor; TBA—thiobarbituric acid. (Adapted from Kitabchi and Stentz [8].)

SUMMARY OF MANAGEMENT OF PATIENTS WITH DIABETIC KETOACIDOSIS

Laboratory evaluation

After a brief history and physical examination, initial laboratory evaluation should include determination of complete blood count, blood glucose, serum electrolytes, blood urea nitrogen, creatinine, serum ketones, osmolality, arterial blood gases, and urinalysis. Admission ECG, chest radiograph, and cultures of blood, urine, and sputum may be ordered if clinically indicated. During therapy, capillary blood glucose should be determined every 1–2 hours at the bedside using a glucose oxidase reagent strip; and blood should be drawn every 4 hours for determination of serum electrolytes, glucose, blood urea nitrogen, creatinine, phosphorus, and venous pH

Fluids

1000 mL normal saline (0.9% sodium chloride) first hour, then normal or 0.45% saline at 250–500 mL per hour depending on serum sodium concentration and hydration status. When plasma glucose < 250 mg/dL, change to D5%1/2NS saline to allow continued insulin administration until ketonemia is controlled, while avoiding hypoglycemia

Insulin

0.1 U/kg body weight as intravenous bolus followed by 0.1 U/kg/h as a continuous infusion. The goal is to achieve a rate of decline of glucose between 50–100 mg per hour. When plasma glucose is < 250 mg/dL, reduce insulin rate to 0.05 U/kg per hour. Thereafter, adjust insulin rate to maintain glucose levels between 150–200 mg/dL until ketoacidosis is resolved. In patients with mild to moderate diabetic ketoacidosis, subcutaneous regular insulin or rapid-acting insulin analogs may be an alternative to intravenous insulin [37,38]

Potassium

Serum K⁺ > 5.0 mEq/L; no supplementation is required.

Serum K⁺ = 4–5 mEq/L; add 20 mEq/L to each L of replacement fluid

Serum K⁺ = 3-4 mEq/L; add 40 mEq/L to each L of replacement fluid

Serum K⁺ < 3 mEq/L; hold insulin and give 10–20 mEq per hour until K⁺ > 3.3, then add 40 mEq/L to each L of replacement fluid

Bicarbonate

Arterial pH < 7.0 or bicarbonate < 5 mEq; 50 mEq/L in 200 ml of H_2O over 1 hour until pH increases to > 7.0. Do not give bicarbonate if pH > 7.0

Phosphate

If indicated (serum levels < 1 mg/dL), 20–30 mmol potassium phosphate over 24 hours. Monitor serum calcium level

Transition to subcutaneous insulin

Insulin infusion should be continued until resolution of ketoacidosis (glucose < 200 mg/dL, bicarbonate > 18 mEq/L, pH > 7.30). When this occurs, start subcutaneous insulin regimen.

To prevent recurrence of diabetic ketoacidosis during the transition period to subcutaneous insulin, intravenous insulin should be continued for 1–2 hours after subcutaneous insulin is given [28]

FIGURE 4-25. Summary of management of patients with diabetic ketoacidosis [28, 37,38].

References

1. Turnebum A: Of the causes and signs of acute and chronic disease, 1554. Reynolds TF, translator. London: William Pickering, 1837.

2. Faich GA, Fishbein HA, Ellis SE: The epidemiology of diabetic acidosis: a population-based study. Am J Epidemiol 1983, 117:551.

3. Fishbein HA, Palumbo PJ: Acute Metabolic Complications in Diabetes. Diabetes in America (National Diabetes Data Group). Bethesda, MD: National Institutes of Health; 1995. NIH Publication 95-1468.

4. Jain SK, McVie R, Jackson R, et al.: Effect of hyperketonemia on plasma lipid peroxidation levels in diabetic patients. Diabetes Care 1999, 22:1171–1175.

5. Jain SK, Kannan K, Lim G, et al.: Elevated blood interleukin-6 levels in hyperketonemic type 1 diabetic patients and secretion by acetoacetate-treated cultured U937 monocytes. Diabetes Care 2003, 26:2139–2143.

6. Stentz FB, Umpierrez GE, Cuervo R, Kitabchi AE: Proinflammatory cytokines, markers of cardiovascular risks, oxidative stress, and lipid peroxidation in patients with hyperglycemic crises. Diabetes 2004, 53:2079–2086.

7. Stentz FB, Kitabchi AE: De novo emergence of growth factor receptors in activated human CD4+ and CD8+ T-lymphocytes. Metabolism 2004, 53:117–122.

8. Kitabchi AE, Stentz FB, Umpierrez GE: Diabetic ketoacidosis induces in vivo activation of human T-lymphocytes. Biochem Biophys Res Commun 2004, 315:404–407.

9. Kitabchi AE, Umpierrez GE, Murphy MB, et al.: Management of hyperglycemic crises in patients with diabetes. Diabetes Care 2001, 24:131–153.

10. Umpierrez GE, Kelly JP, Navarrete JE, et al.: Hyperglycemic crises in urban blacks. Arch Int Med 1997, 157:669–675.

11. Kitabchi AE, Fisher JN: Insulin therapy of diabetic ketoacidosis: physiologic versus pharmacologic doses of insulin and their routes of administration. In Handbook of Diabetes Mellitus, vol 5. Edited by Brownlee M. New York: Garland ATPM Press; 1981:95–149.

12. Carroll P, Matz R: Uncontrolled diabetes mellitus in adults: experience in treating diabetic ketoacidosis and hyperosmolar coma with low-dose insulin and uniform treatment regimen. Diabetes Care 1983, 6:579–585.

13. Kitabchi AE, Fisher JN, Murphy MB, Rumbak MJ: Diabetic ketoacidosis and the hyperglycemic hyperosmolar nonketotic state. In Joslin's Diabetes Mellitus, edn 13. Edited by Kahn CR, Weir GC. Philadelphia: Lea & Febiger; 1994:738–770.

14. Javor KA, Kotsanos JG, McDonald RC, et al.: Diabetic ketoacidosis charges relative to medical charges of adult patients with type 1 diabetes. Diabetes Care 1997, 20:349–354.

15. Orci L: A fresh look at the interrelationships within the islets of Langerhans. Diabetes Research Today. Stuttgart: Meeting of the Minkowski Prizewinners. Symposium Capri, FK Schattauer, Verlag; 1976.

16. Orci L, Baetens D, Rufener C, et al.: Hypertrophy and hyperplasia of somatostatin-containing D-cells in diabetes. Proc Natl Acad Sci USA 1976, 73:1338–1342.

17. Kitabchi AE, Wall BM: Diabetic ketoacidosis. Med Clin North Am 1995, 79:9–37.

18. Morris LE, Kitabchi AE: Coma in the diabetic. In Diabetes Mellitus: Problems in Management. Edited by Schnatz JD. Menlo Park, CA: Addison-Wesley; 1982:234–251.

19. DeFronzo RA, Matsuda M, Barrett E: Diabetic ketoacidosis. A combined metabolic-nephrologic approach to therapy. Diabetes Review 1994, 2:209–238.

20. Miles JM, Rizza RA, Haymond MW, Gerich JE: Effects of acute insulin deficiency on glucose and ketone body turnover in man: evidence for the primacy overproduction of glucose and ketone bodies in the genesis of diabetic ketoacidosis. Diabetes 1980, 29:926–930.

21. McGarry JD, Woeltje KF, Kuwajima M, Foster DW: Regulation of ketogenesis and the renaissance of carnitine palmitoyl transferase. Diab Metab Rev 1989, 5:271–284.

22. Kitabchi AE, Rumbak MJ: Management of diabetic emergencies. Hosp Pract 1989, 24:129–160.

23. Myer C, Stumvolle M, Nadkarni V, et al.: Abnormal renal and hepatic glucose metabolism in type 2 diabetes mellitus. J Clin Invest 1998, 102:619–624.

24. Chupin M, Charbonnel B, Chupin F: C-peptide levels in ketoacidosis and in hyperosmolar non-ketotic diabetic coma. Acta Diabet 1981, 18:123–128.

25. Schade DS, Eaton RP: Dose response to insulin in man: differential effects on glucose and ketone body regulation. J Clin Endocrinol Metab 1977, 44:1038–1053.

26. Alberti KGMM, Hockaday TDR, Turner RC: Small doses of intramuscular insulin in the treatment of diabetic coma. Lancet 1973, 5:515–522.

27. Kitabchi AE, Ayyagari V, Guerra SMO, Medical House Staff: The efficacy of low dose versus conventional therapy of insulin for treatment of diabetic ketoacidosis. Ann Intern Med 1976, 84:633–638.

28. Fisher JN, Shahshahani MN, Kitabchi AE: Diabetic ketoacidosis: low-dose insulin therapy by various routes. N Engl J Med 1977, 297:238–247.

29. Kitabchi AE, Young RT, Sacks HS, Morris L: Diabetic ketoacidosis: reappraisal of therapeutic approach. Ann Rev Med 1979, 30:339–357.

30. Fisher JN, Kitabchi AE: A randomized study of phosphate therapy in the treatment of diabetic ketoacidosis. J Clin Endocrinol Metab 1983, 57:177–180.

31. Matz R: Diabetic acidosis: rationale for not using bicarbonate. NY State J Med 1977, 76:1299–1303.

32. Morris LR, Murphy MB, Kitabchi AE: Bicarbonate therapy in severe diabetic ketoacidosis. Ann Intern Med 1986, 105:836–840.

33. Kitabchi AE, Umpierrez GE, Murphy MB, et al.: Hyperglycemic crises in patients with diabetes mellitus. American Diabetes Association position statement. Diabetes Care 2004, 27:594–5102.

34. Waldhausl W, Kleinberger G, Korn A, et al.: Severe hyperglycemia: effects of hydration on endocrine derangements and blood glucose concentration. Diabetes 1979, 28:577–584.

35. Hillman K: Fluid resuscitation in diabetic emergencies: a reappraisal. Intensive Care Med 1987, 13:4–8.

36. Kitabchi AE, Matteri R, Murphy MB: Optimum insulin delivery in diabetic ketoacidosis and hyperglycemic hyperosmolar nonketotic coma. Diabetes Care 1982, 5:78–87.

37. Umpierrez GE, Cuervo R, Karabell A, et al.: Treatment of diabetic ketoacidosis with subcutaneous insulin aspart. Am J Med 2004, 117:291–296

38. Umpierrez GE, Latif K, Stoever J, et al.: Efficacy of subcutaneous insulin lispro versus continuous intravenous regular insulin for treatment of diabetic ketoacidosis. Diabetes Care 2004, 27:1873–1878.

TYPE 1 DIABETES

Mark A. Atkinson and Jay S. Skyler

5

Type I diabetes is a chronic disorder resulting from autoimmune destruction of the insulin-producing pancreatic β cells. The epidemiologic features of type 1 diabetes are described, and the possible contributions of genetics and environment to its development are illustrated. In addition, based on improved knowledge of the immunopathogenesis of this disorder, we report on work that holds promise for future interventions aimed at prevention.

The exact cause or causes of type 1 diabetes remain unclear [1]. It occurs most frequently in whites of Northern European descent, with more than a 40-fold difference observed in disease incidence rates based on geographic location. Environmental factors such as diet, stress, and viruses have been proposed to play a modifying and perhaps even a primary role in the development of type 1 diabetes. Thus, these factors may contribute to its varying prevalence. The disorder was once termed *juvenile diabetes* and thought to occur predominantly in persons under 18 years of age. However, more recent evidence suggests that the number of new cases may be equal in those over and under 30 years of age.

Susceptibility to type 1 diabetes is inherited, and increased risk is associated with being a first-degree relative to a person with a diabetic proband. However, approximately 85% of new cases show no such familial lineage. The major genetic region associated with predisposition to the disease is the one that encodes genes for the highly polymorphic human leukocyte antigens (HLAs). However, nearly 20 other loci have been proposed as contributing from 50% to 70% of the total genetic susceptibility.

Multiple lines of evidence support the theory that type 1 diabetes has an autoimmune nature. The evidence includes the aforementioned association with HLA, presence of a lymphocytic infiltrate within the pancreatic islet cells (*ie*, insulitis), and expression of islet reactive autoantibodies. Although once viewed as an acutely developing illness, today it is known that the natural history of type 1 diabetes is that of a chronic autoimmune process. In most patients the disease exists for months to years in a preclinical, asymptomatic phase. Many improvements in our knowledge of the pathogenesis of type 1 diabetes derive from investigations of two spontaneous animal models for the disease (*ie*, BioBreeding rats and nonobese diabetic mice).

Although it remains unclear which immune system component or mechanism plays the major role in β-cell destruction, most studies point toward the cellular immune system as providing a key role. Furthermore, multiple interrelated flaws in immunoregulation may underlie the failure to form a tolerance to self-antigens that results in type 1 diabetes. A large number of islet cell antigens have been associated with type 1 diabetes. Their biochemical identification has led to improved markers for predicting future cases and provided the potential to design antigen-specific therapies aimed at prevention. Numerous intervention studies have been directed toward patients with new-onset type 1 diabetes (predominantly involving immunosuppression), with disappointing degrees of success in terms of disease reversal. Improvements have been made in the ability to predict future cases of type 1 diabetes and assess metabolic activity. Therefore, the more recent clinical trials have sought to use alternatives such as nicotinamide and insulin that are much less likely to have such serious side effects as immunosuppressive agents, thus providing a safe and effective means of disease prevention. Unfortunately, these trials have not been successful.

Clinical Description

COMPARISON OF CLINICAL, GENETIC, AND IMMUNOLOGIC FEATURES OF TYPE 1 AND TYPE 2 DIABETES

Characteristic	Type 1	Type 2
Onset	Abrupt	Progressive
Endogenous insulin	Low to absent	Normal, elevated, or depressed
Ketosis	Common	Rare
Age at onset	Any age	Vast majority in adults
Body mass	Usually nonobese	Obese or nonobese
Treatment	Insulin	Diet, oral hypoglycemics, insulin
Family history	10%–15%	30%
Twin concordance	30%–50%	70%–90%
Human leukocyte antigen (HLA) association	HLA-DR, HLA-DQ	Unrelated
Autoantibodies	Present in most (> 85%)	Absent, except in patients with coincident type 1 disease

FIGURE 5-1. Comparisons of clinical, genetic, and immunologic features of type 1 and 2 diabetes. The terms applied to the subgroup of disorders known collectively as diabetes mellitus are useful. However, they often break down in practice owing to confusion regarding the age at diagnosis or to an overlap or absence of the indicated features normally associated with the specific disorder. In many instances, the terms *type 1 diabetes* and *insulin-dependent diabetes* are used interchangeably, as are the terms *type 2 diabetes* and *non–insulin-dependent diabetes*. However, enthusiasm has grown for the terms *type 1 diabetes* or *immune-mediated diabetes* (IMD) to identify the forms of diabetes involving an autoimmune destruction of the insulin-producing pancreatic β cells.

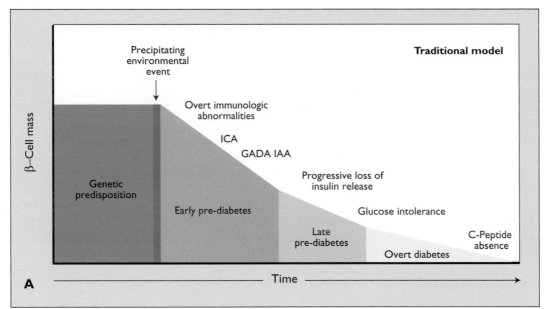

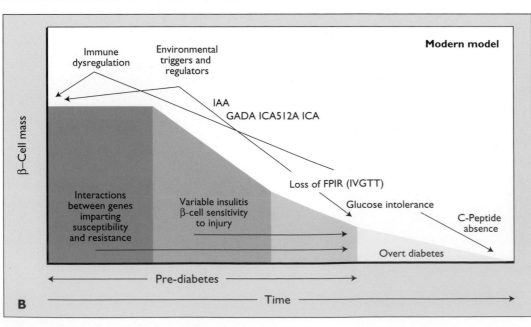

FIGURE 5-2. Traditional and modern models of the pathogenesis and natural history of type 1 diabetes. The traditional model (**A**) provided represents common features cited in numerous publications and presentations from 1986 to date. The modern model (**B**) expands and updates the traditional model by inclusion of information gained through an improved understanding of the roles of genetics, immunology, and environment in the natural history of type 1 diabetes. In the modern model, the natural history of type 1 diabetes has been modeled into a disease comprised of four stages. Stage 1 includes genetic susceptibility and resistance (major histocompatibility complex [MHC] and non-MHC) with intact β-cell mass. The interaction between the genetics surrounding this disorder, immune dysregulation, and environmental encounters results in stage 2, a process that in some cases can begin in the first few months or years of life. At that time, insulitis is initiated and again, owing to a genetic predisposition that does not properly regulate immune responses, the process of β-cell destruction begins. Autoantibodies to islet cell antigens develop, marking the autoimmune disease process; however, no measurable β-cell dysfunction occurs at this stage. In stage 3, a gradual decline in β-cell mass occurs, with the slope being highly variable between persons (*ie*, months to years). Incipient β-cell damage is first detectable as an abnormal intravenous glucose tolerance test with a deficient first-phase insulin response. In stage 4, an advanced degree of β-cell damage, hyperglycemia symptomatic of type 1 diabetes onset (with minimal C peptide), and exogenous insulin dependence occur. With complete β-cell destruction, the C peptide becomes undetectable and autoantibody markers of disease disappear. IAA—insulin autoantibodies; ICA—islet cell autoantibodies; FPIR—first phase insulin response; GADA—glutamic acid decarboxylase autoantibodies; IVGTT—intravenous glucose tolerance test. (*Adapted from* Atkinson [1], Eisenbarth [2], and Devendra *et al.* [3].)

Epidemiology

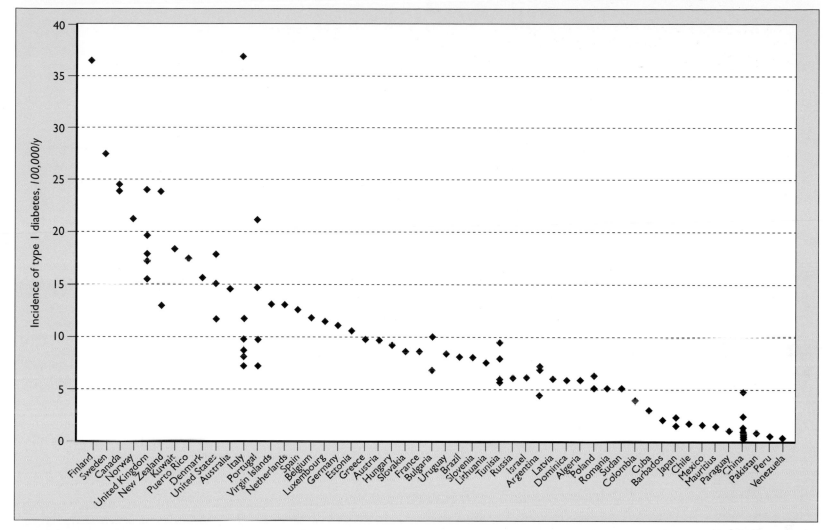

FIGURE 5-3. Variations in the incidence of type I diabetes based on geographic location. This disease predominantly affects populations with a substantial white genetic admixture. In Finland the incidence rate approaches 40 cases per 100,000 persons per year, whereas in Korea and Mexico the rate approximates 0.6 per 100,000 per year. In Europe the incidence is highest in the northern regions and generally declines in countries that lie in the south. Exceptions do exist, especially in the case of Sardinia, Italy, where the incidence rate approximates that of Finland. Furthermore, the disease incidence in Iceland is only one third that of Finland. Multiple studies suggest a continuing increase in the incidence of the disease, reporting regional increases of 6% to 20% per decade. (*Adapted from* Karvonen *et al.* [4].)

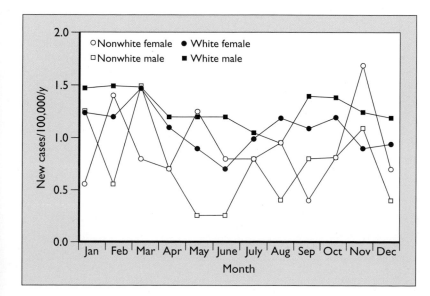

FIGURE 5-4. Variations in the frequency of diagnosing type I diabetes as a function of season. Data from Allegheny County, Pennsylvania, show a decline in newly diagnosed cases in the summer months. Additional studies confirm and expand on this finding, with reports of bimodal peaks in the late winter and early spring. Historically, such findings often have been considered as supporting an environmental agent in the pathogenesis of this disease. (*Adapted from* LaPorte *et al.* [5].)

ENVIRONMENTAL AGENTS AND LIFESTYLE PRACTICES PURPORTED TO INFLUENCE THE INCIDENCE OF HUMAN TYPE I DIABETES

Class	Specific Agent
Viruses	Coxsackie B
	Cytomegalovirus
	Echo
	Encephalomyocarditis
	Epstein-Barr
	Mumps
	Rotaviruses
	Rubella (congenital)
Diet	Cow's milk and cow's milk–based infant formulas
	Caffeine
	Nitrates (N-nitroso compounds)
	Duration of breast-feeding
Lifestyle	Exposure to β-cell toxins (eg, pyriminil)
	Stress
	Quantitative or qualitative exposure to viral and bacterial agents

FIGURE 5-5. Environmental agents and practices purported to influence the incidence of type I diabetes. Numerous epidemiologic studies and case reports have associated viral infections or local epidemics with type I diabetes. Likewise, epidemiologists have provided conflicting reports associating specific dietary practices with the disorder. However, when these practices are identified, their association (in terms of relative risk) usually is modest. Indeed, the collective literature to date has not demonstrated a diabetogenic agent that would represent a single major agent responsible for type I diabetes.

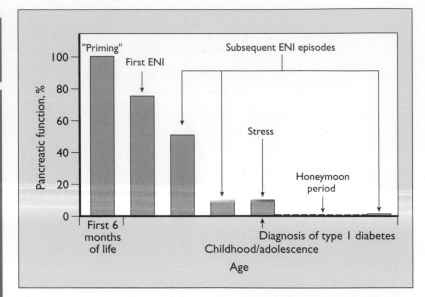

FIGURE 5-6. Multihit nature of action in type I diabetes. Thus far, no single agent has been associated exclusively with the disorder. Therefore, recent models associating environmental agents with type I diabetes have proposed a multihit nature of action. The primary "triggers" for type I diabetes could be those involving a yet to be identified interaction between an enterovirus and a nutritional factor. Subsequent enteroviral-nutritional interactions (ENI) could lead to further destruction of the pancreas. This situation would go unnoticed until there is not enough insulin-producing capability to respond to stress. Indeed, a stressful life event (eg, trauma, other infection, pubescent growth spurt, pregnancy) could cause a person to exceed the insulin-producing capacity of the pancreas and lead to the clinical diagnosis of type I diabetes. (Adapted from Hawkins [6].)

Genetics

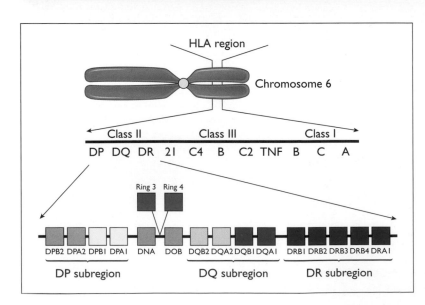

FIGURE 5-7. Genetics of type I diabetes. The human leukocyte antigen (HLA) region located on the short arm of chromosome 6. This region is approximately 3.5 centimorgans long and includes classes I, II, and III loci. Class I gene products (ie, HLA-A, HLA-B, and HLA-C) are expressed on all nucleated cells and serve as the classic transplantation antigens. These proteins present antigenic peptides to CD8+ T cells. Class II gene products are restricted in expression to antigen-presenting cells (eg, macrophages, dendritic cells, and B cells) and function to present peptides to CD4+ T cells. Class III gene products include complement proteins (eg, B, C2, and C4) and tumor necrosis factor (TNF).

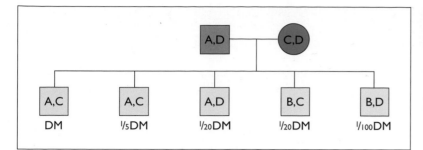

FIGURE 5-8. Familial risk of developing type I diabetes as a function of the relationship to the disease proband. The prevalence of disease (DM) is 30% to 50% in twins (not shown), 20% in human leukocyte antigen (HLA–) identical siblings (patient A,C), 5% in haploidentical siblings (A,D; B,C), and 1% in non-identical siblings (B,D). The mode of inheritance remains an enigma. Both dominant and recessive patterns of inheritance have been proposed; however, neither model adequately addresses type I diabetes. This line of investigation is further complicated by the potential interactions between genes and environmental factors, as well as evidence of the polygenic nature (ie, currently 20 additional loci) of the disorder. Furthermore, the risk of developing diabetes is higher in offspring of a father with type I diabetes than in offspring of a mother with the disorder. The lifetime risk for first-degree relatives is 5% to 8%. The probability is shown relative to inheritance of HLA haplotypes, which is indicated as A, B, C, D.

HLA-DR AND HLA-DQ TYPES AND THE RISK FOR TYPE I DIABETES

Risk	Genotype	Risk	Genotype
Susceptible	DR3	Resistant	DR2
	DR4		DR5 (< DR2)
	DR1 (< DR3 or DR4)		DQB1*0602
	DQA1*0301		DQB1*0301
	DQA1*0501		
	DQB1*0201		
	DQB1*0302		

FIGURE 5-9. Human leukocyte antigen (HLA)-DR and HLA-DQ types and the risk for type I diabetes. Note that these associations are representative of those most often observed in whites with a strong Northern European genetic influence. Interestingly, variance in susceptibility and resistance of human leukocyte antigen (HLA) types have been noted with type I diabetes in patients of different ethnic admixtures, especially those of Asian descent. Approximately 95% of whites with type I diabetes have either HLA-DR3 or HLA-DR4. However, susceptibility appears to reside predominantly in the HLA-DQ alleles under influence of HLA-DR. Furthermore, depending on the specific haplotype inherited, risk can be modified by the presence of a strong susceptibility or resistance allele, eg, DQB1*0602.

LOCATION, CANDIDATE GENES, AND MARKERS FOR REPORTED SUSCEPTIBILITY LOCI FOR HUMAN TYPE I DIABETES IN VARIOUS CAUCASIAN POPULATIONS FROM A VARIETY OF GEOGRAPHIC POPULATIONS

Locus	Chromosome region	Candidate genes	Markers
IDDM1	6p21.3	HLA DR/DQ	HLA-DRB1, DQB1, DQA1
IDDM2	11p15.5	INSULIN VNTR	—
IDDM3	15q26		D15S107
IDDM4	11q13.3	MDUI, ZFM1, RT6, ICE, LRP5, FADD, CD3	FGF3, D11S1917
IDDM5	6q25	SUM04, MnSOD	ESR, a046Xa9
IDDM6	18q12-q21	JK (Kidd), ZNF236	D18S487, D18S64
IDDM7	2q31-33	NEUROD, HOXD8	D2S152, D2S1391
IDDM8	6q25-27		D6S281, D6S264, D6S446
IDDM9	3q21-25		D3S1303, D10S193
IDDM10	10p11-q11		D10S565
IDDM11	14q24.3-q31	ENSA, SEL-1L	D14S67
IDDM12	2q33	CTLA-4	(AT)n 3' UTR, A/G exon 1
IDDM13	2q34	IGFBP2, IGFBP5, NEUROD, HOXD8	D2S137, D2S164, D2S1471
IDDM15	6q21		D6S283, D6S434, D6S1580
IDDM16	14q32	IGH	D14S542
IDDM17	10q25		D10S1750, D10S1773
IDDM18	5Q31.1-33.1	IL12B	IL12B
PTPN22	1p13	LYP=PTPN22	Snp=R620W T allele 1858[C]
	1q42		
	16p11-13		
	17q25		
	16q22-24		D16S3098
	19q11		

FIGURE 5-10. Location and markers for reported susceptibility intervals for human type I diabetes. Studies over the past 2 decades have suggested that a large number of genes or genetic intervals may be implicated in the pathogenesis of type I diabetes [7,8]. These genes are referred to as *susceptibility genes* that, by definition, increase or modify disease risk. Susceptibility genes are neither necessary nor sufficient for disease development. Therefore, some gene carriers may never develop the disease, whereas some noncarriers may develop type I diabetes. The IDDM1 loci (containing the HLA-DR and HLA-DQ regions) is the only major susceptibility interval, accounting for 30% to 50% of the total aggregated risk for type I diabetes.

Pathology

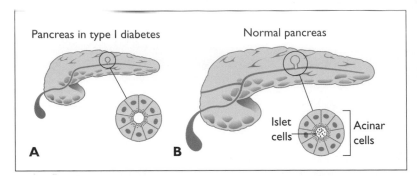

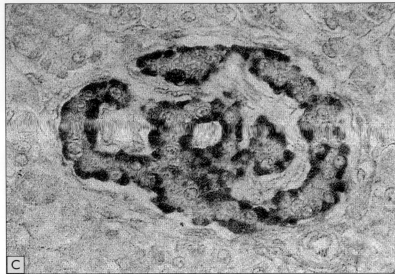

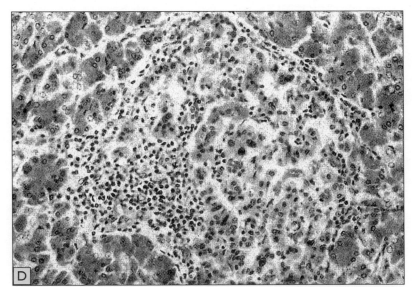

FIGURE 5-11. (*See* Color Plate) The effect of type I diabetes on the pancreas and islet cells. The pancreas of a person with type I diabetes (**A**) is often smaller and weighs less (*ie*, approximately 50% of total organ weight and 30% of endocrine weight) than its healthy counterpart (**B**). This difference is a consequence of the progressive atrophy of exocrine tissue that comprises about 98% of the total pancreatic volume. **C** and **D** demonstrate the pathology of pancreatic specimens from a patient with recent-onset type I diabetes. *Panel C,* Insulin-deficient islet stained for glucagon, somatostatin, and pancreatic polypeptide. All endocrine cells appear to have been stained, confirming the lack of β cells. *Panel D,* Insulitis. A chronic inflammatory cell infiltrate is centered on the islet. Insulitis is an elusive lesion to detect in the human pancreas, with only rare detection after I year of overt type I diabetes. With prolonged duration of disease, a progressive distortion of islet architecture develops, with a tendency for α and δ cells to leave the islet and spread as single cells into the exocrine parenchyma. (*Panel C,* immuno-alkaline phosphatase stain, ×1150; *panel D,* hematoxylin-eosin stain, ×300.) (*Panels C and D from* Foulis [9]; with permission.)

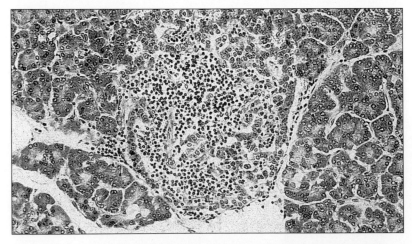

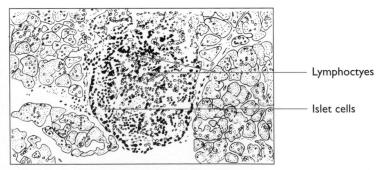

FIGURE 5-12. (*See* Color Plate) Islet of a patient recently diagnosed with type I diabetes demonstrating a diffuse lymphocytic infiltration (insulitis) with onset of atrophy of the islet cords. (Hematoxylin-eosin stain, ×300.) (*From* Foulis [9]; with permission.)

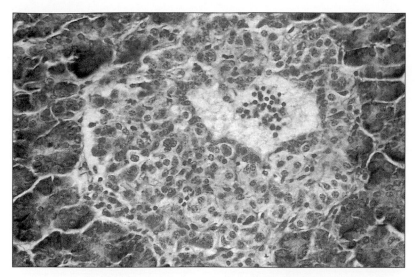

FIGURE 5-13. (*See* Color Plate) Pathology of a regenerating islet in the pancreas of a patient recently diagnosed with type I diabetes. Newly formed islet cells are derived from the epithelium of a duct. Lymphocytes are present in the lumen of the duct and in some places at the periphery. Evidence of such regeneration is rare in the pancreatic organs of patients with type I diabetes and is usually limited to those who die shortly after disease onset. (Hematoxylin-eosin stain, ×400.) (*From* Foulis [9]; with permission.)

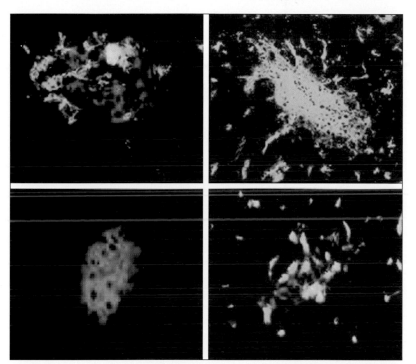

FIGURE 5-14. The cellular composition of the insulitis lesion in human type I diabetes before the symptomatic onset of disease. One of the earliest pieces of evidence suggestive of an autoimmune pathogenesis for type I diabetes was the finding of lymphocytic infiltration of the pancreatic islet cells; findings that were derived predominantly from studies of autopsy specimens from subjects after disease onset. A strength of animal models of the disease (*eg*, BioBreeding rats, nonobese diabetic mice) has been that the natural history and composition of the insulitis lesion can be analyzed at any time including that before disease onset. Only recently have there been attempts in human beings to obtain biopsies of the pancreas—of patients with recent onset diabetes and persons at increased risk for the disease. Shown in this figure are photomicrographs of pancreatic biopsy specimens from such a study involving analysis of subjects with type I diabetes of recent onset. T-cell–predominant infiltration to islets and hyperexpression of major histocompatibility complex class I antigens on islet cells were the two major findings observed in 17 of 29 recent-onset type I diabetic patients. CD3+ T-cells (shown in green) are infiltrating into the islet (insulin-containing pancreatic β-cells are shown in red) in one patient (*top left*), but are not observed in another patient (*bottom left*). Expression of major histocompatibility complex class I antigens were increased in one patient (*top right*), but did not increase in another patient (*bottom right*). Original magnification: ×3280 (*panels top left, bottom left,* and *bottom right*) and ×3200 (*panel top right*). (*From* Imagawa *et al.* [10]; with permission.)

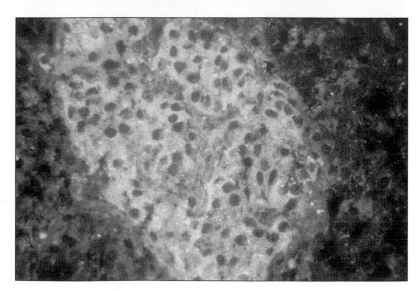

FIGURE 5-15. (*See* Color Plate) Islet cell autoantibodies (ICA). Islet cell autoantibodies are present in the serum of approximately 75% of persons at the onset of type I diabetes versus 0.4% of healthy persons. The first autoantibody ascribed to type I diabetes, the presence of islet cell autoantibodies is identified by indirect immunofluorescent assay using human blood group O pancreas. Islet cell autoantibodies specific for β cells have been identified. However, the autoantibodies react with all cells within the islet, including those that secrete insulin (β cells), glucagon (α cells), somatostatin cells (δ cells), and pancreatic polypeptide (PP cells). Autoantigens thus far ascribed to be responsible for the ICA reaction include sialoglycolipids, glutamic acid decarboxylase, and ICA512/IA-2.

AUTOANTIBODY MARKERS OF ISLET IMMUNITY IN HUMAN TYPE I DIABETES

Described in the 1970s
  Islet cell cytoplasmic autoantibodies
  Islet cell surface autoantibodies
Described in the 1980s
  64kD autoantibodies
  Carboxypeptidase-H autoantibodies
  Heat shock protein autoantibodies
  Insulin autoantibodies
  Insulin receptor autoantibodies
  Proinsulin autoantibodies

Described in the 1990s
  37kd/40kD tryptic fragment autoantibodies
  52kD rat insulinoma autoantibodies
  51kD aromatic-L-amino-acid decarboxylase
    autoantibodies
  128kD autoantibodies
  152kD autoantibodies
  Chymotrypsinogen-related 30 kD pancreatic
    autoantibodies
  DNA topoisomerase II autoantibodies
  Glucose transporter 2 autoantibodies
  Glutamic acid decarboxylase 65 autoantibodies
  Glutamic acid decarboxylase 67 autoantibodies
  Glima 38 autoantibodies
  Glycolipid autoantibodies
  GM2-1 islet ganglioside autoantibodies
  ICA512/IA-2 autoantibodies
  IA-2 autoantibodies
  Phogrin autoantibodies
Described in 2000s
  Carbonic anhidrase I autoantibodies
  Carbonic anhidrase II autoantibodies
  SOX-13 autoantibodies

FIGURE 5-16. Autoantibody markers of islet immunity in human type I diabetes. Since the first description of islet cell autoantibodies (ICAs) in 1974 (see Fig. 5-15), many new autoantibody markers of anti-islet immunity have been identified in patients with type I diabetes. In addition to their presence at disease onset, many of these markers have proved useful in identifying patients in the presymptomatic period, months to years before the clinical onset of type I diabetes. Of these, four markers have gained the most acceptance owing to scientific confirmation, high frequency of expression, and superior disease sensitivity and specificity: ICA, insulin autoantibodies, glutamic acid decarboxylase, and IA-2 autoantibodies.

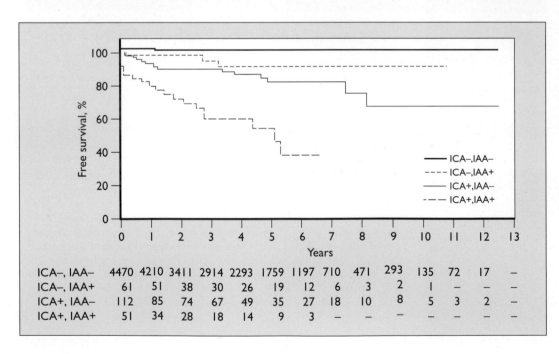

	0	1	2	3	4	5	6	7	8	9	10	11	12	13
ICA–, IAA–	4470	4210	3411	2914	2293	1759	1197	710	471	293	135	72	17	–
ICA–, IAA+	61	51	38	30	26	19	12	6	3	2	1	–	–	–
ICA+, IAA–	112	85	74	67	49	35	27	18	10	8	5	3	2	–
ICA+, IAA+	51	34	28	18	14	9	3	–	–	–	–	–	–	–

FIGURE 5-17. Using autoantibodies to islet cell autoantigens to predict future cases of type I diabetes. This life-table analysis indicates the probability of remaining disease-free, stratified by the appearance of islet cell cytoplasmic autoantibodies (ICA) and insulin autoantibodies (IAA) in relatives of probands with the disease. The number of relatives followed since identification of the autoantibody is displayed at the bottom for each group. As can be observed, the probability of developing type I diabetes is highest in those persons with two autoantibodies, with approximately half of these persons developing the disease within 4 years. (*Adapted from* Krischer et al. [11].)

PREVALENCE OF GLUTAMIC ACID DECARBOXYLASE AUTOANTIBODIES AND THEIR POTENTIAL USE IN IDENTIFYING AUTOIMMUNE ACTIVITY

Subject Group	Autoantibody Frequency, %
Healthy control group	0.3–0.6
First-degree relatives of patients with type I diabetes	3–4
Patients with other autoimmune endocrine disorders	1–2
Patients with newly diagnosed type I diabetes	55–85
Patients with type 2 diabetes	10–15
Patients with gestational diabetes	10

FIGURE 5-18. Prevalence of glutamic acid decarboxylase autoantibodies and their potential use in identifying autoimmune activity. Glutamic acid decarboxylase (GAD) autoantibodies serve as a marker for predicting future cases and diagnosing new cases of type I diabetes. Recent investigations summarized in representative form here indicate that GAD autoantibodies may also be useful in identifying autoimmunity in persons diagnosed with other forms of diabetes. These identifications may be useful in terms of imparting appropriate diabetes management and clinical care.

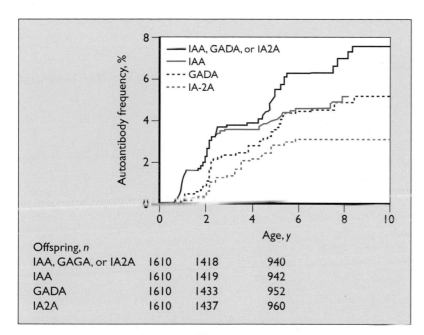

Offspring, n			
IAA, GAGA, or IA2A	1610	1418	940
IAA	1610	1419	942
GADA	1610	1433	952
IA2A	1610	1437	960

FIGURE 5-19. The ontogeny of anti-islet immunity in newborns and young children who were offspring of probands with type I diabetes. Over the past decade, multiple studies have been organized to analyze early events in the pathogenesis and natural history of time. Examples of these events would include but not be limited to breast-feeding, introduction of solid foods, viral infections, and infant immunization practices. When does anti-islet autoimmunity begin? For practical, technical, and ethical reasons, we are currently limited to ascertainment of indirect markers of anti–β-cell autoimmunity, namely type I diabetes–associated autoantibodies. This figure displays findings from one large German study of newborns and children who are the offspring of parents with type I diabetes, "BabyDiab". In this figure, the frequency of at least one autoantibody (autoantibodies to insulin [*IAA*], glutamic acid decarboxylase [*GADA*] or protein tyrosine phosphatase-like molecule IA-2 [*IA-2A*]) is indicated. Life-table islet autoantibody frequencies were 1.4% by 9 months, 3.6% by 2 years, 5.9% by 5 years, and 7.5% by 8 years of age. In terms of the order of autoantibody appearance in this study, this outcome related to the time of first autoantibody appearance. As suggested by this figure, almost all (93%) offspring who developed islet autoantibodies by age 2 years had IAA in their first sample, a number far greater than GADA or IA-2A. (*Adapted from* Hummel *et al.* [12].)

THE NONOBESE DIABETIC MOUSE MODEL OF TYPE I DIABETES

Characteristic	Nonobese Diabetic Mice
Disease onset	Spontaneous, 13–30+ weeks of age
Gender bias	Female predominance
Disease frequency	Strong intercolony variation, 50%–80% female, 20%–50% male, typical rates at 26 weeks of age
Clinical presentation	Hyperglycemia, mild ketosis, polydipsia, polyuria, weight loss, insulin dependency
Additional disease model	Thyroiditis, sialoadenitis (Sjögren syndrome), deafness
Insulitis	Appears in nondestructive (5–12 wk) and destructive (13+ wk) phases; macrophages, dendritic cells, T and B lymphocytes, NK cells
Genetic susceptibility	Major histocompatibility complex (MHC) plus >15 non-MHC loci
Immune markers	Autoantibodies, autoreactive T cells

FIGURE 5-20. The nonobese diabetic mouse model of type I diabetes.

THE BIOBREEDING RAT MODEL OF TYPE I DIABETES

Characteristic	BioBreeding Rats
Disease onset	Spontaneous, 8–14 weeks of age
Gender bias	None
Disease frequency	Minor intercolony variation, 40%–70% at 12 weeks of age
Clinical presentation	Hyperglycemia, mild ketosis, polydipsia, polyuria, weight loss, insulin dependency
Additional disease model	Thyroiditis, T-cell lymphopenia
Insulitis	Rapidly progressive; appears near time of disease onset; macrophages, dendritic cells, T and B lymphocytes, NK cells
Genetic susceptibility	Major histocompatibility complex (MHC) plus *Lyp* (T-lymphopenia) locus (chromosome 4)
Immune markers	Autoantibodies, autoreactive T cells

FIGURE 5-21. The BioBreeding rat model of type I diabetes.

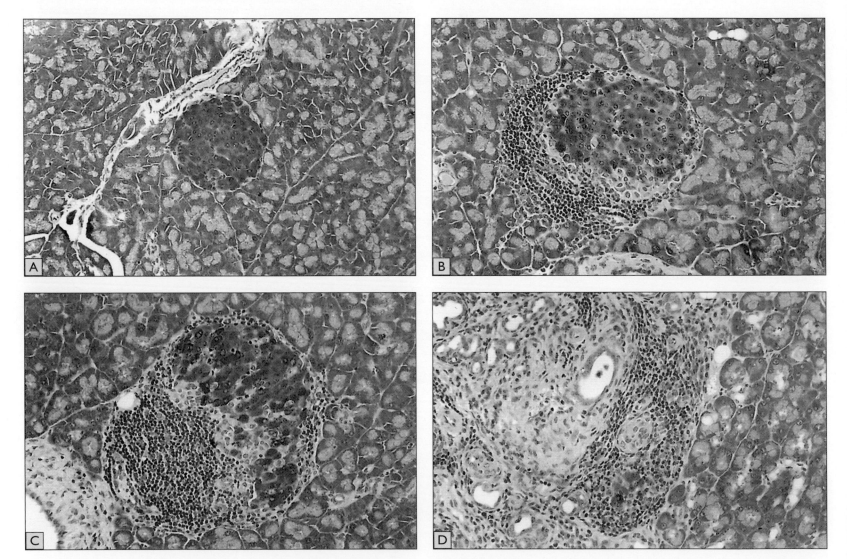

FIGURE 5-22. (See Color Plate) Developmental stages of the insulitis lesion in nonobese diabetic mice. Pathology of pancreatic specimens from a normal islet cell devoid of leukocytic infiltrate (**A**) and at various stages of infiltration (**B** to **H**).

(*Continued on next page*)

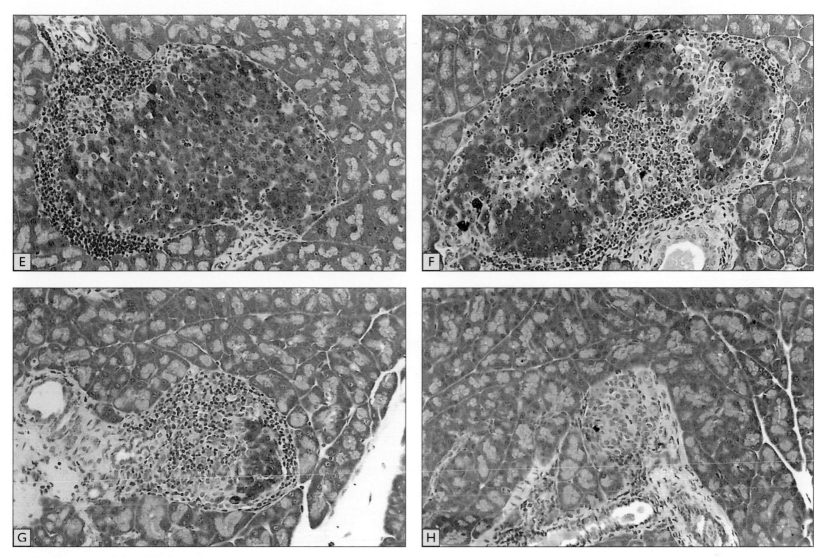

FIGURE 5-22. (*Continued*) Beginning at 5 to 7 weeks of age, leukocytes surround and eventually infiltrate the islets in increasing numbers. Beginning at 12 to 14 weeks, this early insulitis (often termed *nondestructive*) is replaced with an insulitis that destroys the insulin-producing β cells. When the islet is devoid of β cells the leukocytic infiltrate disappears, leaving only α, τ, and δ cells (*panel H*). (Hematoxylin-eosin stain followed by counterstaining with anti-insulin antibody and avidin-biotin, ×300.) (*Courtesy of* A. Peck, University of Florida.)

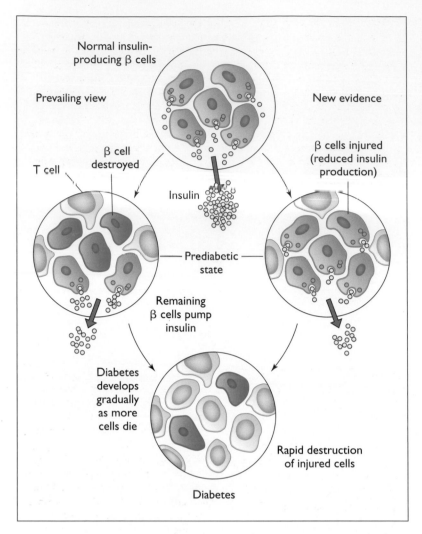

FIGURE 5-23. A new model showing rapid destruction of β cells in the pathogenesis of type 1 diabetes. Until recently, most models assessing the rate of β-cell destruction have presumed a gradual (*ie*, modified linear; *see* Fig. 5-2) endocrine cell loss characterized by small periods of "waxing and waning" in the immune response. However, recent investigations of nonobese diabetic mice have suggested that actual β-cell destruction occurs in a very limited time period immediately before symptomatic onset. The composition of the insulitic lesion, destructive activity, or both before this event would be of nondestructive or limited destructive capacity. Although limited evidence exists for this model in terms of human type 1 diabetes, it is the subject of ongoing investigation.

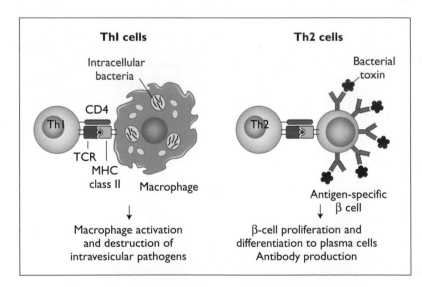

FIGURE 5-24. Th1/Th2 model for immune regulation. Both *in vivo* and *in vitro* studies have supported the notion that activities of CD4+ "helper-T" cells may directly or indirectly relate to the production of specific cytokines. Evolutionary immunologists indicate that the compartmentalization of such responses provides for a more efficient development of an immune response against pathogens of divergent origins and modes of evasion. Although somewhat of an overgeneralization, Th1 cytokines are viewed as enhancing cellular immune activities, whereas Th2 cytokines support those of humoral immunity. Specifically, Th1 activity appears to be enhanced by production of the lymphokines interferon γ (IFN-γ), interleukin 2 (IL-2), and IL-12. Conversely, Th2 augmentation of humoral immunity occurs through the release of IL-4 and IL-10. Note that IL-4 appears to be a strong inhibitor of Th1 immunity. The production of specific cytokines, both systemic and at the site of pancreatic inflammation, may have important implications for the pathogenesis of diabetes as well as the potential for developing methods aimed at disease prevention. MHC—major histocompatibility complex; TCR—T-cell receptor.

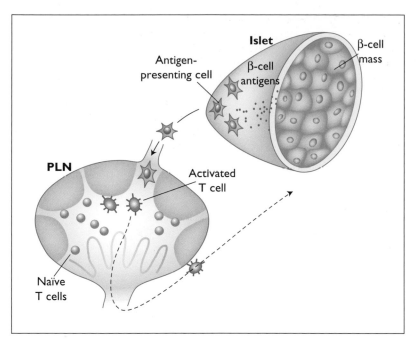

FIGURE 5-25. Hypothetical model for the initiation of type I diabetes. Native T cells circulate through the blood and lymphoid organs, including pancreatic lymph nodes (PLN). In the nodes, they encounter antigen-presenting cells (most likely mature dendritic cells) displaying on their surface major histocompatibility complex (MHC) molecules carrying antigens in the form of peptide fragments. In this case, the antigens derive from proteins synthesized by pancreatic islet β-cells, picked up (in soluble form, as cell bits or as apoptotic cells) when the antigen-presenting cells resided in the islets. A minute fraction of the naive T cells recognize MHC molecule/β-cell antigen complexes, become activated, and then access tissues including the pancreas, where they re-encounter cognate antigen, are reactivated, and are retained. (*Adapted from Mathis et al.* [13].)

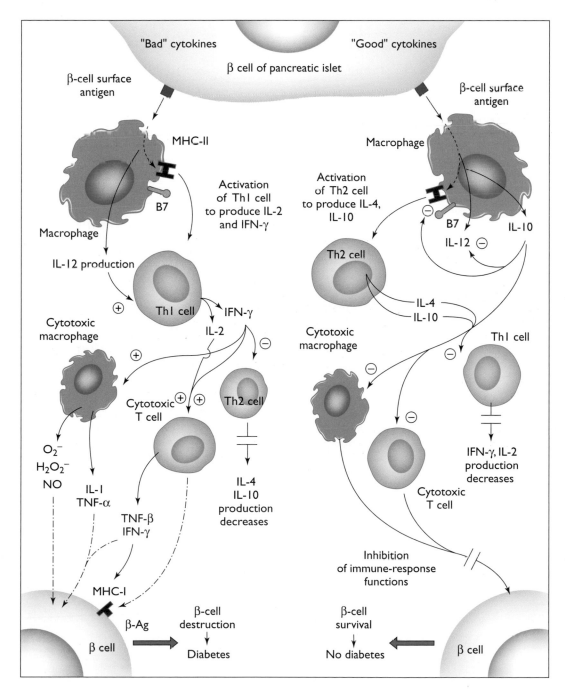

FIGURE 5-26. The "good and bad" cytokine model for the pathogenesis of type I diabetes. As modeled in accordance with Figures 5-24 and 5-25, production of Th2 cytokines would be viewed as providing a pathway of avoidance of β-cell destruction (hence the label "good" cytokine). Production of interleukin-4 (IL-4) and IL-10 would block the destructive actions of the cellular immune response. By contrast, immune responses characterized by "bad" Th1 cytokines would be considered as promoting β-cell destruction through enhancement of actions ascribed to cytotoxic T cells or macrophages (through oxygen radical–mediated damage). Ag—antigen; H_2O_2—hydrogen peroxide; IFN—interferon; MHC—major histocompatibility complex; minus sign—inhibitory pathway; NO—nitric oxide; O_2^-—oxygen free radical; plus sign—promoting pathway; TNF-α—tumor necrosis factor-α.

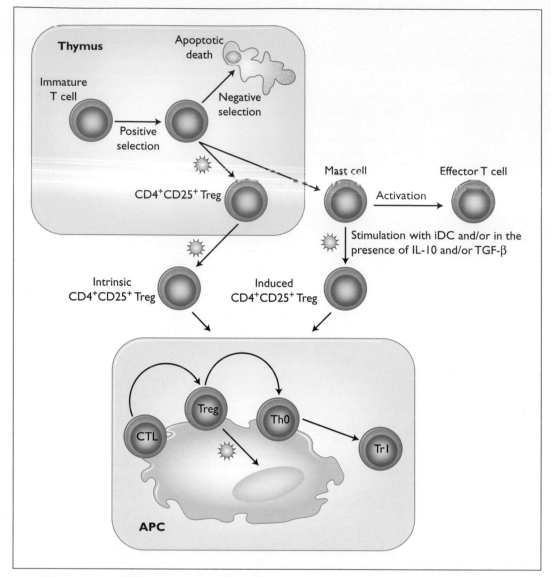

FIGURE 5-27. Two modes for development of regulatory T cells and their modes of action in modulating the immune response (inset). Regulatory T cells are thought to develop in two locations; from cells emanating directly from the thymus as well as those directed into this phenotype from the periphery. For years, immunologists have worked with a model in which positive selection ensures that only T-cells bearing a relevant T-cell receptor (capable of interacting with self–major histocompatibility complex [MHC] molecules) develop and migrate into the periphery. In contrast, negative selection eliminates T-cells bearing high-affinity T-cell receptors for peptide-MHC complexes, thereby preventing these cells from entering the periphery and causing autoimmune diseases including type 1 diabetes. More recently, studies of thymectomized mice have indicated that the thymus also generates cells having a regulatory capacity, so-called T-reg cells. T-reg cells generated in the thymus recognize self-peptide–MHC complexes with high affinity T-cell receptors and escape the fate of apoptotic death that occurs during negative selection. These T-cells differentiate into the naturally occurring (intrinsic) T-reg cells, a population phenotypically characterized by their co-expression of CD4 and CD25. Naïve cells can also differentiate into T-reg cells by a process that requires immature dendritic cells (as a source of antigen-presenting cells [APC]) during the priming of an immune response. Additionally, this process can be promoted by the cytokines interleukin-10 (IL-10) and transforming growth factor-β (TGF-β). Without such activation, these cells have the potential to generate into effector T-cells. In terms of their immune modulating capabilities, T-reg cells that recognize antigen presented by APC suppress other lymphocytes, for example, cytotoxic T lymphocytes (CTL), and helper T-cells (Th cells) through a mechanism that requires direct cell-cell contact. In terms of their importance to type 1 diabetes formation, studies from nonobese diabetic mice have supported the notion that such cells do have the capacity to prevent diabetes and in addition, many forms of therapy capable of interrupting disease in this animal model are associated with the production of CD4+ CD25+ T-cells. In humans, we and others have associated type 1 diabetes with abnormal function of these regulatory T-cells. Although premature to speculate how these cells may in actuality influence the development of type 1 diabetes, a picture is rapidly emerging in the field that understanding T-reg function may provide important clues to aspects ranging from pathogenesis to therapy. (*Adapted from* Sutmuller *et al.* [14].)

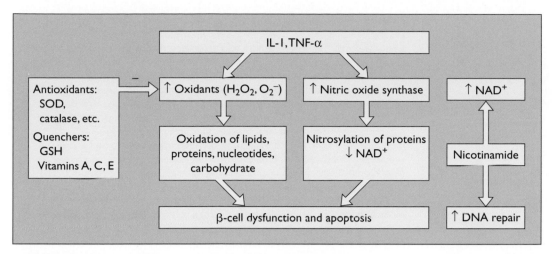

FIGURE 5-28. The lymphokine model for β-cell destruction in type I diabetes. Under this scenario, lymphokines produced in response to a nonspecific infection would, by their mode of action, impart a limited degree of initial β-cell destruction owing to an unusual susceptibility of β cells to such agents. The predominant lymphokines cited in this model are those produced by macrophages and include tumor necrosis factor-α (TNF-α) and interleukin I (IL-I). Despite the benefits of recovery from infection, this process of anti–β-cell immunity would result in those genetically susceptible to the disease. The continuing process of β-cell destruction would occur through the action of various cytotoxic agents (eg, oxidants and nitric oxide) as well as a lack of activity of numerous compounds associated with cellular or DNA repair mechanisms (eg, anti-oxidants). GSH—glomerulus-stimulating hormone; H₂O₂—hydrogen peroxide; NAD+—oxidized nicotinamide adenine dinucleotide; O₂−—oxygen free radical; SOD—superoxide dismutase. (*Adapted from* Kolb and Kolb-Bachofen [15].)

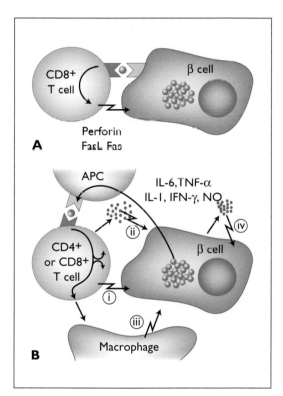

FIGURE 5-29. Proposed mechanisms of β-cell death. **A,** In a recognition-based model, a CD8+ T cell is activated by direct recognition of islet β-cell antigen (*circles*) presented by major histocompatibility complex molecules on β cells. Activation provokes killing of the β cell through cell/cell contact using various pathways (*eg,* Fas/FasL, perforin). **B,** In an activation-based model, a T cell (either CD4+ or CD8+) recognizes β-cell antigens presented indirectly by antigen-presenting cells (APC) located in the vicinity of the islet. The resulting activation provokes β-cell death by (*i*) surface receptors (*eg,* Fas/FasL), (*ii*) soluble mediators from T cells, (*iii*) activation of macrophage cytocidal activities, or (*iv*) activation of death signals in β cells. IFN—interferon; IL—interleukin; NO—nitric oxide. (*Adapted from* Mathis et al. [13].)

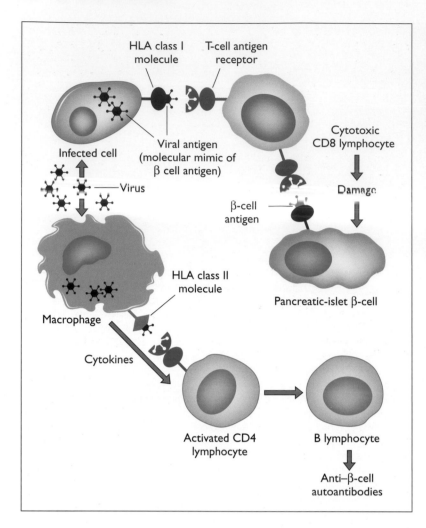

FIGURE 5-30. Potential role for viruses in the pathogenesis of type I diabetes: the molecular mimicry model. In this model, the autoimmune process begins after a "normal" immune response to a cell infected with a virus whose proteins share a similar sequence to that of a β-cell protein. The infected cells display processed viral antigens (by way of Class I molecules) to CD8+ T cells. Macrophages having phagocytosed and processed virus present the viral peptides to CD4+ T cells through Class II molecules. The CD4+ T cells amplify the actions of the CD8+ T cells to become cytotoxic effector cells that can kill β cells that express a peptide common to the viral protein. Despite exhaustive research efforts to demonstrate molecular mimicry as an underlying cause of type I diabetes, it remains an unproved model. Contemporary support predominantly derives from studies demonstrating amino acid sequence similarity between β-cell proteins (eg, glutamic acid decarboxylase and IA-2) with those of viruses (eg, Coxsackie and Rotavirus) and the ability of human lymphocyte antigen (HLA) molecules with susceptibility and resistance to type I disease to bind these regions of mimicry. Studies, in particular those of cellular immunity, of the natural history of diabetes in humans and nonobese diabetic mice have failed to elevate this model beyond the hypothetical stage. (*Adapted from* Atkinson and Eisenbarth [1].)

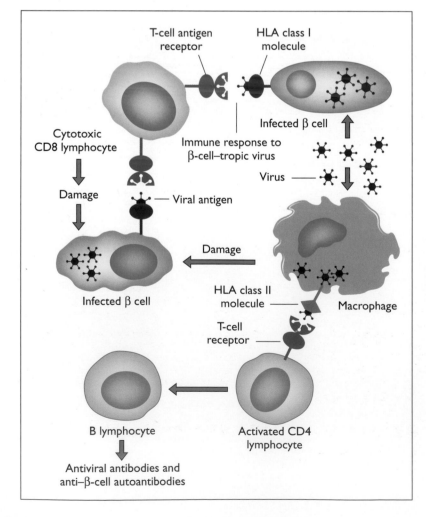

FIGURE 5-31. Potential role for viruses in the pathogenesis of type I diabetes: β-tropic virus–viral superantigen models. In these models, initiation of the autoimmune process follows direct viral infection of β cells or the expression in β cells of a virus acting as a superantigen. In both situations, leukocytes are recruited to pancreatic islets. Recruitment increases the release of cytokines (eg, interferon-α) and adhesion of leukocytes within the pancreatic islets. In the β-cell tropic model, the infected β cell is susceptible to direct attack by antiviral cytotoxic lymphocytes. In both models, cytokines and free radicals produced by macrophages activated within the islet cells may augment the cytotoxic response to the β cells; the cytokines also recruit CD4+ T cells to the lesion. Macrophages present autoantigens derived from virus-damaged β cells, thus leading to the development of lymphocytes and autoantibodies that react with β-cell proteins. Support for both of these models exists, yet they remain hypothetical. Whereas viruses capable of β-cell destruction have been isolated from an extremely limited number of human pancreatic organs, examination of a large number of these tissues from patients with type I diabetes has failed to reveal the presence of such viruses. Support for the superantigen model exists through the identification of T cells characteristic of superantigen activation in the pancreatic organs of a limited number of patients with new-onset type I diabetes. To date, however, no such viral superantigen has been unequivocally identified. HLA—human leukocyte antigen. (*Adapted from* Atkinson and Eisenbarth [1].)

THERAPIES DELAYING OR PREVENTING THE ONSET OF TYPE I DIABETES IN THE NONOBESE DIABETIC MOUSE MODEL

Adeno-associated virus murine interleukin (IL)-10

Adeno-associated virus rat preproinsulin gene (vLP-1)

Adenovirus expressing mIL-4

Aerosol insulin

Allogenic thymic macrophages

Alpha-galactosylceramide

Alpha-interferon (rIFN-α)

Alpha/beta T-cell receptor thymocytes

Aminoguanidine

Androgens

Anesthesia

Antioxidant MDL 29,311

Antisense glutamic acid decarboxylase (GAD) mRNA

Azathioprine

Anti-B7-1

Bacille-Calmette Guérin

Baclofen

Bee venom

Biolistic-mediated IL-4

Blocking peptide of major histocompatibility complex (MHC) class II

Bone marrow transplantation

Castration

Anti-CD3

Anti-CD4

CD4+CD25+ regulatory T cells

Anti-CD8

Anti-CD28 MAb

Cholera toxin B subunit-insulin protein

Class I–derived self-I-A beta(g7) (54-76) peptide

Cold exposure

Anticomplement receptor

Complete Freund's adjuvant

Anti–cytotoxic T lymphocyte antigen (CTLA)-4

Cyclic nucleotide phosphodiesterases

Cyclosporin

Dendritic cells (DC) deficient in nuclear factor κB

DC from pancreatic lymph node

DC with IL-4

Deflazacort

Deoxyspergualin

Dexamethasone/progesterone/ growth hormone/estradiol

Diazoxide

1,25 dihydroxycholecalciferol

Elevated temperature

Emotionality

Encephalomyocarditis virus

Essential fatty acid deficient diets

FK506

FTY720 (myriocin)

GAD 65 peptides in utero

Anti-GAD monoclonal antibody

Galactosylceramide

Glucose (neonatal)

Glutamic acid decarboxylase (intraperitoneal, intrathymic, intravenous, oral)

Glutamic acid decarboxylase 65 T helper 2 cell clone

Glutamic acid decarboxylase peptides (intraperitoneal, intrathymic, intravenous, oral)

Gonadectomy

Guanidinoethyldisulphide

Heat shock protein 65

Heat shock protein peptide (p277)

Hematopoietic stem cells encoding proinsulin

Housing alone

Human insulin growth factor (IFG-1)

I-A beta g7(54-76) peptide

Anti-I-A monoclonal antibodies

Anti- intercellular adhesion molecule -1

Immunoglobulin G-2a antibodies

Immobilization

Inomide

Anti-integrin α4

Insulin (intraperitoneal, oral, subcutaneous, nasal)

Insulin B chain (plasmid)

Insulin B chain/B chain amino acids 9-23 (intraperitoneal, oral, subcutaneous, nasal)

Insulin-like growth factor I

Interferon-α (oral)

Interferon-γ

Anti–interferon-γ

Interferon-γ receptor/immunoglobulin G-1 fusion protein

IL-1

IL-4

IL-4–immunoglobulin fusion protein

IL-4-plasmid

IL-10

IL-10-plasmid DNA

IL-10-viral

IL-11-human

IL-12

Intrathymic administration of mycobacterial heat shock protein 65

Intrathymic administration of mycobacterial heat shock peptide p277

Islet cells-intrathymic

L-Selectin (MEL-14)

Lactate dehydrogenase virus

Large multilamellar liposome

Lazaroid

Anti-leukocyte function–associated antigen

Anti-leukocyte function–associated antigen -1

Linomide (quinoline-3-carboxamide)

Lipopolysaccharide-activated B cells

Lisofylline

Lymphocyte choriomeningitis virus

Antilymphocyte serum

Lymphoctyte vaccination

Lymphocytic choriomeningitis virus

Anti-L-selectin

Lymphotoxin

LZ8

MC1288 (20-epi-1, 25-dihydroxyvitamin D3)

MDL 29311

Metabolically inactive insulin analog

Anti-MHC class I

Anti-MHC class II

MHC class II derived cyclic peptide

Mixed allogeneic chimerism

Mixed bone marrow chimeras

Monosodium glutamate

Murine hepatitis virus

Mycobacterium avium

Mycobacterium leprae

Natural antibodies

Natural polyreactive autoantibodies

Neuropeptide calcitonin gene-related peptide

Nicotinamide

Nicotine

Ninjin-to (Ren-Shen-Tang), a Kampo (Japanese traditional) formulation

Natural killer T cells

NY4.2 cells

OK432

Overcrowding

Pancreatectomy

Pentoxifylline

Pertussigen

Poly [I:C]

Pregestimil diet

Prenatal stress

Preproinsulin DNA

Probucol

Prolactin

Rampamycin

Recombinant vaccinia virus expressing GAD

Reg protein

Rolipram

Saline (repeated injection)

Schistosoma mansoni

Semipurified diet (eg, AIN-76)

Short-term chronic stress

Silica

Sirolimus/tacrolimus

Sodium fusidate

Soluble interferon-γ receptor

Somatostatin

Nonspecific pathogen-free conditions

Streptococcal enterotoxins

Streptozotocin

Sulfatide (3'sulfogalactosylceramide)

Superantigens

Superoxide dismutase-desferrioxamine

Anti–T-cell receptor

Transforming growth factor-β-1 somatic gene therapy

T helper 1 clone specific for heat shock protein 60 peptide

Anti-thy-1

Thymectomy (neonatal)

Tolbutamide

Tolerogenic dendritic cells induced by vitamin D receptor ligands

Top of the rack housing

Treatment combined with a 10% w/v sucrose-supplemented drinking water

Tumor necrosis factor-alpha

TX527 (19-nor-14,20-bisepi-23-yne-1,25(OH)(2)D(3))

Vitamin E

Anti–very late antigen-4

FIGURE 5-32. Therapies delaying or preventing the onset of type 1 diabetes in the nonobese diabetic mouse model.

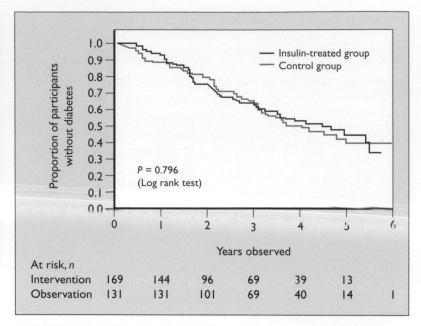

RESULTS OF STUDIES TO PREVENT HUMAN TYPE 1 DIABETES IN THOSE AT INCREASED RISK FOR THE DISEASE

	Parenteral insulin	Nicotinamide	Oral insulin
	At 5 years	At 4 years	At 5 years
Control	61%	24%	35%
Treated	50%	27%	33%

Approximate percentage of subjects developing type 1 diabetes in three large multicenter prevention trials; based on survival curves.

FIGURE 5-33. Results of two large clinical trials designed to prevent the development of type 1 diabetes in humans. The Diabetes Prevention Trial (DPT-1) addressed this goal through administration of parenteral insulin and oral insulin, whereas the European Nicotinamide Diabetes Intervention Trial (ENDIT) utilized nicotinamide. Both studies analyzed relatives of patients with type 1 diabetes, and through a combination of genetic, immunologic, and metabolic markers, identified subjects at increased-risk of developing the disease. Each trial posed the question of whether the given therapy could delay the onset of type 1 diabetes. In the case of DPT-1, based on the degree of risk—high or intermediate—study subjects were placed onto parenteral or oral insulin, respectively. More detailed results of the DPT-1 parenteral insulin trial and the ENDIT study are shown in subsequent figures. (*Adapted from* Skyler and Marks [16].)

FIGURE 5-34. Kaplan-Meier curves showing the proportion of subjects without type 1 diabetes during the Diabetes Prevention Trial-1 parenteral insulin trial, by treatment assignment. The insulin-treated group is depicted by the *solid line*, whereas the control group is indicated by the *dotted line*. There is no difference between the two curves in terms of the rate of progression to overt type 1 diabetes. The proportion of subjects without type 1 diabetes is indicated on the y-axis, whereas the x-axis depicts the number of at risk subjects (intervention-top and observation-bottom) observed for a given duration in years. (*Adapted from* Diabetes Prevention Trial Type 1 Diabetes Study Group [17].)

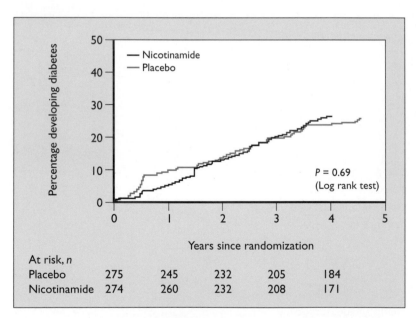

FIGURE 5-35. The cumulative incidence of type 1 diabetes in the European Nicotinamide Diabetes Intervention Trial in relatives at increased risk of type 1 diabetes, by treatment assignment. The placebo curve is *blue*, the nicotinamide curve is *green*. The proportion of subjects with type 1 diabetes is indicated on the y-axis, whereas the time since randomization (in years) and the number of placebo- and nicotinamide-treated subjects are reported on the x-axis. There is no difference between the curves in terms of the rates of progression to type 1 diabetes. (*Adapted from* European Nicotinamide Diabetes Intervention Trial [18].)

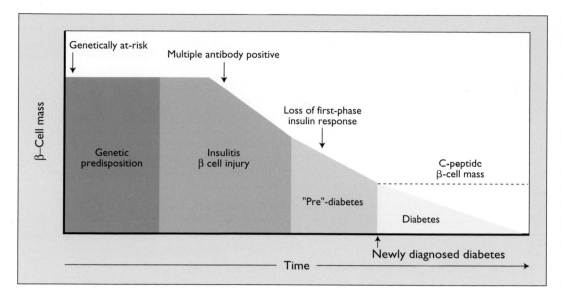

Genetically at-risk

Multiple antibody positive

Loss of first-phase insulin response

β—Cell mass

Genetic predisposition

Insulitis β cell injury

C-peptide β-cell mass

"Pre"-diabetes

Diabetes

Newly diagnosed diabetes

Time

FIGURE 5-36. Potential timing of interventions to interdict the type I diabetes disease process. Through a combination of analyzing previous studies involving humans and animal models of type I diabetes (*ie*, nonobese diabetic mice), a model has recently emerged supporting specific "windows of opportunity" for interventions aimed at type I diabetes prevention. These would include studies at the time of diagnosis, aimed at preserving β-cell function, as measured by C-peptide; studies in "pre-diabetes" in multiple autoantibody positive individuals or in those who have lost first phase insulin response or have some glucose abnormality already—to prevent diabetes; and studies in those genetically at-risk—to prevent autoimmunity. Key principles to this model include that of matching risk versus reward (*ie*, more benign therapies in newborns in which progression to type I diabetes is less certain), and the utilization of agents when they may provide the most therapeutic effectiveness. (*Adapted from* Skyler [19].)

FIGURE 5-37. Interventions that have been studied, are being studied, or are planned to be studied in human type I diabetes, at the various stages discussed in Figure 5-33. Compare this list with that in Figure 5-29, which enumerates the many successful interventions in nonobese diabetic mice.

INTERVENTIONS STUDIED IN HUMAN TYPE I DIABETES

New-onset diabetes: to preserve β-cell function

Completed studies with suggestion of metabolic benefit

Cyclosporin

Azathioprine with glucocorticoids

Anti-CD5 monoclonal antibody with ricin-A chain (immunotoxin)

Insulin-intensive therapy

Nicotinamide

Plasmapheresis

Anti-CD3 monoclonal antibody

Heat-shock protein-60 (hsp60) p277 peptide

Completed studies without benefit

Bacille-Calmette Guérin

Intravenous immune globulin

Oral insulin

Studies in progress or planned

Anti-CD3 (repeated doses)

Anti-CD25 monoclonal antibody (daclizumab)

Oral interferon

Insulin B9-23 altered peptide ligand

GAD vaccine

Vitamin D

Vitamin E

Mycophenolate mofetil alone and with anti-CD25 antibody (daclizumab)

Anti-CD20 monoclonal antibody (rituxamab)

Thymoglobulin

Interleukin-2 plus rapamycin (sirolimus)

Anti-CD3 plus exenatide

Antibody-positive relatives at risk

Completed studies without benefit

Parenteral insulin

Nicotinamide

Oral insulin (except suggested benefit in a subgroup)

Studies in progress or planned

Nasal insulin

Oral insulin

Anti-CD3

Exenatide

Newborns or neonates to prevent autoimmunity and diabetes

Studies in progress or planned

Nasal insulin

Omission of cow milk protein

Omega-3-fatty acids

References

1. Atkinson M, Eisenbarth G: Type 1 diabetes: new perspectives on disease pathogenesis and treatment. *Lancet* 2001, 358:221–229.

2. Eisenbarth GS: Type 1 diabetes mellitus. A chronic autoimmune disease. *N Engl J Med* 1986, 314:1360–1368.

3. Devendra D, Liu E, Eisenbarth GS: Type 1 diabetes: recent developments. *BMJ* 2004, 328:750–754.

4. Karvonen M, Tuomilehto J, Libman I, LaPorte R: WHO Diamond Project Group: a review of the recent epidemiological data on incidence of type 1 (insulin-dependent) diabetes mellitus worldwide. *Diabetologia* 36:883–892.

5. LaPorte RE, Matsushima M, Chang Y-F: Prevalence and incidence of insulin dependent diabetes. In *Diabetes in America*. Edited by Harris M. Bethesda, MD: NIH Publications; 1995:37–46.

6. Hawkins HW: Could the aetiology of IDDM be multifactorial? *Diabetologia* 1997, 40:1235–1240.

7. She JX: Susceptibility to type 1 diabetes: HLA-DQ and DR revisited. *Immunol Today* 1996, 17:323–329.

8. Field LL: Genetic linkage and association studies of Type 1 diabetes: challenges and rewards. *Diabetologia* 2002, 45:21–35.

9. Foulis AK: In *Textbook of Diabetes*. Vol. 1. Edited by Pickup J, Williams G. Oxford, England: Blackwell Scientific; 1991.

10. Imagawa A, Hanafusa T, Tamura S, *et al.*: Pancreatic biopsy as a procedure for detecting in situ autoimmune phenomena in type 1 diabetes: close correlation between serological markers and histological evidence of cellular autoimmunity. *Diabetes* 2001, 50:1269–1273.

11. Krischer JP, Schatz D, Riley WJ, *et al.*: Insulin and islet cell autoantibodies as time-dependent covariates in the development of insulin-dependent diabetes. *J Clin Endocrinol Metab* 1993, 77:743–749.

12. Hummel M, Bonifacio E, Schmid S, *et al.*: Brief communication: early appearance of islet autoantibodies predicts childhood type 1 diabetes in offspring of diabetic parents. *Ann Intern Med* 2004, 140:882–886.

13. Mathis D, Vence L, Benoist C: Beta-cell death during progression to diabetes. *Nature* 2001, 414:729–798.

14. Sutmuller RPM, Offringa R, Mellet CJM: Revival of the regulatory T cell: new targets for drug development. *Drug Discov Today* 2004, 9:310–317.

15. Kolb H, Kolb-Bachofen V: Nitric oxide in autoimmune disease: cytotoxic or regulatory mediator? *Immunol Today* 1998, 19:556–561.

16. Skyler JS, Marks JB: Immune intervention. In *Diabetes Mellitus: A Fundamental and Clinical Text*, edn 3. Edited by LeRoith D, Taylor SI, Olefsky JM. Philadelphia: Lippincott Williams & Wilkins; 2004:701–709.

17. Diabetes Prevention Trial Type 1 Diabetes Study Group: Effects of insulin in relatives of patients with type 1 diabetes mellitus. *N Engl J Med* 2002, 346:1685–1691.

18. European Nicotinamide Diabetes Intervention Trial (ENDIT): A randomized controlled trial of intervention before the onset of type 1 diabetes. *Lancet* 2004, 363:925–931.

19. Skyler JS: Immunotherapy for interdicting the type 1 diabetes disease process. In *Textbook of Diabetes*, edn 3. Edited by Pickup J, Williams G. Oxford, UK: Blackwell Publishing Ltd.; 2003:74-1–74-12.

MANAGEMENT OF TYPE 1 DIABETES

Irl B. Hirsch and Jay S. Skyler

6

The treatment of type 1 diabetes has a relatively short history; the disease was uniformly fatal before the discovery of insulin in 1922. It is interesting to note that by the late 1920s, it was observed that insulin tended to make "fat people fatter," but it was not until the mid-1930s that some of the basic differences in the two major types of diabetes were noted. Insulin therapy, although it allowed the avoidance of certain death in type 1 diabetes, brought on a new era of problems not formally appreciated. This "era of complications" was notable for the grim realization that approximately half of patients developed proliferative diabetic retinopathy and between 30% and 40% developed diabetic nephropathy. One of the most important scientific debates of the 20th century was the relationship of diabetic complications and glycemic control. By the 1980s, new tools such as home self-monitoring of blood glucose (SMBG), assessment of integrated glycemic control by glycated hemoglobin HbA_{1c} (A_{1c}), continuous subcutaneous insulin infusion (CSII), and human insulins made it possible to attempt near normal glycemic control. The announcement of the results of the Diabetes Control and Complications Trial (DCCT) in 1993 ended the debate by demonstrating a strong relationship between blood glucose control and the microvascular and neuropathic complications of type 1 diabetes. Since then, the goals have been to further improve our tools for the management of type 1 diabetes and to develop new strategies for the treatment of diabetes-related complications after they develop.

Rationale for Improved Glycemic Control

Several small studies in the 1980s suggested that "intensive therapy" with improved glycemic control could reduce the risk of the development of the microvascular complications of diabetes. Despite this long-standing debate dating back decades, it was not until the 1980s that this question could be adequately addressed. During the early part of that decade, there was a dramatic change in the management tools for type 1 diabetes. SMBG, A_{1c}, purified insulins, and CSII therapy were all being routinely (although not necessarily widely) used in the management of this patient population.

The landmark study that ended all of the debate was the DCCT. Starting in 1982 and ending in 1993, this study of 1441 subjects addressed the fundamental question about the relationship between glycemic control and microvascular and neuropathic complications. Follow-up examinations occurred after a mean of 6.5 years. The DCCT actually asked two questions: 1) does an intensive therapy program prevent the appearance of microvascular disease (primary prevention) and 2) does this therapy retard the progression of early preexisting disease (secondary intervention)? "Intensive therapy" was defined as a multiple daily injection regimen (at least three injections per day) or CSII, in combination with a minimum of premeal and bedtime SMBG measurements, monthly clinic visits, and psychologic and nutritional support.

This intensive therapy resulted in a mean A_{1c} difference of approximately 2% over the course of the study. When compared with conventional therapy for primary prevention and secondary intervention, intensive therapy reduced the development of early and later manifestations of diabetic retinopathy, microalbuminuria, clinical grade proteinuria, and peripheral and autonomic neuropathy. However, in this young population of subjects with type 1 diabetes, the reduction in cardiovascular events—few in number—did not reach statistical significance. Intensive therapy did result in a threefold increased risk of severe hypoglycemia (requiring the assistance of another person) and in weight gain. No cognitive impairment was found in those with severe hypoglycemia. It is important to note that the DCCT ended before the introduction of insulin analogues.

Subjects from the DCCT have had continued follow-up in a study known as the Epidemiology of Diabetes Interventions and Complications (EDIC). After the formal DCCT was completed, the two treatment groups had a merging of A_{1c} levels to approximately 8%. Despite that, there appeared to be a "metabolic memory" in that over the next 8 years, the progression of retinopathy, nephropathy, and even carotid artery intimal thickness was reduced in the group previously randomized to intensive therapy. Although the mechanism of "metabolic memory" is unknown, because the DCCT population initiated the study with disease durations of approximately 2.5 years (primary prevention) and 8.7 years (secondary intervention), it is clear that early and aggressive glycemic management is critical.

Available Forms of Insulin

When insulin therapy became available in the 1920s, preparations were somewhat crude, required reasonably large volumes, and were relatively short acting. This resulted in most patients receiving insulin being treated with three or more daily injections. In the 1930s and 1940s, protein chemists modified the existing soluble (regular) insulin with the goal of prolonging its duration of action, thus making insulin therapy less cumbersome. The result was the development of protamine zinc insulin (PZI); neutral protamine Hagedorn (NPH) or isophane insulin; globin insulin; and the Lente series if insulins (SemiLente, Lente, and UltraLente) [1]. By the 1960s, several clinicians realized that convenience resulted in a deterioration of glycemic control, and the classical "split-mix" program of twice-daily NPH and regular insulin was popularized [2]. Although this was an improvement in physiologic insulin replacement, this insulin regimen was still far from perfect.

The quantity of insulin impurities declined, and human insulin was introduced in 1982 [3]. The introduction of purified human insulin did not alter the treatment of diabetes as much as some had predicted, but this was the first example of recombinant DNA technology's having a major impact in the pharmacologic treatment of a disease.

Traditionally, insulin has been classified based on its pharmacokinetic characteristics as short, intermediate, and long acting. By understanding pharmacokinetics (the appearance of insulin into the blood) and pharmacodynamics (the time of insulin action on blood glucose levels), it is quite clear that the traditional classification strategy based on time actions is problematic. A better way to conceptualize insulin is by considering its physiologic role. "Basal insulin" is the insulin injected to suppress hepatic glucose production overnight and between meals. "Prandial insulin" (also know as "bolus" or mealtime insulin) is insulin injected to minimize glucose excursions after food ingestion. Classifying insulin in this way, it is clear why the older nomenclature is problematic. The standard insulins available today—regular NPH, Lente, and UltraLente—have prandial and basal components because of their peaks and long durations of action [4]. The implications of the pharmacodynamics of these insulins are important to appreciate. Regular insulin, for example, has a pharmacodynamic peak long after carbohydrate is consumed, but more importantly, the long "tail" of action of regular insulin necessitates a snack or meal to be consumed after the previous meal is digested. NPH insulin, on the other hand, has a peak that has traditionally been used for lunchtime insulin coverage, but its insulin action profile, especially when combined with regular insulin, causes the two preparations to overlap (also termed *insulin stacking*), aggravating the need for frequent snacks to avoid hypoglycemia.

Although the evolution of multiple daily injections and even CSII improved some of the problems with insulin stacking, the real seminal change in the treatment of type 1 diabetes occurred with the introduction of insulin analogues. The three prandial insulin analogues—insulin lispro, insulin aspart, and insulin glulisine—more selectively match prandial insulin requirements. The two basal insulins—insulin glargine and insulin detemir—are true basal insulin preparations in that, if they are dosed correctly, they do not require additional snacking. However, for someone using prandial and basal analogues, snacking usually requires an additional injection of prandial insulin.

The major advantage of the analogues compared with standard insulins is that less hypoglycemia has been consistently seen with all of the analogues. Although some of this is related to the fact that each analogue has a single function, in general, these insulins are also less variable in their absorption than their standard insulin comparators [5].

There is one other insulin category: "correction dose" or supplemental insulin [4]. This is insulin used to correct hyperglycemia regardless of the time in relation to the meal, although it is usually provided with the prandial insulin. There have been no studies comparing rapid-acting insulin analogues (lispro, aspart, glulisine) with regular insulin for correction dose insulin, although the analogues would be expected to correct the hyperglycemia more quickly and provide less risk of insulin stacking than regular insulin.

The goal of modern insulin replacement in type 1 diabetes is to provide physiologic insulin replacement to maintain near-normal glycemia. Current goals for this include maintaining A_{1c} below 7% with preprandial and postprandial glucose targets of 90 to 130 mg/dL and less than 180 mg/dL, respectively [6].

One strategy for achieving these goals is to provide insulin injections in a physiologic replacement manner. The two components to doing this are replacing basal insulin, usually with insulin glargine or detemir, and providing prandial insulin, usually with insulin lispro, insulin aspart, or insulin gllisine. In occasional situations, one may opt for use of a standard insulin instead of an analogue. This may include using regular insulin at lunch time for the school-aged child to provide greater insulinemia in the late afternoon for an afternoon snack; using regular insulin for meals low in carbohydrate and high in protein and fat, when prolonged action is desired; or adding a dose of bedtime NPH when significant early morning insulin resistance is present (the "dawn phenomenon").

Another strategy for physiologic insulin replacement to achieve the glycemic goals is CSII. Insulin pump therapy has been an option since 1980, and it has slowly gained in popularity. Basal and prandial insulin are provided by a subcutaneous pump that is connected to a catheter that is changed every 2 or 3 days. Not surprisingly, the insulin analogues have resulted in better glycemic control than regular insulin when used in pumps [7]. A meta-analysis comparing CSII with multiple injections in 12 randomized, controlled trials showed an improvement in A_{1c} with CSII [8]. The authors concluded that even this relatively small improvement (equivalent to an A_{1c} of 0.51%) will significantly reduce the risk of microvascular complications. The major risks of CSII include unexplained hyperglycemia or ketoacidosis and skin infection. Both of these can be minimized with strict attention to detail.

It needs to be emphasized that for any insulin regimen to be successful sufficient, SMBG is required. Specific recommendations are difficult because the ideal frequency of blood glucose testing has never been studied. At the least, before-meal and bedtime SMBG are recommended for type 1 diabetes, but between-meal tests are also suggested, particularly if it is unknown how much insulin should be injected for a food not usually consumed or to confirm that adequate insulin had been given for the treatment of premeal hyperglycemia.

The other critical factor required to ensure success is a basic understanding of prandial insulin dosing for a meals. Trial and error based on SMBG is attempted by some, but a more quantitative strategy often proves to be more successful. This is best accomplished with the assistance of a nutritionist, and several methods have been tested. One popular approach is the "carbohydrate counting" method. With this, carbohydrate is quantified, by estimating the number of grams of carbohydrates in a portion of food (*eg*, one piece of bread is 15 g of carbohydrate) or noting how much carbohydrate is present in a serving based on package information. Many patients learn this by actually weighing their food in their initial education. The "carbohydrate ratio" then refers to the number of grams of carbohydrate required for one unit of insulin. For example, a carbohydrate ratio of 1/15 refers to one unit of insulin injected for every 15 g of carbohydrate. The ratio can then be altered based on frequent SMBG results.

New Tools for the Management of Type 1 Diabetes

Although there have been tremendous advances with the development of insulin analogues, several new developments will likely further improve the management of type 1 diabetes.

The first new tool is the development of the analogue of the naturally occurring hormone amylin called pramlintide [9]. Native amylin is co-secreted with insulin and appears to improve glycemia by inhibiting the paradoxical increase in postprandial glucagon concentrations that occur in type 1 diabetes. It also appears to have a direct effect on modulating gastric emptying. Thus, the net effect is a reduction of postprandial hyperglycemia. Small but consistent weight loss has been observed with pramlintide.

There also is continued interest with the development of pulmonary inhaled insulin. This mode of delivery eliminates the needs for prandial injections, and it can be used to replace these in type 1 diabetes without deterioration in glycemic control [10].

One of the other goals of new technology in type 1 diabetes is the development of a real-time continuous glucose sensor. The first continuous glucose monitoring system was introduced in 2000 [11]. This device measures interstitial fluid glucose from a subcutaneous glucose sensor. Glucose readings can then be retrospectively reviewed after a download into a computer. The goal for the future is for real-time glucose sensor readings to replace capillary blood glucose testing, and at least one such implantable glucose sensor has been described [12]. Furthermore, the continuous sensor could then be in communication with an external or even an internal insulin pump, creating the potential of glucose-controlled insulin infusion [13].

Conclusions

The changes in the management of type 1 diabetes in a relatively short period of time have been dramatic. Less than 100 years ago, children diagnosed with diabetes rarely lived more than a few months, and even those who lived longer had a poor quality of life. The current tools allow most patients to live relatively normal lives, although teaching patients and providers how to use these tools has proven to be a challenge. The translation of the DCCT has not been as smooth as was originally predicted. However, the future for the treatment of type 1 diabetes appears even brighter, and the practical goal for patients and providers will be to extrapolate the research and use the new tools as efficiently as possible so that the morbidity and early mortality of this once fatal disease can be eliminated.

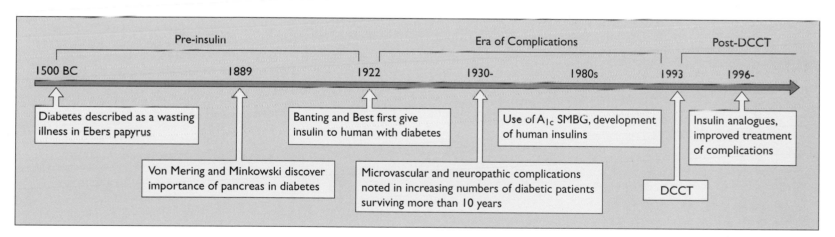

FIGURE 6-1. The three eras in the history of type 1 diabetes. The history of type 1 diabetes can be divided into three distinct eras. In the pre-insulin era, diabetes was usually fatal within 1 to 2 years of its development. In the era of complications, acute mortality was almost eliminated, but chronic complications were first noted. The Diabetes Control and Complications Trial (DCCT) [14] proved that intensive diabetes therapy with a multidisci-plinary team, frequent self-monitoring of blood glucose (SMBG), and an insulin regimen consisting of multiple injections or continuous subcutaneous insulin infusion could dramatically reduce the appearance and progression of microvascular and neuropathic complications. In the post-DCCT era, newer tools have been developed for the management of hyperglycemia and its complications.

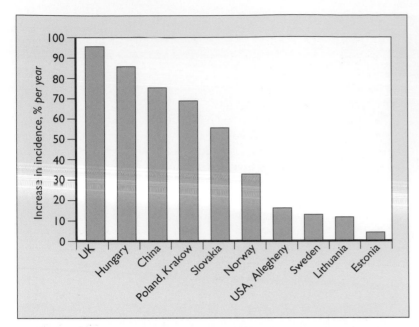

FIGURE 6-2. Relative increase in type 1 diabetes for children younger than age 14 years. There is a large international variation in type 1 diabetes incidence, and the increase is similar to what is being reported for type 2 diabetes. (*From* Devendra *et al.* [15]; with permission.)

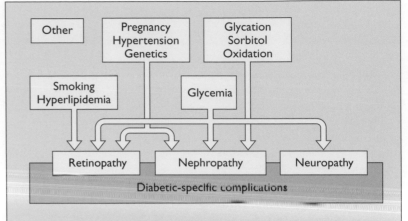

FIGURE 6-3. Pathogenesis of complications. The specific mechanism or mechanisms that cause the microvascular and neurologic complications of diabetes remain unidentified. Several obvious contributing factors, however, have been noted in epidemiologic studies, animal models, and interventional studies. Although no single mechanism is likely to explain the myriad complications, glycemia appears to be an underlying cause for all of them, as demonstrated in interventional studies such as the Diabetes Control and Complications Trial [14]. It is probable that different clinical stages of specific complications, for example, nonproliferative and proliferative retinopathy, have different causes. Genetic susceptibility to retinopathy and neuropathy is suggested by familial clustering [16]. Hypertension and pregnancy are well known to accelerate the development of retinopathy and neuropathy. In addition, interventional studies using the antihypertensive agents, and especially angiotensin-converting enzyme inhibitors, have demonstrated attenuation of the otherwise inexorable progression of neuropathy [17–19].

LONG-TERM COMPLICATIONS OF TYPE 1 DIABETES AND THE RISK OF DEVELOPING CLINICAL MANIFESTATIONS OF SPECIFIED COMPLICATIONS

Cataract: 25% to 30% lifetime risk with 3% to 5% requiring cataract extraction

Glaucoma (open angle): 10% risk after 30 years

Retinopathy: 90% develop some degree over lifetime; 40% to 50% require laser and 3% to 5% are blind after 30 years' duration

Adhesive capsulitis: frozen shoulder, prevalence 10%

Coronary artery disease: major cause of mortality

Gastroparesis: 1% to 5% develop symptoms—lifetime risk

Carpal tunnel syndrome: 30% with electrophysiologic evidence; 9% with symptoms (prevalence)

Nephropathy: 35% develop endstage renal disease over lifetime

Trigger finger, DuPuytren's contractures: 10% prevalence

Autonomic neuropathy (prevalence): bladder, 1% to 5% with dysfunction; impotence, 10% to 40%; diarrhea, 1%

Peripheral vascular disease

Peripheral neuropathy: 54% lifetime risk; 2% to 3% foot ulcers/y

FIGURE 6-4. Long-term complications of type 1 diabetes and the risks of developing clinical manifestations of specified complications. Data for some complications are sparse. The estimates provided reflect the era before the Diabetes Control and Complications Trial. Intensive therapy of type 1 diabetes is anticipated to reduce the lifelong development of retinopathy, nephropathy, and neuropathy by 50% to 80%. The overall effect of diabetic complications results in a substantial 15-reduction in the life span, predominantly owing to the development of nephropathy and cardiovascular disease.

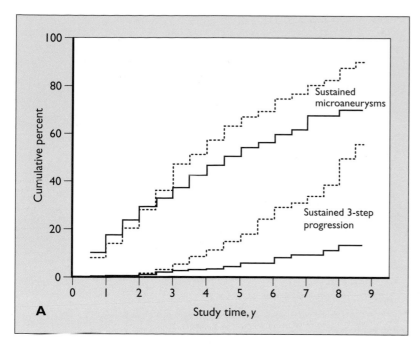

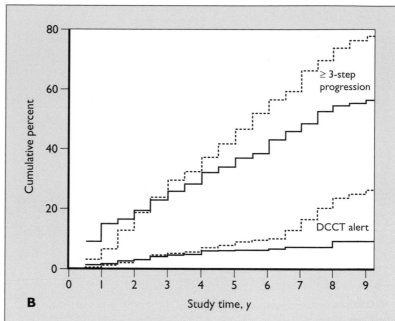

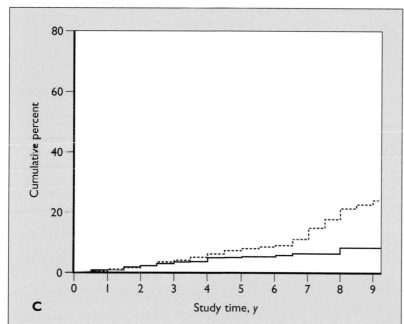

FIGURE 6-5. In the Diabetes Control and Complications Trial (DCCT), retinopathy measured in 18,000 sets of photographs with seven-field stereoscopic fundus photography performed every 6 months. The development and progression of retinopathy at virtually every stage were decreased by intensive therapy. **A,** The primary prevention cohort had 1 to 5 years' duration of diabetes and no retinopathy at baseline. In the primary cohort, the development of sustained microaneurysms, defined as one or more microaneurysm detected at two consecutive 6-month examinations, and of sustained three-step or greater progression according to the Early Treatment of Diabetic Retinopathy Study scale, were decreased by 27% and 76% (P < 0.002), respectively. **B,** The secondary intervention cohort was defined as having 1 to 15 years' duration of diabetes and at least one microaneurysm in either eye at baseline. In the secondary intervention cohort, intensive therapy was highly effective at reducing the progression to more severe levels of retinopathy, including a 34% reduction in three-step or greater progression (P < 0.02) (DCCT alert). **C,** The development of even more severe retinopathy, defined as neovascularization on the disc or elsewhere, was reduced by 48% (P < 0.02). (*Adapted from* DCCT Research Group [20].)

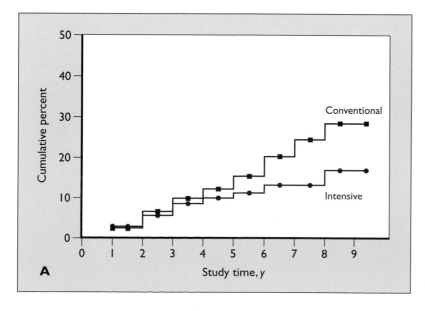

FIGURE 6-6. Nephropathy. Nephropathy in patients with type 1 diabetes progresses through several stages, usually over 15 to 25 years. The development of microalbuminuria, defined as between 20 and 40 mg of albumin excretion per 24 hours, is the first detectable stage, progressing to clinical albuminuria (> 300 mg albumin excretion per 24 h), usually over more than a decade. Albumin excretion progresses to the level consistent with nephrotic syndrome followed by decreasing glomerular filtration rate and culminating in endstage renal disease. Hypertension uniformly accompanies the development of nephropathy. Treatment of hypertension, especially with angiotensin-converting enzyme (ACE) inhibitors, and use of ACE inhibitors during the microalbuminuric stage, even in the absence of hypertenThe Diabetes Control and Complications Trial (DCCT) demonstrated a uniformly beneficial effect of intensive therapy on the development of microalbuminuria (40 mg/24 h). **A,** In patients with primary prevention, a 34% risk reduction (P = 0.04).

(Continued on next page)

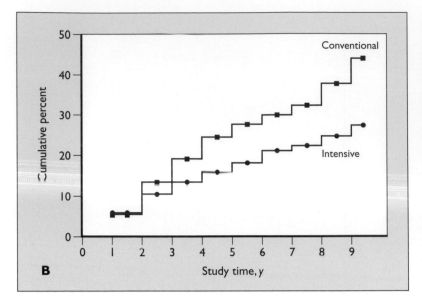

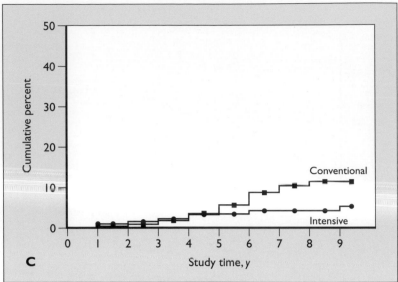

FIGURE 6-6. (Continued) **B,** In patients with secondary prevention, a 43% reduction (*P* < 0.001). **C,** A 56% reduction in the development of more

advanced stages of nephropathy, such as clinical albumiunuria (*P* < 0.01). (*Adapted from* DCCT Research Group [21].)

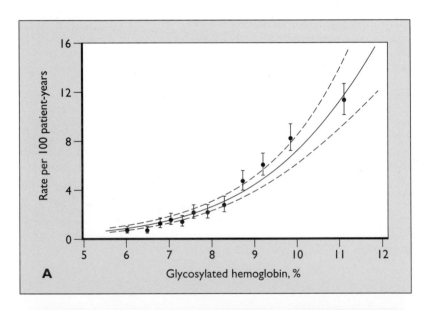

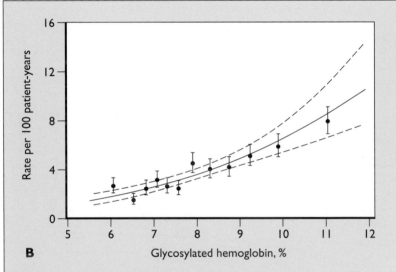

CALCULATED RELATIVE RISK REDUCTIONS ASSOCIATED WITH 10% LOWER MEAN HEMOGLOBIN A$_{1C}$

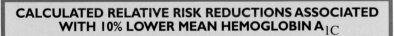

Complication	Risk Reduction, %*
Retinopathy	
Onset	35
Sustained progression	39
Severe nonproliferative	37
Nephropathy	
Microalbuminuria (40 mg/24 h or greater)	25
Microalbuminuria (100 mg/24 h or greater)	39
Albuminuria (300 mg/24 h or greater)	34
Neuropathy	30

*Calculated reduction in risk for every 10% lowering of HbA$_{1C}$.

FIGURE 6-7. Glycemia and complications. The Diabetes Control and Complications Trial (DCCT) performed primary analyses comparing the effects of intensive and conventional therapy on long-term complications. In addition, the DCCT performed secondary analyses examining the relationship of glycemia (mean of all hemoglobin A$_{1C}$ [HbA$_{1C}$] values for each subject during the trial) and the development or progression of complications, independent of treatment assignment. These analyses provide an assessment of the expected risk for different complications based on HbA$_{1C}$ achieved. **A,** Rate of retinopathy progression in combined treatment groups. **B,** Rate of development of microalbuminuria (> 40 mg/24 h) in combined treatment groups. In addition, the risk reduction for a specified decrease in HbA$_{1C}$ can be calculated (**C**). (*Adapted from* DCCT Research Group [22].)

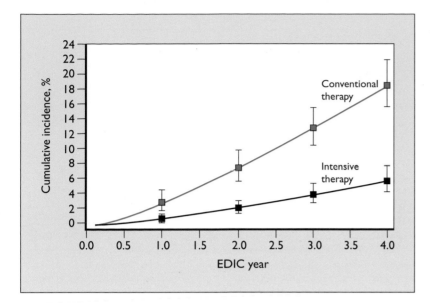

FIGURE 6-8. Cumulative incidence of further progression of retinopathy in the former conventional therapy and intensive therapy groups. EDIC— Epidemiology of Diabetes Interventions and Complications (*Adapted from* DCCT/EDIC Research Group [23]; with permission.)

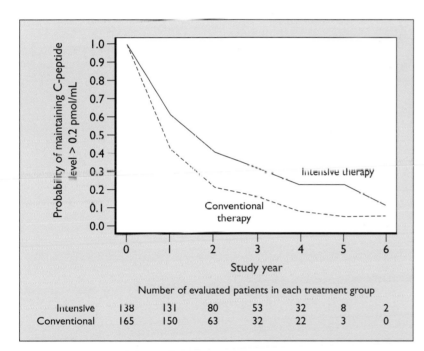

FIGURE 6-9. Preservation of endogenous insulin secretion with intensive therapy. In the Diabetes Control and Complications Trial (DCCT), patients with less than 5 years' duration of diabetes could have a modest degree of residual insulin secretion (C-peptide level 0.2–0.5 pmol/mL 90 min after a standardized meal). Of the patients, 303 fulfilled this criteria; 138 were randomly assigned to intensive therapy and 165 to conventional therapy. During the DCCT, repeated tests of endogenous insulin secretion were performed. As shown, intensive therapy was more likely to preserve endogenous secretion of insulin than was conventional therapy, extending the residual secretion by at least 2 years. Compared with patients having intensive treatments without residual insulin secretion, those having intensive treatment with residual insulin secretion maintained lower hemoglobin A_{1C} levels with less exogenous insulin and had less frequent severe hypoglycemia and a lower risk of retinopathy progression. Thus, preservation of endogenous insulin secretion is clinically important, facilitating the safe implementation of intensive therapy. Intensive therapy should be initiated as early as possible in the course of type I diabetes. (*Adapted from* DCCT Research Group [24].)

FIGURE 6-10. Classification of insulin preparations and insulin analogues. NPH—neutral protamine Hagedorn.

CLASSIFICATION OF INSULIN PREPARATIONS AND INSULIN ANALOGUES

Insulin	Onset	Peak	Effective Duration, h
Rapid	5–15 min	30–90 min	5
Insulin lispro			
Insulin aspart			
Insulin glulisine			
Short	30–60 min	2–3 h	5–8
Regular			
Intermediate			
NPH	2–4 h	4–10 h	10–16
Lente	2–4 h	4–12 h	12–18
Long			
UltraLente	6–10 h	10–16 h	18–24
Glargine	2–4 h	None	20–24
Detemir	2–4 h	4–12 h	14–20

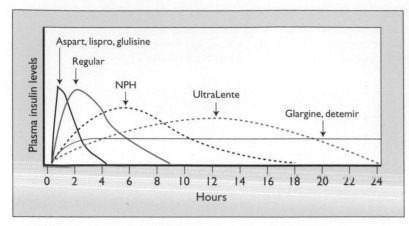

FIGURE 6-11. Idealized insulin appearance curves after subcutaneous injection. NPH—neutral protamine Hagedorn.

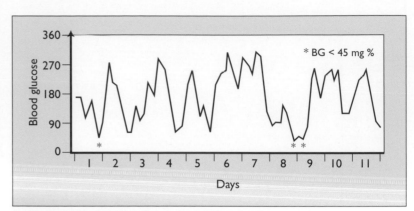

FIGURE 6-12. Blood glucose (BG) levels over 11 days in a patient with type 1 diabetes receiving twice-daily neutral protamine Hagedorn insulin. Note that using the NPH to contribute to prandial and basal need blood glucose results in extremely variable glycemia. In this study, blood glucose measurements were obtained eight times every day. (*From* Lauritzen *et al.* [25]; with permission.)

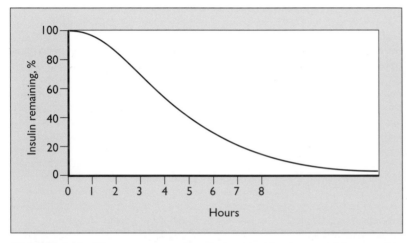

FIGURE 6-13. The appearance of insulin into the blood stream (pharmacokinetic) is different than the measurement of insulin action (pharmacodynamic). This figure is a representation of the timing of insulin action for insulin aspart from euglycemic clamp (0.2 U/kg into the abdomen). Using this graph assists patients in avoiding "insulin stacking." For example, 3 hours after administration of 10 U of insulin aspart, one can estimate that there is still 40% of the 10 U, or 4 U of insulin remaining. By way of comparison, the pharmacodynamics of regular insulin is approximately twice that of insulin aspart or insulin lispro. Currently used insulin pumps keep track of this "insulin on board" to avoid insulin stacking. (*Adapted from* Mudaliar *et al.* [26]; with permission.)

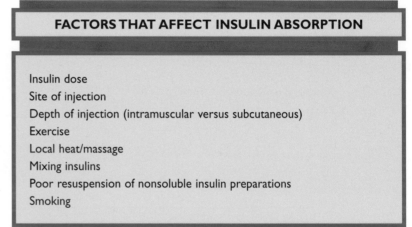

FACTORS THAT AFFECT INSULIN ABSORPTION

Insulin dose

Site of injection

Depth of injection (intramuscular versus subcutaneous)

Exercise

Local heat/massage

Mixing insulins

Poor resuspension of nonsoluble insulin preparations

Smoking

FIGURE 6-14. Factors that affect insulin absorption.

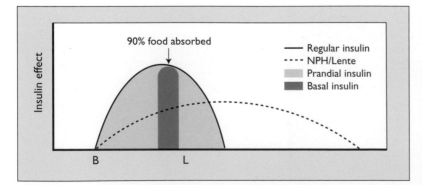

FIGURE 6-15. These idealized insulin action curves for morning neutral protamine Hagedorn (NPH) plus regular insulin demonstrate the problem with these conventional insulins, namely, that each insulin has a prandial and a basal component and neither provides physiologic insulin replacement. B—breakfast; L—lunch.

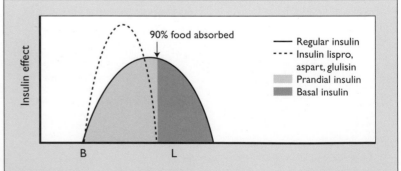

FIGURE 6-16. Idealized insulin action curves for morning regular insulin (*solid line*) and rapid-acting insulin analogues (lispro, aspart, glulisine; *dotted line*). The rapid-acting analogues only contribute to prandial insulin, but the regular insulin contributes to prandial and basal insulin. B—breakfast; L—lunch.

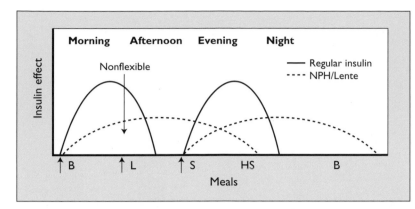

FIGURE 6-17. Idealized insulin curves for a twice-daily "split-mix" neutral protamine Hagedorn (NPH) and regular insulin regimen. Note that the morning regular insulin is a prandial insulin for breakfast and lunch. Furthermore, because of the mid-day regular and NPH stacking, there is little flexibility for the timing of lunch. The NPH insulin is a main insulin component for lunchtime calories. It is difficult, if not impossible, to control fasting hyperglycemia because of the waning dinnertime NPH. Even more problematic is the timing of insulin availability of both insulin components overnight, increasing the risk of nocturnal hypoglycemia. B—breakfast; HS—bedtime; L—lunch; S—supper.

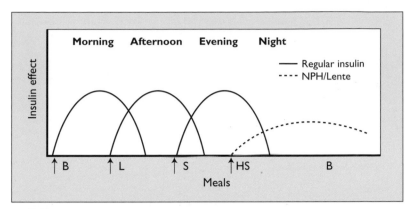

FIGURE 6-18. Idealized insulin curves for prandial regular insulin with bedtime neutral protamine Hagedorn (NPH) insulin. This regimen can be effective if the timing of insulin injections and meals are closely followed. The regular insulin acts as a basal and prandial insulin. B—breakfast; HS—bedtime; L— lunch; S—supper.

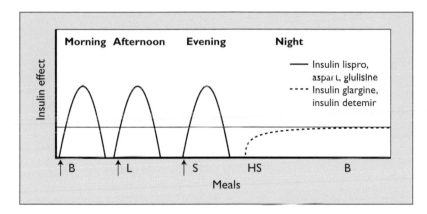

FIGURE 6-19. Idealized insulin curves for prandial insulin with a rapid-acting insulin analogue (lispro, aspart, glulisine) together with basal insulin as insulin glargine. Each insulin is responsible for the prandial or basal component. Some patients find that the insulin glargine does not last the entire 24 hours, and they give the insulin twice daily. Alternatively, giving half on arising and half on retiring adds flexibility in times of arising and retiring. To date, there have been no clinical trials that have tested these points. B—breakfast; HS—bedtime; L—lunch; S—supper.

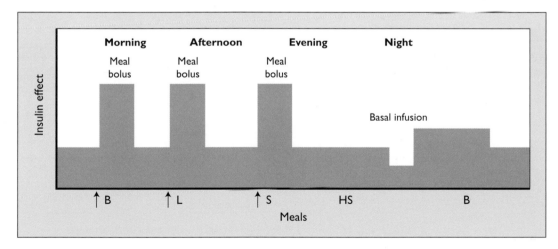

FIGURE 6-20. Idealized insulin curves for continuous subcutaneous insulin infusion with a rapid-acting insulin analogue (lispro, aspart, glulisine). Note that the basal insulin component can be altered based on changing basal insulin requirements. Typically, insulin rates need to be lowered between midnight and 4 AM (predawn sleep hypoglycemia phenomenon) and increased between 4 and 8 AM (dawn phenomenon). The basal rate the rest of the day is usually intermediate to the other two. Modern-day pumps can calculate prandial insulin dose by the patient's entering into the pump the blood glucose concentration and the anticipated amount of carbohydrate to be consumed. The pump calculates how much previous prandial insulin is still available and provides the patient with a final suggested dose, which the patient may activate or override. B—breakfast; HS—bedtime; L— lunch; S—supper.

UNEXPLAINED HYPERGLYCEMIA WITH CSII: FACTORS TO CONSIDER

Pump
1. Basal rate programmed incorrectly
2. Battery discharged
3. Pump malfunction
4. Cartridge does not advance properly

Cartridge
1. Improper placement
2. Insulin depleted
3. Insulin leakage

Infusion set
1. Insulin leakage
2. Dislodged catheter
3. Air in tubing
4. Insulin occlusion
5. Tear in tubing

Infusion site
1. Redness, irritation, inflammation
2. Placement in area of lipohypertrophy

Insulin
1. Expired or exposed to extreme temperature (hot or cold) and is not at normal potency

FIGURE 6-21. Possible causes for unexplained hyperglycemia with continuous subcutaneous insulin infusion (CSII).

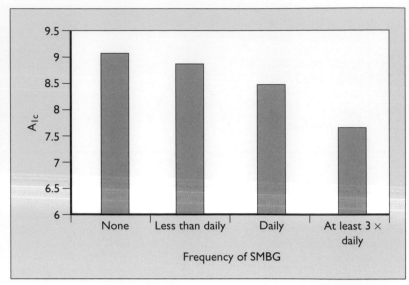

FIGURE 6-22. Estimated A_{1c} for a population (n = 1159) of patients with type 1 diabetes in a large health maintenance organization. As frequency of self-monitoring of blood glucose (SMBG) increased, A_{1c} improved. (*Adapted from* Karter *et al.* [27].)

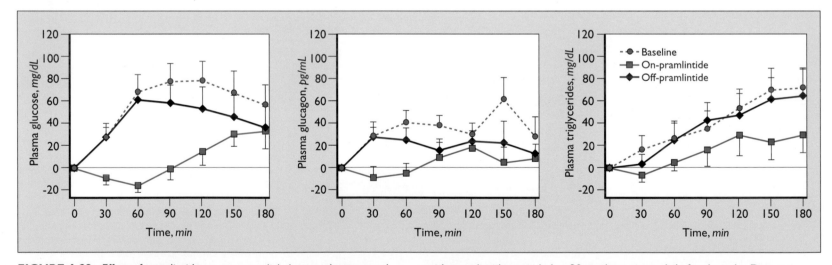

FIGURE 6-23. Effect of pramlintide on postprandial glucose, glucagon, and triglycerides in type 1 diabetes. In this study, there were 18 evaluable patients with pramlintide provided at 30 µg three times daily for 4 weeks. Data are presented as change from baseline. (*Adapted from* Levetan *et al.* [9].)

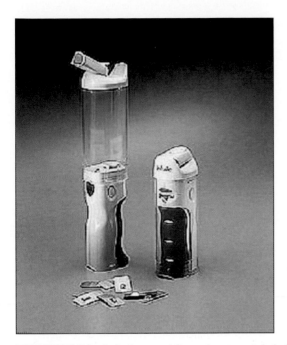

FIGURE 6-24. A device used for pulmonary inhaled insulin. With this device, the powdered insulin is placed in a canister, where it is vaporized before inhalation.

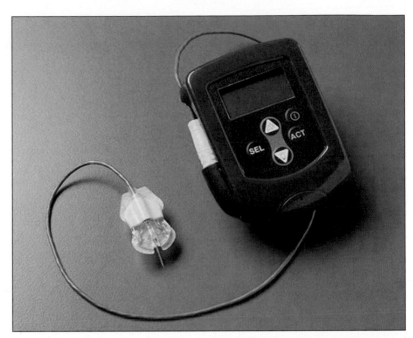

FIGURE 6-25. Continuous glucose monitoring system. The sensor is placed on the tip of the subcutaneous catheter, and the device measures the interstitial fluid glucose level.

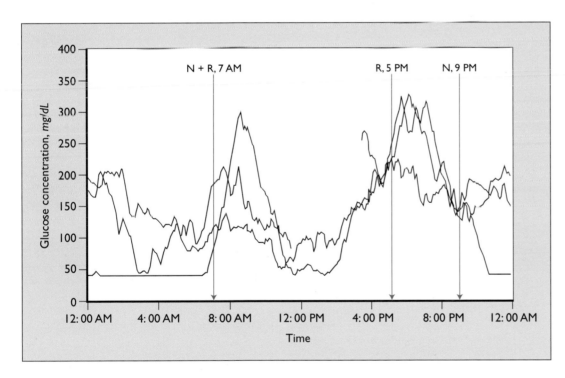

FIGURE 6-26. A continuous sensor tracing of a 16-year-old girl with A_{1c} of 7.3%. She receives neutral protamine Hagedorn (NPH) and regular insulin before breakfast, regular insulin before dinner, and NPH insulin at bedtime. Note the consistent decrease in blood glucose in the late morning, the increase in blood glucose by dinner, and the nocturnal hypoglycemia. This is a frequent pattern with this particular insulin regimen.

References

1. Skyler JS: Insulin pharmacology. *Med Clin North Am* 1988, 72:1337–1354.

2. Jackson RL: Historical background. In *The Physiologic Management of Diabetes in Children*. Edited by Jackson RL, Guthrie RA. New York: Medical Examination Publishing Company; 1986:6–16.

3. Skyler JS: Human insulin of recombinant DNA origin: clinical potential. *Diabetes Care* 1982, 5(suppl 2):181–186.

4. Dewitt DE, Hirsch IB: Outpatient insulin therapy in type 1 and type 2 diabetes mellitus. scientific review. *JAMA* 2003, 289:2254–2264.

5. Lepore M, Pampanelli S, Fanelli C, et al.: Pharmacokinetics and pharmacodynamics of subcutaneous injection of long-acting human insulin analog glargine, NPH insulin, and ultralente human insulin and continuous subcutaneous infusion of insulin lispro. *Diabetes* 2000, 49:2142–2148.

6. American Diabetes Association: Standards of medical care. *Diabetes Care* 2004, 27:(suppl 1):S15–S35.

7. Colquitt J, Royle P, Waugh N: Are analogue insulins better than soluble in continuous subcutaneous insulin infusion? Results of a meta-analysis. *Diabet Med* 2003, 20:863–866.

8. Pickup J, Mattock M, Kerry S: Glycaemic control with continuous subcutaneous insulin infusion compared with intensive insulin injections in patients with type 1 diabetes: meta-analysis of randomized controlled trials. *BMJ* 2002, 324:1–6.

9. Levetan C, Want LL, Weyer C, et al.: Impact of pramlintide on glucose fluctuations and postprandial glucose, glucagon, and triglyceride excursions among patients with type 1 diabetes intensively treated with insulin pumps. *Diabetes Care* 2003, 26:1–8.

10. Skyler JS, Cefalu WT, Kourides IA, et al.: Efficacy of inhaled human insulin in type 1 diabetes mellitus: a randomized proof-of-concept study. *Lancet* 2001, 3:331–335.

11. Skyler JS (ed): Advances in continuous glucose monitoring in diabetes mellitus. *Diabetes Technol Ther* 2000, 2:(suppl 1): S1–S97.

12. Garg SK, Schwartz S, Edelman SV: Improved glucose excursions using an implantable real-time continuous glucose sensor in adults with type 1 diabetes. *Diabetes Care* 2004, 27:634–738.

13. Renard R: Implantable closed-loop glucose-sensing and insulin delivery: the future for insulin pump therapy. *Curr Opin Pharmacol* 2002, 2:708–716.

14. Diabetes Control and Complications Trial Research Group: The effect of intensive treatment of diabetes on the development and progression of long-term complications in insulin-dependent diabetes mellitus. *N Engl J Med* 1993, 329:977–986.

15. Devendra D, Liu E, Eisenbarth GS: Type 1 diabetes: recent developments. *BMJ* 2004, 328:750–754.

16. Diabetes Control and Complications Trial Research Group: Clustering of long-term complications in families with diabetes in the Diabetes Control and Complications Trial. *Diabetes* 1997, 46:1829–1839.

17. Parving HH, Smidt UM, Friisberg B, et al.: A prospective study of glomerular filtration rate and arterial blood pressure in insulin-dependent diabetics with nephropathy. *Diabetologia* 1981, 20:457–461.

18. Klein BEK, Moss SE, Klein R: Effect of pregnancy on progression of diabetic retinopathy. *Diabetes Care* 1990, 13:34–40.

19. Lewis EJ: The effect of angiotensin-converting enzyme inhibition on diabetic retinopathy. *N Engl J Med* 1993, 329:1456–1462.

20. Diabetes Control and Complications Trial Research Group: Progression of retinopathy with intensive versus conventional treatment in the Diabetes Control and Complications Trial. *Ophthalmology* 1995, 102:647–661.

21. Effect of intensive therapy on the development and progression of diabetic nephropathy in the Diabetes Control and Complications Trial (DCCT) Research Group. *Kidney Int* 1995, 47:1703–1720.

22. Diabetes Control and Complications Trial Research Group: The absence of a glycemic threshold for the development of long-term complications. *Diabetes* 1996, 45:1289–1298.

23. DCCT/EDIC Research Group: Retinopathy and nephropathy in patients with type 1 diabetes four years after a trial of intensive therapy. *N Engl J Med* 2000, 342:381–389.

24. Diabetes Control and Complications Trial Research Group: Effect of intensive therapy on residual b cell function in patients with type 1 diabetes in the Diabetes Control and Complications Trial. *Ann Int Med* 1998, 128:517–523.

25. Lauritzen T, Faber OK, Binder C: Variation in 125I-insulin absorption and blood glucose concentration. *Diabetologia* 1979, 17:291–295.

26. Mudaliar S, Lindberg FA, Joyce M, et al.: Insulin aspart (B28 Asp-insulin): a fast-acting analog of human insulin. *Diabetes Care* 1999, 22:1501–1506.

27. Karter AJ, Ackerson LM, Darbinian JA, et al.: Self-monitoring of blood glucose levels and glycemic control: the Northern California Kaiser Permanente Diabetes registry. *Am J Med* 2001, 111:1–9.

7

CHILDHOOD DIABETES
Daina Dreimane and Francine Ratner Kaufman

Diabetes has a unique impact on children and their families. The daily lives of children and youths are affected by the rigors of the diabetes regimen and the need to frequently monitor blood glucose levels, give glucose-lowering agents, and balance the effects of activity and food. Despite this, pediatric patients must still strive to reach the normal developmental milestones of childhood and adolescence, succeed in school, and develop eventual autonomy. To accomplish these tasks, an organized system of diabetes care using a multidisciplinary team versed in pediatric issues must be in place to ensure optimal physical and emotional health for affected children as well as offer support and education for the family, caregivers, and school personnel. In this way, children with type 1 or type 2 diabetes can reach adulthood with as little adverse impact on their well being as possible.

One of the major risks of type 1 diabetes for children is the development of diabetic ketoacidosis (DKA). DKA remains a major source of morbidity and mortality in pediatric patients because of cerebral edema. The treatment of DKA in patients younger than age 20 years involves meticulous rehydration with electrolyte-containing solutions, intravenous insulin administration via a low-dose continuous infusion, avoidance of bolus bicarbonate therapy, and extremely close monitoring of neurologic status. There is increasing evidence that risk factors for cerebral edema include severe dehydration, as evidenced by a high initial blood urea nitrogen concentration and failure of the serum sodium level to increase with therapy. In addition to brain swelling, brain infarction can be a consequence of DKA and its treatment, and it may lead to persistent neurologic deficit. Because it remains unclear how to avoid the neurologic sequelae of DKA-associated cerebral edema, it becomes imperative to avoid DKA altogether. This can be done by giving patients and families detailed sick-day guidelines so that dehydration, acidosis, and severe hyperglycemia can be avoided during intercurrent illness or when diabetes management is less than appropriate.

Since the completion of the Diabetes Control and Complications Trial, the benefits of following a system of intensive diabetes management that allows for optimal glycemia has become increasingly apparent for infants, children, and youths with type 1 diabetes. The benefit not only appears to be immediate but also long term, and the management system should be instituted in prepubertal children as well as in postpubertal children. Despite modern insulin treatment, more than 50% of patients with childhood diabetes develop complications after 12 years of disease. Inadequate glycemic control, including during the first 5 years of diabetes, seems to accelerate time to occurrence of microvascular complications. A side effect of intensive diabetes therapy is an increased incidence of hypoglycemia. Frequent hypoglycemia in young children may result in neurocognitive deficits, and it needs to be addressed and treated promptly. Continuous subcutaneous insulin infusion using insulin pump therapy as well as basal–bolus insulin injection regimens with the insulin analogues glargine and lispro or aspart are increasingly and successfully used in order to achieve tight blood glucose control and minimize the frequency and severity of hypoglycemia. Systems of diabetes management that improve glycemic control must be well defined with age-specific targets and must be carefully taught to patients and families using algorithms that allow for flexibility of lifestyle. To assure that targets are being met, glucose levels can be assessed with modalities such as continuous glucose monitoring systems that allow for pattern identification. The diabetes regimen can then be altered to optimize glycemic outcome. However, these continuous glucose-monitoring systems, now limited to only intermittent 3-day use, cannot replace home glucose monitoring. An updated real-time continuous glucose monitoring system is currently in trial. Close multidisciplinary follow-up care with screening for diabetes complications and comorbidities is imperative. Findings such as limited joint mobility, which used to be the most common complication of diabetes in childhood, are decreasing in prevalence, most likely because of improved glycemic outcome. Finally, certain aspects of diabetes care must also be conveyed to school personnel and other caregivers if pediatric subjects are to benefit from an intensive management approach.

The psychological stress of diabetes, with the fear of immediate and long-term complications, must be addressed by providers of pediatric diabetes care. Children and adolescents with diabetes, as well as their family members, including parents and siblings, should be evaluated to assure that there is not a negative effect on family functioning. Quality of life must be an outcome measure. As such, evidence suggests that improved diabetes control, with all of its demands, actually improves quality of life. The developmental capabilities of children must be taken into account. As technology advances and more skills and knowledge are required for diabetes management, a limiting factor might be the cognitive and developmental capabilities of some children and their families. Criteria should be established before technologically difficult management tools, such as insulin pumps, are given to a specific patient and family.

As found in the adult population, type 2 diabetes in children and youths is attributable to the combination of insulin resistance coupled with relative β-cell failure. Although there are significantly higher levels of autoimmune markers present in children with type 1 diabetes mellitus, islet cell autoimmunity is present in up to 35% of pediatric subjects with type 2 diabetes. Genetic testing is now available to differentiate type 2 diabetes from maturity-onset diabetes of youth (MODY). There appears to be a host of potential genetic and environmental risk factors for insulin resistance and limited β-cell reserve, and perhaps the most significant risk factor is being overweight. Overweight in youth has reached epidemic proportions and has caused higher incidence of metabolic syndrome and nonalcoholic fatty liver disease in adolescents. Few studies have been done to determine the most effective treatment regimens for type 2 diabetes in youths and the role that physical activity and nutrition counseling play in improving glycemic outcome. Because fewer than 10% of youths with type 2 diabetes can be treated with diet and exercise alone, pharmacologic intervention is required for these patients to achieve glycemic targets. In most surveys, practitioners use metformin, insulin, another oral agent, or dual-agent therapy. Treatment guidelines have been developed to enable target hemoglobin A_{1c} levels to be met and maintained. A multicenter study sponsored by the National Institutes of Health is currently under way to evaluate efficacy and safety of three available treatment modalities and to assess the natural course and pathophysiology of type 2 diabetes in children. There is increased incidence of dyslipidemias and hypertension in adolescents with type 2 diabetes compared with type 1 diabetes, frequently present at the time of diagnosis. Prompt recognition and treatment of these comorbidities is crucial.

Although diabetes management remains demanding, children and families can succeed in reaching glycemic targets and in achieving phys-ical and psychological well being. A multidisciplinary team, including the primary care provider, that is able to appropriately assess and follow a patient can play a major role in preparing children and youths for as complication free a future as is possible.

Diabetic Ketoacidosis in the Pediatric Population with Type 1 Diabetes

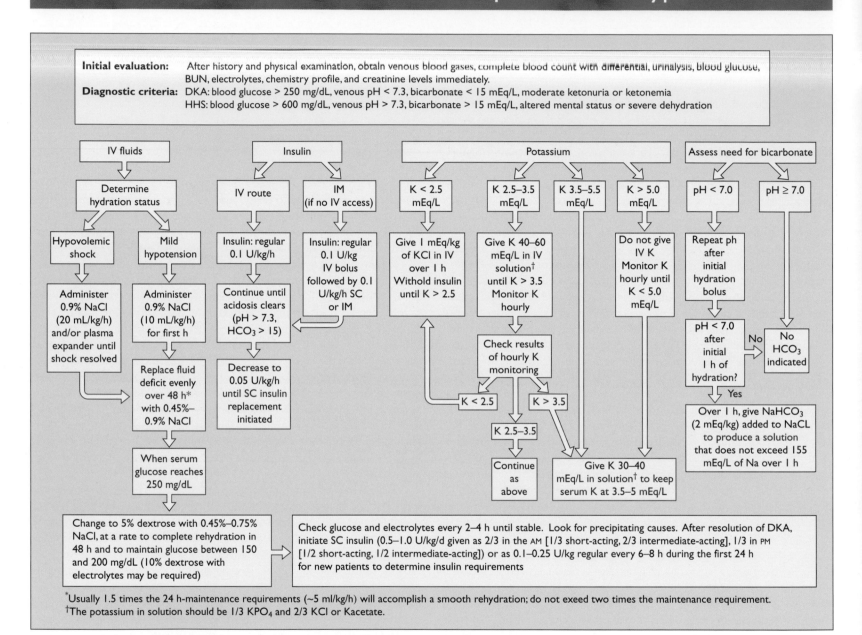

FIGURE 7-1. Management of pediatric patients (younger than age 20 years) with diabetic ketoacidosis (DKA). The protocol for the management of these patients begins with intravenous (IV) fluid therapy to restore circulation. The rate of fluid administration is dependent on the presence or absence of hypovolemic shock. After fluid resuscitation, IV fluid administration is given at a rate that will complete rehydration in 48 hours. The sodium concentration of the fluid replace-ment solution is between 0.45% and 0.75%. Insulin infusion is begun after fluid resuscitation at a rate of 0.1 U/kg/h. Insulin can be administered intramuscularly (IM) if IV access cannot be secured. Potassium is added to the replacement fluids at a variable infusion rate depending on the serum potassium level. Bicarbonate is given only for severe acidosis, pH below 7.0, and it is administered over 1 hour, not as IV bolus therapy. Glucose is added to the IV solution as the serum glucose level decreases. The key to successful management is close monitoring of glucose and electrolyte levels and appropriate level of care to detect and treat early neurologic compromise [1]. BUN—blood urea nitrogen; HHS—hyperglycemic hyperosmolar state; SC—subcutaneous.

CONTRAINDICATIONS TO AMBULATORY INSULIN INITIATION

Very young age (under 2 years)

Ketoacidosis (venous pH 7.3 or less and/or bicarbonate 15 mmol/L or less)

Dehydration (moderate of severe)

Profound grief reaction in family

Geographic isolation

No telephone in home

Language or other communication difficulties

Significant psychologic or psychiatric problems within the family

FIGURE 7-2. Contraindications to ambulatory initiation of insulin therapy. During the past decade, there has been a fundamental shift from inpatient management to outpatient management of children with newly diagnosed type 1 diabetes mellitus. A systematic review and other studies have concluded that in a number of patients, there are no disadvantages of ambulatory management compared with inpatient management of children and adolescents with newly diagnosed type 1 diabetes. Older children and adolescents who are not dehydrated and acidotic may be successfully managed out of hospital if diabetes support teams are available [2,3].

MULTIVARIATE ANALYSIS OF RISK FACTORS FOR CEREBRAL EDEMA*

Variable†	Relative Risk (95% CI)	P Value
Male gender	0.6 (0.3–1.4)	0.27
Age (per 1-y increase)	0.9 (0.6–1.3)	0.53
Initial serum sodium concentration (per increase of 5.8 mmol/L)	0.7 (0.5–1.02)	0.06
Initial serum glucose concentration (per increase of 244 mg/dL)	1.4 (0.5–3.9)	0.58
Initial serum urea nitrogen concentration (per increase of 9 mg/dL)	1.8 (1.2–2.7)	0.008
Initial serum bicarbonate concentration (per increase of 3.6 mmol/L)	1.2 (0.5–2.6)	0.73
Initial partial pressure of arterial carbon dioxide (per decrease of 7.8 mm Hg)	2.7 (1.4–5.1)	0.002
Rate of increase in serum sodium concentration during therapy (per increase of 5.8 mmol/dL/h)	0.6 (0.4–0.9)	0.01
Rate of decrease in serum glucose concentration during therapy (per decrease of 190 mg/dL/h)	0.8 (0.5–1.4)	0.41
Rate of increase in serum bicarbonate concentration during therapy (per increase of 3 mmol/L/h)	0.8 (0.5–1.1)	0.15
Administration of insulin bolus	0.8 (0.3–2.2)	0.62
Treatment with bicarbonate	4.2 (1.5–12.1)	0.008
Rate of infusion of intravenous fluid (per increase of 5 mL/kg of body weight/h)	1.1 (0.4–3.0)	0.91
Rate of infusion of sodium (per increase of 0.6 mmol/kg/h)	1.2 (0.6–2.7)	0.59
Rate of infusion of insulin (per increase of 0.04 U/kg/h)	1.2 (0.8–1.8)	0.30

*The cerebral edema group was compared with the matched control group by means of conditional logistic regression.
†The increase or decrease used in the analysis of each continuous variable (except age) represents a change of 1 SD in the variable in the randomly selected control children with diabetic ketoacidosis.

FIGURE 7-3. Multivariate analysis of risk factors for cerebral edema. In a multi-center study, 61 children who developed symptomatic cerebral edema associated with diabetic ketoacidosis (DKA) were compared with 181 randomly selected children with DKA and 174 children with DKA matched according to age, new-onset versus known case, initial pH, and initial serum glucose concentration [4]. Multivariate statistical methods showed that children with DKA-related cerebral edema had lower initial PCo_2 values and higher serum urea nitrogen concentrations than the control groups. A lesser increase in serum sodium concentration during treatment was seen in those with cerebral edema, although it is unclear whether this was caused by therapy itself or a physiologic response to cerebral injury. The administration of bicarbonate bolus was also associated with the development of cerebral edema, suggesting that bicarbonate therapy, for the most part, is contraindicated in children with DKA. (*Adapted from* Glaser et al. [4].)

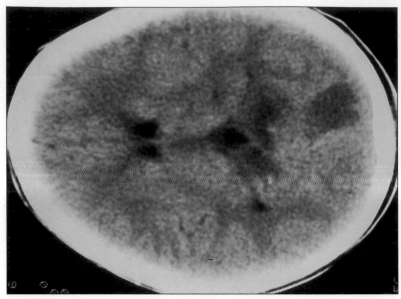

FIGURE 7-4. Magnetic resonance imaging scan of cerebral edema in a 5-year-old boy hospitalized with progressive polyuria and polydipsia. He was found to have a serum glucose level of 1288 mg/dL, sodium level of 136 mEq/L, potassium level of 4.0 mEq/L, total CO_2 level of 14 mEq/L, chloride level of 95 mEq/L, and large ketones. He was started on insulin and fluid therapy and improved over the first 17 hours, at which time he had a generalized convulsion and developed dilated pupils. A computed tomography (CT) scan done 6 hours after the neurologic crisis showed infarction in the distribution of the left posterior cerebral artery, including the occipital pole and the undersurface of the temporal lobe. The geniculate nuclei and the posterior part of the left thalamus were also infarcted. At the time of this CT scan, there was no evidence of cerebral edema. After 2 months, the patient was discharged with a moderate left hemiplegia and was able to do age-appropriate schoolwork. Although it is likely that brain edema may have been present initially and before the time of the CT scan, patients with persistent neurologic deficit may also suffer brain infarction during diabetic ketoacidosis–related cerebral edema. The pathophysiology of infarction remains unclear but may be caused by a combination of factors, including compression of vessels; systemic hypotension and intracranial hypertension; and thrombosis from dehydration, hemoconcentration, and hyperviscosity [5].

Warning signs

Call the health team if:

Vomiting (more than 2 times or longer than 4 h)

Elevated BG level (2 or more readings outside of the target range or > 250 mg/dL)

Presence of blood or large urinary ketones

Weakness, dry mouth, or signs of dehydration, excessive thirst

Heavy breathing, shortness of breath

Abdominal pain, diarrhea

Evidence of bacterial infection

Altered level of consciousness or change in mental status

Never stop insulin

Phone numbers: Pediatrician _____

Diabetes team _____

Emergency # _____

Log sheet

	1st h	2nd h	3rd h	4th h	5th h	6th h	7th h
Blood sugar							
Ketone level							
Temperature							
Fluid input							
Output urine							
Insulin dose							

Principles for high blood sugar

Give extra rapid-acting (or short-acting) insulin every 2 hours

Add extra insulin for each 50 mg/dL above target (200 mg/dL)

For children < 5 years, 0.25 U for each 50 mg/dL

For children ages 5–11 years, 0.5–1.0 U for each 50 mg/dL

For children ages 12–18 years, 1–2 U for each 50 mg/dL

Nonglucose–containing fluids should be given until the blood glucose level reaches 250 mg/dL

Fluids containing sodium and potassium should be used if there is excessive fluid loss

Replacement of fluids is more important than food

Principles for low blood sugar

Glucose-containing fluids should be given in small quantities

Insulin should be decreased by 20%–50%

If persistent hypoglycemia occurs and patients are not able to retain glucose-containing solutions, consider a minidose of glucagon (for children ≤ 2 years, 20 μg or 2 "units" on the insulin syringe; for children > 2 years, 150 μg or 15 "units")

FIGURE 7-5. Sick-day management guidelines for the prevention of diabetic ketoacidosis (DKA). Early signs of DKA need to be treated aggressively, and the results of treatment must be carefully monitored to avoid the development of moderate to severe dehydration, hyperglycemia, and acidosis. Precursors to DKA in children and youths with established diabetes include intercurrent illness, infection, incorrect insulin dosage for the glycemic level, inappropriate insulin administration, omission of insulin, psychologic trauma, and surgery [6]. Patients, parents, babysitters, school personnel, and day care workers need to understand the early signs of DKA and how to access the health care team so that DKA can be reversed. A sick-day management guideline can be useful in promoting the early institution of monitoring and treatment to avoid the need for hospitalization and emergency room visits [7,8]. BG—blood glucose.

SYMPTOMS AND TREATMENT OF HYPOGLYCEMIA IN CHILDREN WITH DIABETES

Severity	Clinical Features	Treatment
Mild	Mild adrenergic and cholinergic symptoms: hunger, shakiness, tremor, nervousness, anxiety, sweatiness, pallor, palpitations, tachycardia. Mild neuroglycopenia: decreased attention and cognitive performance	Juice, soda, hard candy, snacks; for very mild case, bring forward the scheduled meal if within 15–30 minutes of planned mealtime
Moderate	Moderate neuroglycopenia and autonomic symptoms: headache, abdominal pain, behavior changes, aggressiveness, impaired or double vision, confusion, drowsiness, weakness, impaired speech, tachycardia, dilated pupils, pallor, sweatiness	10–20 g carbohydrate (juice, soda) followed by a complex carbohydrate snack
Severe	Severe neuroglycopenia: disorientation, loss of consciousness, focal or generalized seizures	Outside hospital: glucagons IM injection: < 8 y or < 25 g: 0.5 mg > 8 y or > 25 kg: 1.0 mg Repeat in 10 min if no response; continue with oral carbohydrates and monitor blood glucose closely In hospital: 10% dextrose IV bolus 2–5 mL/kg, followed by 5%–10% dextrose infusion as needed

FIGURE 7-6. Symptoms and treatment of hypoglycemia in children with diabetes. Patients should be taught to recognize symptoms of hypoglycemia and know how to treat it. Frequent and severe hypoglycemia (seizures) cause neurocognitive impairment in children who are diagnosed with diabetes younger than age 5 years [9]. Autonomic responses mediated by counterregulatory hormones usually precede neuroglycopenia. Recurrent, short-term hypoglycemia impairs hormonal counterregulation and symptom awareness. Initially, the capacity to release glucagon during hypoglycemia is lost and, as the duration of disease increases, the response of the other major counterregulatory hormone epinephrine may also decrease. Because children exhibit both greater epinephrine responses and at higher blood glucose levels than adults, the impairment of epinephrine release decreases the ability of child to identify hypoglycemia, thus delaying treatment. Avoidance of hypoglycemia restores awareness by increasing β-adrenergic sensitivity [10]. IM—intramuscular; IV—intravenous. (*Adapted from* Clinical Practice Guidelines [2].)

Importance of Intensive Management

DIABETES CONTROL AND COMPLICATIONS TRIAL RESULTS

	Adults		Adolescents	
	Intensive	**Conventional**	**Intensive**	**Conventional**
Glycemia				
Mean BG mg/dL	155 ± 30	231 ± 55	171 ± 31	260 ± 52
HbA$_{1C}$	7.12 ± 0.03	9.02 ± 0.05	8.06 ± 0.03	9.76 ± 0.12
Risk reduction				
Retinopathy	63%		61%	
Microalbuminuria	54%		35%	
Hypoglycemia				
Episodes/100 patient-years	61.2	18.7	85.7	29.6
Relative risk	3.3		2.8	

FIGURE 7-7. Diabetes Control and Complications Trial (DCCT) results of comparison of adults versus adolescents. The DCCT enrolled adolescent patients; 14% were between the ages of 13 and 17 years at the time of entry into the study [11,12]. Patients younger than age 13 years were not enrolled in the study. Compared with adult subjects, the adolescents had higher blood glucose (BG) and hemoglobin A$_{1c}$ (HbA$_{1c}$) levels in the intensive and the conventional groups. Nevertheless, there was still a difference in the mean BG and HbA$_{1c}$ level between the two groups of adolescents. For adolescents, there was a 1.7% + 0.2% decrease in HbA$_{1c}$ in the intensive group compared with the conventional group. The reduction in the development of complications seen in adolescents because of achieving improved glycemia was similar to the reduction appreciated in adults. This reduction was coupled with a greater absolute rate of severe hypoglycemia in adolescents compared with adults.

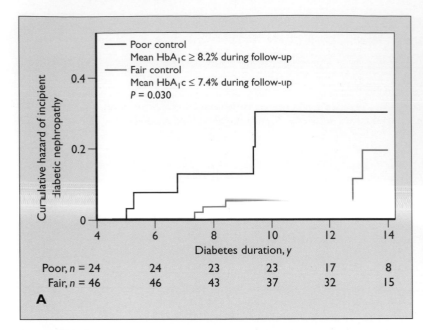

A

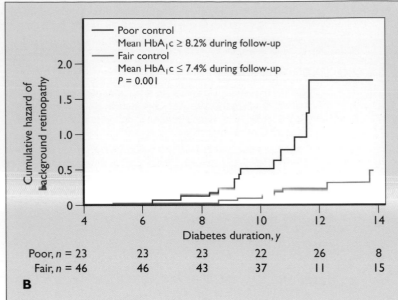

B

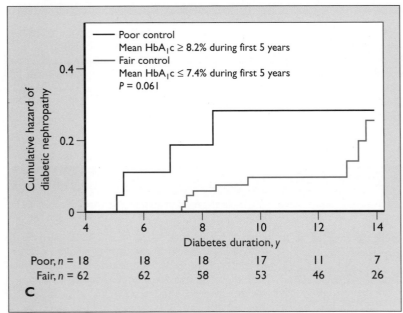

C

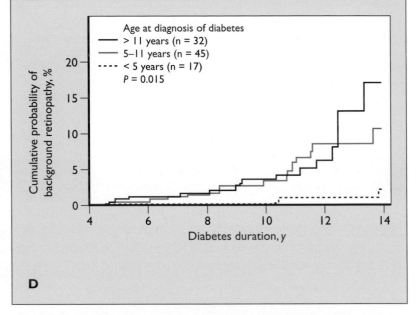

D

FIGURE 7-8. Effect of early glycemic control, age at onset and development of microvascular complications in childhood-onset type 1 diabetes. It has been previously shown that intensive insulin treatment and improved glycemic control delay the onset and slow the progression of diabetes complications. Controversy exists as to the effect of duration of diabetes before puberty versus the effect of diabetes duration in the postpubertal period. Although it is clear that the hormonal changes of puberty, particularly augmentation of the growth hormone–insulin-like growth factor axis, may have a permissive role in the damaging effect of diabetes on the microvasculature, the contribution of prepubertal diabetes duration may be minimal. In a recent study, 94 children diagnosed at age 0 to 14 years in northern Sweden were identified using the Swedish Childhood Diabetes registry. During the follow-up period of 12 ± 4

years, 18% of patients developed microalbuminuria (MA), 48% of patients developed retinopathy (RP), and 52% had either or both complications. As shown in **A** and **B**, poor control (hemoglobin A_{1c} [HbA_{1c}] > 8.2%) significantly increased cumulative hazard rates for MA and RP compared with fair control (HbA_{1c} < 7.4%). More importantly, poor glycemic control early in course (first 5 years) was an important predictor of later development of MA and RP (**C**). This study found that diagnosis of type 1 diabetes before the age of 5 years significantly prolonged time to occurrence of RP, compared with the age groups 5 to 11 and older than 11 years, indicating a protective effect of prepubertal duration (**D**). However, blood glucose control either early or late in course is a powerful predictor for developing complications; therefore, glucose levels should be optimized in all age groups [14].

GLYCEMIC AND HbA₁c TARGETS FOR PEDIATRIC PATIENTS WITH TYPE I DIABETES

	Age of Patient			
Blood glucose	0–2 y	3–6 y	7–12 y	13 y
Premeal, *mg/dL*	100–180	70–150	70–150	70–150
2–3 h postprandial, *mg/dL*	< 200	< 200	< 200	< 180
Before bed, *mg/dL*	100–200	100–180	100–180	80–150
2–4 am, *mg/dL*	> 100	> 100	> 100	> 80
HbA₁c, %	< 9.0	< 8.5	< 8.5	< 7.5

FIGURE 7-9. Glycemic and hemoglobin A_{1c} (HbA$_{1c}$) targets for pediatric type I subjects by age. The management goal for infants, children, and adolescents with type I diabetes is to have blood glucose and HbA$_{1c}$ levels fall within an age-specific target range that takes into account the developmental, cognitive, and communicative abilities and resources of the patient and family [15]. Because it appears that young children are more susceptible to severe hypoglycemia, the target ranges for blood glucose and HbA$_{1c}$ levels are generally higher. However, as children age, the primary concern shifts from avoidance of excessive hypoglycemia to avoidance of hyperglycemia as a means to decrease long-term diabetes complications.

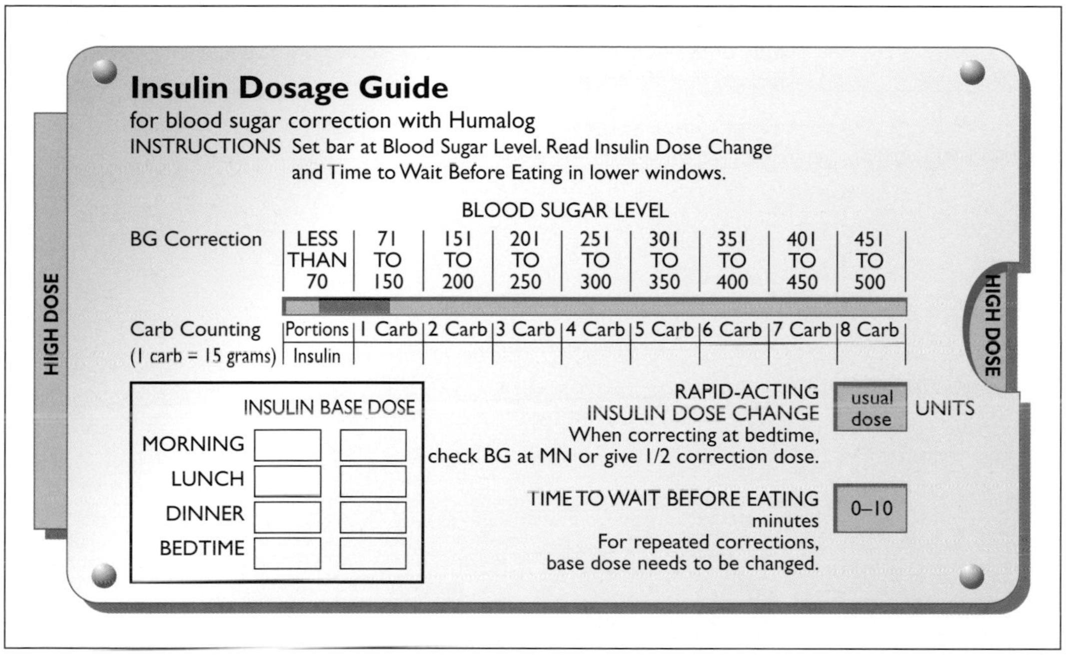

Insulin Dosage Guide
for blood sugar correction with Humalog
INSTRUCTIONS Set bar at Blood Sugar Level. Read Insulin Dose Change and Time to Wait Before Eating in lower windows.

BLOOD SUGAR LEVEL

BG Correction	LESS THAN 70	71 TO 150	151 TO 200	201 TO 250	251 TO 300	301 TO 350	351 TO 400	401 TO 450	451 TO 500

Carb Counting (1 carb = 15 grams)	Portions	1 Carb	2 Carb	3 Carb	4 Carb	5 Carb	6 Carb	7 Carb	8 Carb
	Insulin								

INSULIN BASE DOSE
MORNING
LUNCH
DINNER
BEDTIME

RAPID-ACTING INSULIN DOSE CHANGE
usual dose UNITS
When correcting at bedtime, check BG at MN or give 1/2 correction dose.

TIME TO WAIT BEFORE EATING
0–10
minutes
For repeated corrections, base dose needs to be changed.

HIGH DOSE

FIGURE 7-10. Insulin dosage guide for correction of blood glucose (BG) levels out of the target range. By treating BG levels that are outside of a predetermined age-specific target range with supplemental oral glucose or extra insulin, children and adolescents can minimize episodes of both hypoglycemia and hyperglycemia. However, it is challenging to teach insulin dosage adjustment algorithms designed to normalize elevated BG levels and to compensate for alterations in carbohydrate intake. Even with instruction, many families feel uneasy adjusting insulin dosages on their own because of the complexities of these adjustment algorithms, and they often persist in believing that they must have contact with a health care provider to ensure accuracy. A handheld plastic Insulin Dosage Guide for both rapid- or short-acting insulin in a variety of regimens, including insulin pump therapy, was designed to enable patients to correct abnormal BG levels in a standard, consistent fashion and to determine how much insulin to take if they are practicing carbohydrate counting [16]. In 83 patients with issues concerning glycemic control, mean age 11.4 ± 4.3 years and with a mean diabetes duration of 4.4 ± 3.1 years, there was a reduction in hemoglobin A_{1c} (HbA$_{1c}$) levels from 9.5% ± 2.0% at entry to 8.4% + 1.5% at 3 months ($P = 0.0002$). Improvement was sustained for 12 months ($P = 0.0001$) while using the Insulin Dosage Guide. Inexpensive, portable, and easy-to-use algorithms for insulin dosage adjustment may improve glycemic control in children and youths and allow for flexibility in lifestyle.

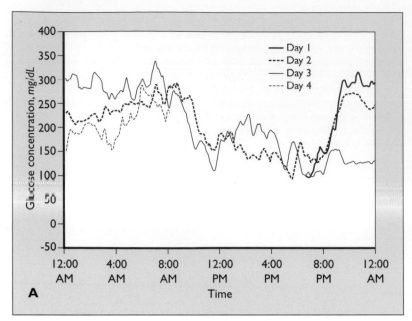

A

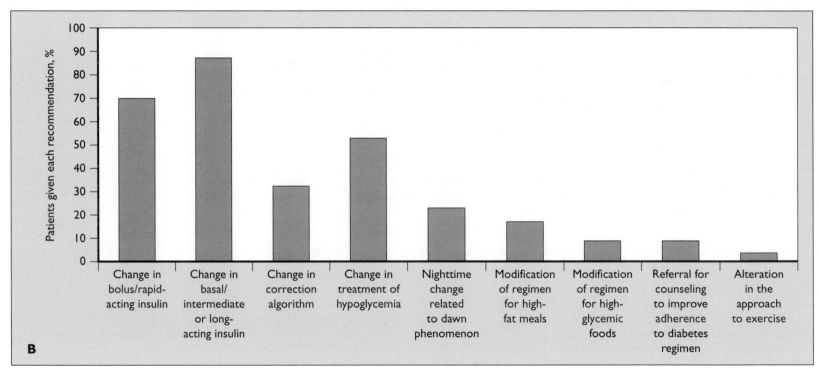

FIGURE 7-11. Continuous glucose monitoring of children with type 1 diabetes. Continuous subcutaneous glucose monitoring with the MiniMed system (CGMS) (Medtronic MiniMed, Northridge, CA) can be used in pediatric subjects to detect unrecognized nocturnal hypoglycemia and other patterns of abnormal glucose control so that alterations of the diabetes regimen can be made to regulate hemoglobin A_{1c} (HbA_{1c}) [17]. **A,** CGMS tracing from a 4-year-old child with a high post-breakfast pattern [18]. **B,** A recent study involving 47 pediatric patients using CGMS with diabetes management problems showed a variety of abnormal glucose patterns [19]. After these patterns were detected, a mean of 3.3 specific alterations of the diabetes regimen were made. This resulted in an overall significant change in HbA_{1c} from 3 months before using CGMS to 6 months after CGMS was begun (analysis of variance, 0.04). Post hoc analysis showed a significant change in HbA_{1c} from 8.6% ± 1.5% at baseline to 8.4% ± 1.3% at 3 months (paired Student's t test, 0.03). A new continuous glucose monitoring system (Paradigm 522; Medtronic MiniMed, Northridge, CA) consisting of a glucose sensor, transmitter, and insulin pump receiver can provide real-time sensor glucose values that correlate well with blood glucose readings and allow patients to deliver insulin more accurately (Halvorson and Kaufman, unpublished data). Using continuous glucose monitoring systems will likely help improve glycemic control in pediatric subjects by allowing for pattern detection and alteration of the diabetes regimen. (Panel A *adapted from* Kaufman *et al.* [18]; panel B *adapted from* Kaufman *et al.* [19].)

B

Diabetes care plan for _____ (name of student) _____ **School** _____ **Effective dates:** _____

To be completed by parents/health care team and reviewed with necessary school staff. Copies should be kept in student's classrooms and school records.

Date of birth: _____ **Grade** _____ **Homeroom teacher:** _____

Contact information _____

Parent/guardian #1: _____ Address: _____

   Telephone-Home: _____ Work: _____ Cell phone: _____

Parent/guardian #2: _____ Address: _____

   Telephone-Home: _____ Work: _____ Cell phone: _____

Student's doctor/health care provider: _____ Telephone: _____

   Nurse educator: _____ Telephone: _____

Other emergency contact: _____ Relationship: _____

   Telephone-Home: _____ Work: _____ Cell phone: _____

Notify parent/guardian in the following situations: _____

Blood glucose monitoring

Target range for blood glucose: _____ mg/dL to _____ mg/dL   Type of blood glucose meter student uses: _____

Usual times to test blood glucose: _____

Times to do extra tests (check all that apply):   _____ Before exercise   _____ When student exhibits symptoms of hyperglycemia

   _____ After exercise   _____ When student exhibits symptoms of hypoglycemia

   _____ Other (explain): _____

Can student perform own blood glucose tests?   Yes   No   Exceptions: _____

School personnel trained to monitor blood glucose level and dates of training: _____

Insulin

Times, types, and dosages of insulin injections to be given during school:

Time   **Type(s)**   **Dosage**

_____   _____   _____

_____   _____   _____

_____   _____   _____

School personnel trained to assist with insulin injection and dates of training: _____

_____

Can student give own injections?   Yes   No

Can student determine correct amount of insulin?   Yes   No

Can student draw correct dose of insulin?   Yes   No

For students with insulin pumps

Type of pump: _____

Insulin/carbohydrate ratio: _____

Correction factor: _____

Is student competent regarding pump?   Yes   No

Can student effectively troubleshoot problems (eg, ketosis, pump malfunction)?   Yes   No

Comments: _____

_____

_____

Meals and snacks eaten at school (The carbohydrate content of the food is important in maintaining a stable blood glucose level.)

    Time   **Food content/amount**

Breakfast _____ _____

AM snack _____ _____

Lunch _____ _____

PM snack _____ _____

Dinner _____ _____

Snack before exercise?

   Yes   No

Snack after exercise?

   Yes   No

Other times to give snacks and content/amount: _____

_____

A source of glucose, such as _____ should be readily available at all times.

Preferred snack foods: _____

Foods to avoid, if any: _____

Instructions for when food is provided to the class, eg, as part of a class party or food sampling _____

Hypoglycemia (low blood sugar)

Usual symptoms of hypoglycemia: _____

_____

Treatment of hypoglycemia: _____

_____

School personnel trained to administer glucagon and dates of training: _____

_____

Glucagon should be given if the student is unconscious, having a seizure (convulsion), or unable to swallow. If required, glucagon should be administered promptly and then 911 (or other emergency assistance) and parents should be called.

Hyperglycemia (high blood sugar)

Usual symptoms of hyperglycemia: _____

_____

Treatment of hyperglycemia: _____

_____

Circumstances when urine ketones should be tested:

_____

_____

Treatment for ketones: _____

_____

Exercise and sports

A snack such as _____ should be readily available at the site of exercise or sports.

Restrictions on activity, if any: _____

Student should not exercise if blood glucose is below _____ mg/dL.

Supplies and personnel

Location of supplies: Blood glucose monitoring equipment: _____   Insulin administration supplies: _____

   Glucagon emergency kit: _____   Ketone testing supplies: _____

   Snack foods: _____

Personnel trained in the symptoms and treatment of low and high blood sugar and dates of training: _____

Signatures

Reviewed by: [student's health provider/date] Acknowledged/received by: [guardian/date] Acknowledged/received by [school representative]

FIGURE 7-12. Diabetes in the school and day care centers. Approximately 125,000 children of school age in the United States have diabetes. For these young people to be able to attend school or day care, the staff must be knowledgeable about diabetes to be able to provide a safe environment. Parents and the health care team must work in concert to give personnel the information, training, and equipment to allow children with diabetes to participate fully and safely in the school experience and to be in compliance with federal laws that protect these children. The Rehabilitation Act of 1973, the Individuals with Disabilities Education Act of 1991, and the Americans with Disabilities Act of 1992 make it illegal for schools to discriminate against children with special needs.

(Continued on next page)

FIGURE 7-12. *(Continued)* Any school that receives federal funding or is considered open to the public must reasonably accommodate the special needs of children with diabetes with as little disruption to the routine of the school and child as possible, allowing for full participation in all school activities. To ensure this, general guidelines explaining the responsibilities of the parent or guardian, the school or day care provider, the health care team, and the student have been put forth in a position statement issued by the American Diabetes Association. Key to the successful implementation of these guidelines is the development of an individualized diabetes care plan that provides specific instructions regarding blood glucose monitoring, insulin administration, recognizing and treating hypoglycemia and hyperglycemia, the meal plan, and testing for ketones. An example of the diabetes care plan is shown to illustrate the complexity of appropriately managing each child with diabetes in the school or day care setting [20].

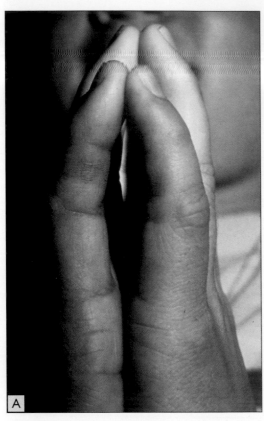

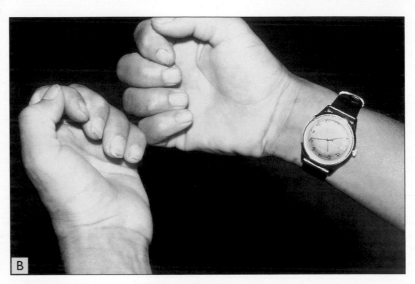

FIGURE 7-13. (See Color Plate) Limited joint mobility (LJM): changes in frequency and severity in children with type 1 diabetes between 1976 and 1978 and in 1998. **A** and **B,** LJM is the earliest long-term complication of type 1 diabetes in children and youths. It is a risk indicator for microvascular complications, and its appearance is primarily affected by long-term metabolic control [21]. Staging for LMJ is as follows: stage 0: no stiffness or contractures; stage 1: stiffness of fingers only; stage 2: stiffness and contractures only of the fifth fingers bilaterally; stage 3: stiffness and contractures of more than just the fifth fingers bilaterally; stage 4: stiffness and contractures of the fingers plus the wrists; and stage 5: spine, neck, and other joints also involved. LJM has decreased in prevalence and severity over the last 20 years. In 1998, 312 subjects, ages 7 to 18 years, were examined using the same methods as the 515 subjects in this age group who were examined between 1976 and 1978 [21]. The 1998 cohort was found to have a greater than fourfold reduction in frequency of LJM (31%) compared with the 1976 to 1978 cohort (7%). There was a decrease in the proportion of patients with moderate or severe LJM as well, from 35% to 9%. This decrease in LJM is most likely the result of improved blood glucose control since the early 1980s [21,22].

COMPONENTS OF THE OUTPATIENT VISIT

Assess

Frequency, causes, and severity of hypoglycemia or hyperglycemia

Results of home glucose monitoring from logbooks and blood glucose meter downloads

Self-adjustments made to diabetes regimen

Integration of home care management behavior, understanding of diabetes management plan and goals

Education assessment and needs

Review of systems for intercurrent problems or diabetes complications

Current medications

Psychosocial issues

Changes in life situations

School performance, after school, weekend, and sports activities

Risk-taking behavior, particularly for adolescents

Physical examination	Frequency/ recommendations
Weight, height, BMI	Every 3 mo, assess changes in percentile
Tanner stage	Every 3 mo, note pubertal progression
Blood pressure	Every 3 mo, target < 90th percentile
Eye	Dilated fundoscopic exam every 12 mo after 5 y of diabetes
Thyroid	Every 3 mo, presence of hepatomegaly, fullness, signs of malabsorption, inflammation
Abdomen	Every 3 mo, inspection; after age 12 y, thorough examination for sensation, pulses, vibration yearly
Foot, peripheral pulses	Every 3 mo, injection sites, joint mobility, lesions associated with diabetes
Skin, joints, injection sites	Every 12 mo, signs of autonomic changes, pain, neuropathy
Neurologic	

Laboratory examination	Frequency
HbA$_{1c}$	Every 3 mo
Microalbuminuria	Every 12 mo after puberty or after 5 y with diabetes
U/A, creatinine	At presentation and with signs or renal problems
Lipid profile	At diagnosis and every 12 mo
Thyroid function tests	Every 12 mo
Celiac screen	At time of diagnosis, if symptoms, at puberty
Islet antibodies	At diagnosis

FIGURE 7-14. Components of the outpatient visit. Pediatric patients with diabetes should have comprehensive, multidisciplinary outpatient visits at regular intervals [23,24]. The purpose of these visits is to assess their health status, adjust the diabetes regimen as indicated, promote diabetes knowledge and competency, and motivate patients and families to improve short- and long-term outcomes. Diabetes health care providers should ensure that patients receive routine pediatric care to diagnose and treat other medical and psychological problems and to administer immunizations and anticipatory guidance. At quarterly visits, hemoglobin A$_{1c}$ (HbA$_{1c}$) levels should be measured. The results should be available at the time of the clinic visit to allow for a face-to-face discussion if glycemic targets are not met. Thyroid function testing should be done yearly. Thyroid autoantibodies are present in 20% to 30% of pediatric patients with type 1 diabetes; however, overt hypothyroidism occurs in 1% to 5% and compensated hypothyroidism in 5% to 10%. A fasting lipid profile that includes total cholesterol, high- and low-density lipoprotein cholesterol, and triglyceride levels should be obtained in children and adolescents after glucose control has been established. Microalbumin levels can be measured using a random microalbumin-to-creatinine ratio, timed overnight microalbumin assay-to-albumin excretion rate assessment, or 24-hour timed urinary microalbumin-to-albumin excretion rate measurement.

Celiac disease has been reported to occur 10 to 50 times more often in children with diabetes compared with the general population. Depending on the study, celiac disease may be present in 1% to 10% of children and adolescents with type 1 diabetes. A diagnosis of celiac disease should be considered in children and youth with gastrointestinal symptoms such as diarrhea, pain, flatulence, dyspepsia, or aphthous ulcers. Unexplained hypoglycemia, dermatitis herpetiformis, and delayed growth or pubertal development can also be associated with celiac disease. A celiac screen, including anti-endomysial IgA antibody quantitation, should be obtained. At the time of diagnosis, patients should have liver function tests, a serum creatinine test, and urinalysis. Assessment of islet autoimmunity should be made by obtaining specific antibodies to islet antigens. BMI—body mass index.

Adjustment to Childhood Diabetes

PSYCHOSOCIAL ISSUES IN PEDIATRIC DIABETES

Psychsocial Factors Affecting Initial Diabetes Management

Patient's and family's adjustment to losses and uncertainties inherent in diagnosis

Cultural and health beliefs competing with treatment requirements

Emotional reactions to diabetes-specific tasks and complications (fear of injections, BGM, responses to hypo- and hyperglycemia, long-term complications)

Psychiatric and social problems preceding diagnosis

Community and social support surrounding the family

Relationship and communication with health care team

Financial resources for treatment and access to good caretakers

Important Factors in Psychosocial Management

Self-care tasks appropriate to maturity rather than age

Complete supervision in children, discrete supervision in adolescents

Avoidance of extremes of overprotection or total independence

Clear attribution and sharing of responsibilities among family members and patients

Realistic treatment goals according to the patient's acceptance

Empathic understanding of the stresses of living with diabetes

Encouragement of open communication and venting of negative feelings about diabetes

Recognition of diabetes burnout

Problem-solving skills practiced regularly

Help from mental health professionals if necessary

Focus on overall success: age-appropriate developmental skills, adequate social and family relationships, good glycemic control

FIGURE 7-15. Psychosocial issues in pediatric diabetes. The majority of patients diagnosed with diabetes exhibit mild depression, anxiety, and somatic complaints at the time of diagnosis [25]. In most cases, these symptoms are usually self-limited and resolve within 6 to 9 months. However, in a subset of patients, depressive symptoms increase over time and anxiety worsens, more often in girls than boys. Patient adjustment to diabetes at the time of diagnosis predicts later adjustment. The psychosocial factors that affect initial diabetes management are shown. Family characteristics have a major influence on adjustment to diabetes, self-management, and quality of life. Children and adolescents living in families with a high degree of conflict or with parents who are less caring have less optimal metabolic control. To improve psychological stability and glycemic control, early assessment of family dynamics and, when appropriate, intervention should be done by a multidisciplinary diabetes team equipped to provide social and psychological support. BGM—blood glucose monitoring.

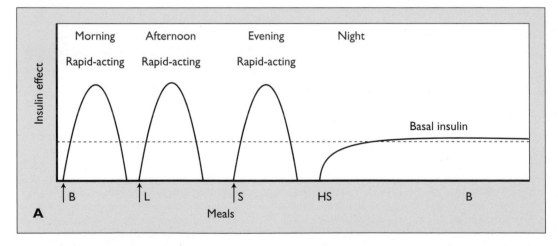

A

FIGURE 7-16. Basal–bolus treatment with rapid-acting and long-acting insulin analogues. Conventional intermediate and long-acting insulin preparations for basal therapy have insulin peaks 4 to 6 hours after injection, durations of action of less than 24 hours, and a large variability of absorption. A new long-acting insulin, glargine, has been developed with a peakless, prolonged time–action profile that enables glargine to provide sufficient basal insulin over 24 hours. In combination with a pre-meal rapid-acting insulin analogue, it can produce more physiological insulin pharmacokinetics (**A**). In a randomized cross-over study, 28 adolescents with type 1 diabetes on multiple injection therapy received either insulin glargine before bedtime plus lispro preprandially or NPH insulin before bedtime plus regular human insulin preprandially for 16 weeks.

(Continued on next page)

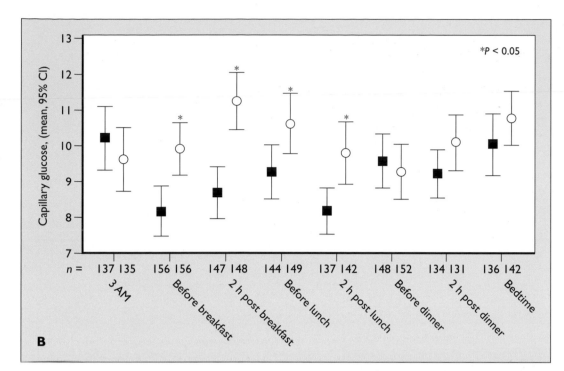

FIGURE 7-16. *(Continued)* Although there was no difference in hemoglobin A_{1c} (HbA$_{1c}$) between groups, lispro/glargine was associated with lower mean blood glucose levels versus NPH/regular and with 43% lower incidence of nocturnal hypoglycemia. Total insulin dose to achieve target blood glucose control was lower with lispro/glargine (**B**) [26].

B

A. SKILLS, KNOWLEDGE, AND ATTITUDES NEEDED TO USE CSII, BY AGE*

Age, y	Skills	Knowledge/attitude
6–10	Insert pump catheter, wear pump with help	Agree to wear the pump
	Unhook and rehook with help	Know how to protect the pump during activity
	Activate bolus with supervision	
10–12	Protect pump during daily activities without help	Know how to do carbohydrate count
		Understand role of exercise
	Unhook and rehook without help	Start to circulate correction dose
	Activate bolus without assistance	
12–14	Suspend basal dose	Calculate and deliver bolus dose
	Program basal rates with assistance	Understand need for temporary basal change
	Suspend basal dose	
	Program basal rates with assistance	
15–18	Program change in basal rate	Determine factors that affect basal/bolus, use algorithms
		Understand sick-day protocol

All patients using CSII must monitor BG three to four times per day, use insulin algorithms, perform carbohydrate counts, and try the infusion catheter.

B. CSII THERAPY IN PEDIATRICS

Time	Mean HbA$_{1c}$, %	P Value
Pump initiation	8.4 ± 1.8	
3 mo	7.8 ± 1.2	0.006
1 y	8.2 ± 0.9	0.05
2 y	8.1 ± 1.1	0.04

FIGURE 7-17. Continuous subcutaneous insulin infusion (CSII) in pediatrics. CSII has been found to be of benefit to children and youths with diabetes [18,21]. **A,** Criteria for initiating CSII vary at different pediatric centers, but the major criterion for adolescents is the desire to maximize basal–bolus therapy with CSII. Other reasons include frequent hypoglycemia, the "dawn" phenomenon, desire for lifestyle flexibility, recurrent diabetic ketoacidosis, and diabetes that is difficult to control with conventional therapy. To successfully use pump treatment, patients and families must have sufficient knowledge and skills and the appropriate attitudes to manage the technology [27]. In preschool and early school-aged children, the tasks required are done by the parent or guardian. As the child matures, pump management is gradually assumed by the patient so that by late adolescence, the child can assume responsibility for CSII. **B,** A decrease in hemoglobin A_{1c} (HbA$_{1c}$) can be expected in pediatric subjects on insulin pump therapy. In a cohort of 83 patients on insulin pump therapy with a mean age of 13.6 ± 3.9 years and mean diabetes duration of 5.3 ± 3.2 years, a significant decrease in HbA$_{1c}$ after 3 months of pump therapy was sustained for 1 and 2 years [28]. (*Panel A adapted from* Kaufman and Halvorson [18].)

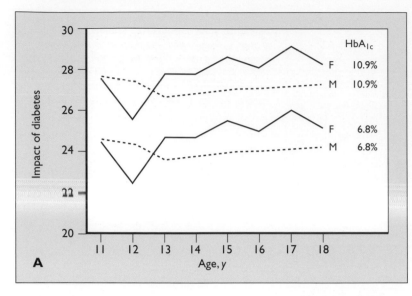

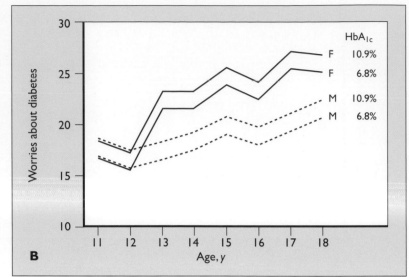

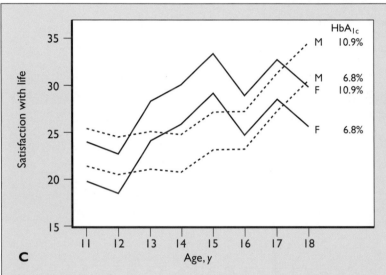

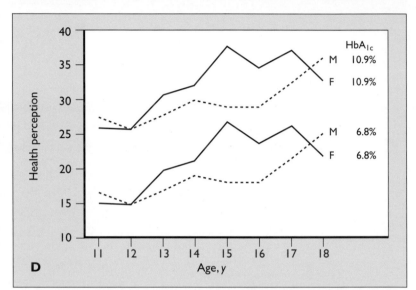

FIGURE 7-18. Metabolic control and quality of life. It is unclear whether the demands of good metabolic control or the consequences of poor control have a greater influence on the quality of life of adolescents with type 1 diabetes. The Diabetes Quality of Life (DQOL) questionnaire was given to 2101 patients, ages 10 to 18 years, to measure the impact of diabetes, worries about diabetes, satisfaction with life, and health perception [27]. **A–D,** The mean hemoglobin A_{1c} (HbA_{1c}) of the group was 8.7%, but those with lower HbA_{1c} were found to be

less impacted by diabetes ($P < 0.0001$) and have fewer worries ($P < 0.05$), greater satisfaction ($P < 0.0001$), and better health perception ($P < 0.0001$). Girls demonstrated increased worries ($P < 0.01$), less satisfaction ($P < 0.01$), and poorer health perception ($P < 0.01$) earlier than boys. Lower HbA_{1c} was significantly associated with better adolescent-rated quality of life; therefore, improved glycemic control should be encouraged as not only a means to prevent the long-term complications of diabetes but also to lessen the psychologic burden of the disease.

Type 2 Diabetes in Children and Youths: A New Epidemic

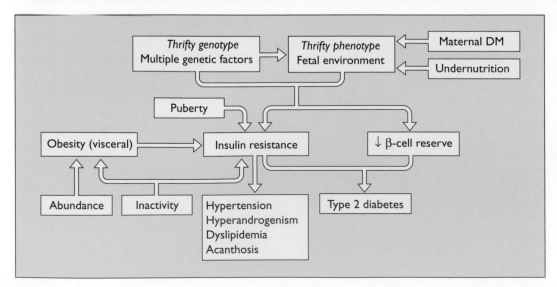

FIGURE 7-19. Associations between insulin resistance and type 2 diabetes in children. Type 2 diabetes in children and adolescents is attributable to insulin resistance and puts subjects at risk for hyperandrogenism (polycystic ovary syndrome), hypertension, dyslipidemia, and other atherosclerosis risk factors [29,30]. Risk factors for type 2 diabetes include obesity, family history, diabetic gestation, and being underweight or overweight for gestational age. Limited β-cell reserve plays a role in progression to frank diabetes. DM—diabetes mellitus [31].

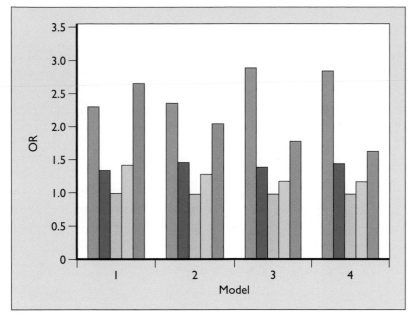

FIGURE 7-20. Effect of birth weight on risk of type 2 diabetes in the children. Several studies have suggested that for both men and women, those born with low birth weight were at an elevated risk for type 2 diabetes during adulthood. In Pima Indians, however, studies revealed U-shaped relationship between birth weight and risk for diabetes. A study conducted in Taiwan involved a mass screening program for detecting diabetes and renal disease. All schoolchildren (~ 3,000,000 for each semester) ages 6 to 18 years underwent urine testing for glycosuria, followed by fasting blood glucose, if the test result was positive. A total of 1966 cases of diabetes was identified. Data on birth weight and gestational age in weeks were obtained from Taiwan's Birth Registry; families were interviewed by phone. After adjusting for age, gender, body mass index (BMI), family history of diabetes, and socioeconomic status, the risk for type 2 diabetes remained significantly high for the low birth weight(< 2500 g) and high birth weight (> 4500 g) groups compared with those with birth weights between 2500 and 4000 g. This study confirms the U-shaped relationship between birth weight and risk for type 2 diabetes. In addition, type 2 diabetic subjects born with high birth weight had higher BMIs, higher diastolic blood pressures, and a higher incidence of family history of diabetes compared with those with low birth weight [32]. Different birth weight categories are shown in *vertical bars* with a 500-g increment from < 2500 to > 4000 g.

TESTING FOR TYPE 2 DIABETES IN CHILDREN

Criteria

Overweight (BMI > 85th percentile for age and gender, weight for height > 85th percentile, or weight > 120% ideal for height)

Plus

Any two of the following risk factors:

Family history of type 2 diabetes in first- or second-degree relative

Race/ethnicity (American Indian, black, Hispanic, Asian/Pacific islander)

Signs of insulin resistance or conditions associated with insulin resistance (acanthosis nigricans, hypertension, dyslipidemia, PCOS)

Age of initiation

Age 10 years or at onset of puberty if puberty occurs at a younger age

Frequency

Every 2 years

Test

Fasting plasma glucose preferred

FIGURE 7-21. Case finding for type 2 diabetes in children. The American Diabetes Association consensus statement for type 2 diabetes in children and adolescents, which was endorsed by the American Academy of Pediatrics, recommended that overweight children and adolescents with two or more risk factors for type 2 diabetes be tested every 2 years beginning at age 10 years or at the onset of puberty [30]. BMI—body mass index; PCOS—polycystic ovary syndrome.

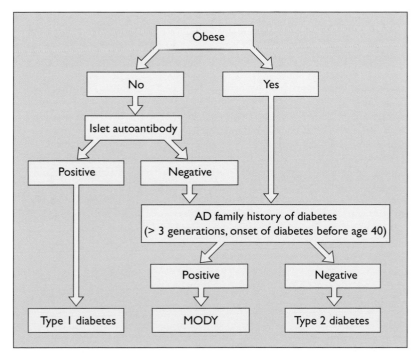

FIGURE 7-22. Research schema for classification of diabetes in children and adolescents to determine the presence of type 2 diabetes. Between 50% to 90% of youths with type 2 diabetes have a body mass index greater than 27 kg/m^2 or are above the 85th percentile for age. Children who are overweight and have a high fasting C peptide or insulin level are presumed to have type 2 disease. Autoantibodies should be measured in overweight children with low fasting C peptide or insulin levels. If they are present, the patient likely has type 1 diabetes. If autoantibodies are absent, the patient could have idiopathic diabetes or maturity-onset diabetes of youth (MODY). In nonobese children and adolescents, the presence of autoantibodies indicates type 1 diabetes. Nonobese children with absent antibodies should have their C peptide and insulin levels assessed. If these levels are high, the patient likely has type 2 diabetes; if these levels are low, the patient may have idiopathic diabetes or MODY. The final diagnostic classification may require following the patient's clinical course for a few years after diagnosis [30]. AD—autosomal dominant.

SEPARATING MATURITY-ONSET DIABETES OF YOUTH FROM TYPE 2 DIABETES IN CHILDREN

	Type 2 Diabetes	MODY
Age of onset	Middle/old age	Childhood/adolescence/young adulthood
Disease-related mortality	High	Variable
Availability of multiple affected three-generation families	Very rare	Frequent
Role of environment	Considerable	Minimal
	Frequently obese	Rarely obese
Pathophysiology	β-cell dysfunction and insulin resistance	β-cell dysfunction
Inheritance	Polygenic	
	Heterogeneous	Monogenic
		Autosomal dominant
		Homogeneous (within a pedigree)

FIGURE 7-23. Separating maturity-onset diabetes of youth ([MODY] positive hepatocyte nuclear factor-1α gene [HNF1-α] mutation) from type 2 diabetes in children. MODY represents a group of monogenic causes of β-cell dysfunction presenting in the second to fourth decades of life. These patients have a different disease profile from type 2 diabetes, being lean and insulin sensitive with high rather than low high-density lipoprotein (HDL) cholesterol, and they progress more rapidly to insulin treatment. Most of the monogenic forms of diabetes present in the same age group as type 2 diabetes. The most common form is caused by mutations in the HNF1α, accounting for about 65% of the cases in the United Kingdom. Finding a specific cause allows individualization of management and gives patients more certain prognosis. HNF1α gene testing should be considered in any type 2 child who is not obese, does not have acanthosis nigricans, or has low HDL, especially if the child is white. (*Adapted from* Hattersley [33].)

A. CLINICAL AND AUTOIMMUNE CHARACTERISTICS OF PATIENTS WITH TYPE 2 DIABETES

Variable	Type 2	Type 1	P Value
BMI (kg/m^2)	31.24 ± 8.83	17.9 ± 3.87	0.74
Acanthosis nigricans	37%	0	
DKA at diagnosis	33.3%	53.3%	0.142
C-peptide at diagnosis	2.2 ± 2.2	1.8 ± 3.5	0.647
Positive ICA	8.1%	71.1%	0.001
Positive GAD	30.3%	75.7%	0.001
Positive IAA	34.8%	76.5%	0.009

B. DIABETES AUTOIMMUNE MARKERS IN NONINSULIN REQUIRING PATIENTS WITH TYPE 2 DIABETES MELLITUS

	Percentage with positive titer	Percentage with negative titer
GAD	18.75	81.25
IAA	37.5	62.5
ICA	0	100

FIGURE 7-24. Clinical and autoimmune characteristics of type 2 diabetes in the pediatric population. The differential diagnosis between types 1 and 2 diabetes in children is complicated and relies heavily on clinical criteria, such as Hispanic or black ancestry, family history, obesity, evidence of insulin resistance, absent or milder than expected blood glucose fluctuations, or ketosis or hypoglycemic reactions to insulin. The presence of any of the autoimmune β-cell markers was used to exclude type 2 diabetes in children; however, it had been well documented in adults with type 2 diabetes. There is evidence, that islet cell cytoplasmic autoantibodies (ICAs) positivity predict future insulin requirement. Hathout et al. [34] reported that in a cohort of 48 children with type 2 diabetes aged 9.7 to 17.9 years, compared with 39 randomly selected children with type 1 diabetes, there were significantly more Hispanics and fewer whites, and higher frequency of type 2 diabetes in first-degree relatives, higher body mass index, and exclusive presence of acanthosis nigricans. The incidence of diabetic ketoacidosis and hemoglobin A$_{1c}$ (HbA$_{1c}$) at the time of diagnosis was lower in type 2 diabetes group, but the difference was not statistically significant. Although there were significantly higher levels of autoimmune markers present in children with type 1 diabetes, positive ICA was reported in 8.1%, positive glutamic acid decarboxylase in 30.3%, and positive insulin autoantibodies in 34.8% subjects with type 2 diabetes (**A**). One year after diagnosis, 50% of type 2 diabetes patients were doing well off insulin, and none of those had ICA at diagnosis; however, all type 2 diabetes patients with ICA present required insulin therapy 1 year after onset (**B**). The data confirm that absence of diabetes autoimmune markers is not a prerequisite for the diagnosis of type 2 diabetes in children [34]. GAD— glutamic acid decarboxylase; IAA—insulin autoantibody.

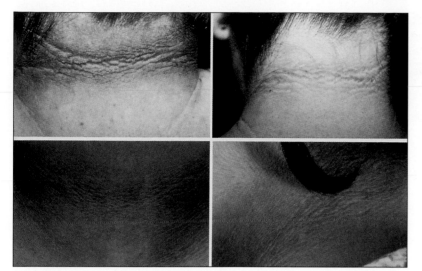

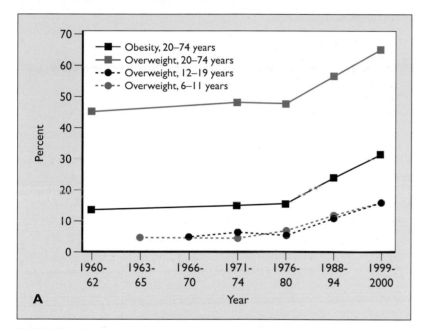

FIGURE 7-25. (See Color Plate) Acanthosis nigricans. This condition is a marker of insulin resistance frequently associated with type 2 diabetes; 60% to 90% of youths with type 2 diabetes have acanthosis nigricans. The skin is hyperpigmented in intertriginous areas. In a survey by Stuart *et al.* [35] of 1412 students, 7.1% had acanthosis nigricans. The prevalence was highest in black students (13.3%), followed by Hispanics (5.5%) and whites (0.5%). Acanthosis nigricans is highly associated with obesity. The prevalence of diabetes is six times higher in black patients with acanthosis nigricans than it is in blacks without this skin lesion. Because acanthosis nigricans is associated with diabetes so highly, it may be used as a screening tool to help identify those at high risk for type 2 diabetes. (*From* Stuart *et al.* [35]; with permission.)

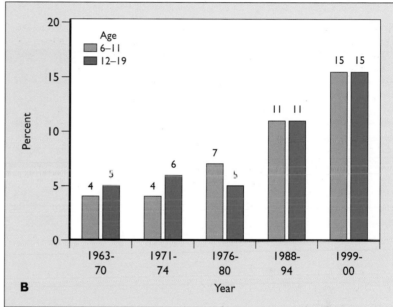

FIGURE 7-26. Prevalence of overweight and obesity in different age groups. **A,** Overweight and obesity by age: United States, 1960 to 2000. Overweight in adults is defined as body mass index (BMI) above 25 kg/m² and obesity as body mass index (BMI) above 30 kg/m². **B,** Prevalence of overweight in children and adolescents. There has been a marked increase in the prevalence of overweight and at risk for overweight in girls and boys across all ethnic groups, except white girls, since 1966. The increase in type 2 diabetes in youths mirrors the increase in obesity. Overweight is in children is defined as BMI at or above the gender- and age-specific 95th percentile and at risk for overweight is defined as BMI in the 85th to 95th percentile [36].

PREVALENCE OF INDIVIDUAL METABOLIC SYNDROME RISK FACTORS AMONG US ADOLESCENTS 12 TO 19 YEARS OF AGE: NHANES III

	Percentage (95% CI)				
	Abdominal Obesity	High Glucose Level	High Triglyceride Levels	Low HDL-C Level	Elevated BP
Total	9.8 (8.2–11.4)	1.5 (0.1–2.8)	23.4 (19.9–27.0)	23.3 (20.6–26.0)	4.9 (3.4–6.4)
Gender					
Male	10.2 (8.0–12.4)	2.4 (0.0–4.9)	24.7 (18.9–30.5)	31.2 (27.1–35.3)	6.7 (4.1–9.4)
Female	9.4 (6.9–11.8)	0.5 (0.2–0.8)	22.1 (17.6–26.6)	15.1 (11.9–18.3)	3.0 (1.8–4.2)
Race/ethnicity					
White	9.3 (6.9–11.7)	1.6 (0.0–3.6)	25.5 (20.7–30.3)	26.1 (22.5–29.7)	5.2 (3.1–7.3)
Black	12.2 (9.6–14.8)	1.7 (0.6–2.8)	10.5 (8.0–14.5)	11.7 (9.0–14.5)	6.2 (4.4–8.1)
Mexican American	13.0 (9.4–16.5)	1.6 (0.7–2.4)	24.7 (21.0–28.4)	20.2 (15.5–24.9)	5.1 (3.2–6.9)
BMI status, percentile					
Normal (< 85th)	0.3 (0.0–0.6)	0.7 (0.0–1.4)	17.6 (13.9–21.2)	17.7 (14.7–20.8)	3.2 (2.2–4.3)
At risk (85th to < 95th)	11.5 (5.4–17.8)	4.5 (0.0–9.5)	33.5 (23.9–43.0)	32.3 (24.0–40.5)	8.6 (2.8–14.4)
Overweight (95th or higher)	74.5 (67.1–81.8)	2.6 (0.0–6.3)	51.8 (40.7–62.9)	50.0 (42.3–57.8)	11.2 (5.7–16.8)

FIGURE 7-27. Prevalence of a metabolic syndrome phenotype in adolescents. The metabolic syndrome is a constellation of metabolic derangements that include obesity, insulin resistance, dyslipidemia, and hypertension, and the syndrome predicts both type 2 diabetes mellitus and premature coronary artery disease. Substantial percentage of overweight children and adolescents may be affected by metabolic syndrome. Cook *et al.* [37] analyzed cross-sectional data obtained from the Third National Health and Nutrition Examination Survey (NHANES III, 1988 to 1994). Sample consisted of 2430 subjects aged 12 to 19 years. Metabolic syndrome was defined as waist circumference greater than 90% for age and gender for the study population; blood pressure at or above 90% for age, gender, and height, fasting glucose level above 110 mg/dL; and high-density lipoprotein cholesterol (HDL-C) and triglyceride levels above 90% for age. Overall prevalence of the metabolic syndrome in adolescents was 4.2%. It was more common in boys (6.1%) than girls (2.1%) and was more frequent in Mexican Americans (5.6%) and whites (4.8%) than black subjects (2.0%). Almost half of subjects (41%) had one or more risk factors, and 14% of subjects had two or more. The distribution of each element of the metabolic syndrome is shown in this figure. High triglyceride levels and low HDL cholesterol levels were most common, and high fasting glucose levels were the least common. Adolescent subjects who manifest this risk profile may constitute a subgroup of overweight teenagers to target for lifestyle behavior changes [37]. BMI—body mass index; BP—blood pressure. (*Adapted from* Cook *et al.* [37].)

FIGURE 7-28. Treatment of type 2 diabetes in children. The treatment of type 2 diabetes in pediatric patients must include diabetes education for the family and patient, with emphasis on the importance of regular exercise and appropriate nutrition. Glycemic targets should be established. Maintaining hemoglobin A_{1c} (HbA_{1c}) below 7.0% and fasting plasma glucose levels as near to 126 mg/dL as possible is difficult in adolescents [31,38].

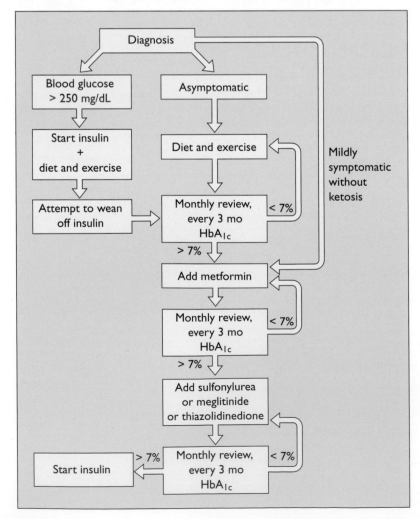

USE OF METFORMIN IN PEDIATRIC PATIENTS WITH TYPE 2 DIABETES

	Metformin	Placebo	Difference (Metformin vs Placebo)
Baseline mean FPG (mmol/L)	9.0 ± 2.7	10.7 ± 2.7	-3.6 ± 0.8
Last double-blind visit mean FPG (mmol/L)	7.0 ± 2.2	11.5 ± 4.5	5.1 to -2.0
Adjusted mean* FPG change from baseline (mmol/L)	-2.4 ± 0.5	1.2 ± 0.5	< 0.001‡
95% CI	-3.5 to -1.3	0.1 to 2.3	-1.2 ± 0.2
$p†$	8.2 ± 1.3	8.9 ± 1.4	(-1.6 to -0.7)
Baseline mean HbA$_{1c}$, %	7.2 ± 1.2	8.9 ± 1.6	< 0.001
Adjusted mean* HbA$_{1c}$, %	7.5 ± 0.2	8.6 ± 0.2	
95% CI	(7.2–7.8)	(8.3–9.0)	
$p§$			

*Mean adjusted for baseline FPG or for baseline HbA1C.

†The P value is based on an ANCOVA, comparing metformin to placebo using baseline FPG as the covariate and treatment as the main effect.

‡Significance level P < 0.03355, in which the testwise critical value was adjusted for an 8-week interim analysis of FPG, to preserve an overall a level of 0/05 or less using the O'Brien-Fleming method with an a of 0.025 at the interim analysis.

§P value is based on an ANCOVA, comparing metformin to placebo using baseline HbA1C as the covariate and treatment as the main effect.

FIGURE 7-29. Use of metformin in pediatric patients with type 2 diabetes. Metformin is the first oral agent to be proven safe and effective for the treatment of type 2 diabetes in pediatric subjects. It is the first oral hypoglycemic agent to gain Food and Drug Association approval for type treatment of type 2 diabetes in children. A multicenter study evaluated 82 patients with doses of metformin up to 1000 mg twice daily. Subjects were between 10 and 16 years of age and were treated for up to 16 weeks in a randomized, double-blind, placebo-controlled trial. Entry criteria were a fasting plasma glucose (FPG) of 126 or higher and 240 mg/dL or lower; hemoglobin A$_{1c}$ (HbA$_{1c}$) of 7.0% or greater; and C peptide of 0.5 nmol/L or greater. Subjects had a body mass index above the 50th percentile for age. Metformin showed a beneficial effect compared with placebo. Improvement in fasting plasma glucose occurred in both genders and all race groups. Metformin did not have a negative impact on body weight or lipid profile, and the adverse events were similar to those seen in adults [38].

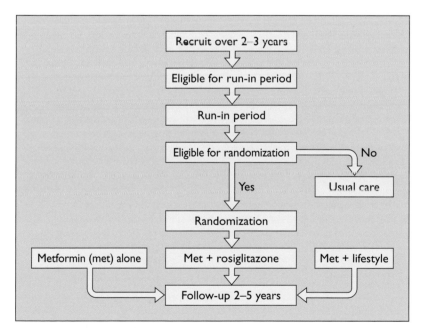

FIGURE 7-30. Study to treat or prevent pediatric type 2 diabetes. Despite the dramatic increase in the number of cases of type 2 diabetes in pediatric patients, there have been no published large-scale studies investigating the pathophysiology, treatment, and complications of this disorder in children and youths. Patients with type 2 diabetes have dual abnormalities of insulin resistance and insulin deficiency. It is hypothesized that to achieve the level of glycemic control required to optimize long-term outcome and decrease or prevent microvascular complications, treatment regimens should be designed to improve insulin sensitivity and preserve residual β-cell function. The available antidiabetic agents have not been adequately evaluated in pediatric patients with regard to using combination therapy to improve glycemic control or lifestyle interventions aimed at obesity and sedentary behavior. The national Institute of Diabetes and Digestive and Kidney Diseases (NIDDK) of the National Institutes of Health (NIH) has sponsored a collaborative multicenter trial titled Study to Treat or Prevent Pediatric Type 2 Diabetes (STOPP-T2D). This will include Treatment of Type 2 Diabetes in Adolescents and Youth (TODAY) and a school-based primary prevention trial of type 2 diabetes in children and youths. The primary objective of the TODAY trial is to compare the efficacy of the three treatment modalities (metformin alone, metformin and rosiglitazone, and metformin plus intensive lifestyle modification). The secondary aims are to evaluate safety of three study arms and to compare the effects of the pathophysiology of type 2 diabetes in youths, including β-cell function, insulin resistance, body composition, nutrition, fitness, cardiovascular risk factors, macrovascular complications, quality of life, and psychological outcomes. In addition, the study will evaluate the influence of individual and family behavior on treatment response and assess the relative cost effectiveness of the three treatment arms. The multicenter study recruits patients over a 3-year period and follows patients for a minimum of 2 years. The qualifying patients are enrolled in a run-in phase to be weaned from insulin, thiazolidinediones, or sulfonureas and to titrate metformin dose to maximum 2000 mg/d. Run-in is also used to assess adherence. The anticipated duration of trial is 7 years [39].

A. ONGOING EVALUATION AND MONITORING AFTER DIAGNOSIS: LABORATORY EVALUATION*

Test	Frequency	Recommendations
Self-monitoring blood glucose test	Fasting and 2-h postprandial glucose daily	Individualized
Fasting plasma glucose test	Initially and ongoing	
2-h postprandial glucose test	At diagnosis and as needed	
Hemoglobin A$_{1C}$	Every 3 mo	
Urinalysis	Every 12 mo	
Microalbuminuria	Every 12 mo	
Creatinine	At diagnosis	And per protocol, if there is hypertension, microalbuminuria, or ACE inhibitor treatment
Lipid profile	At diagnosis and every 12 mo	
Liver function test	At diagnosis	Before initiating oral hypoglycemic agents

*More frequent monitoring at diagnosis, during initiation of new treatment, and during metabolic changes (illness, stress, increased activity, and growth).

B. MANAGEMENT OF DYSLIPIDEMIA IN CHILDREN/ADOLESCENTS WITH DIABETES

Screening
After glycemic control is achieved
Type 1
  Obtain lipid profile at diagnosis and then, if normal, every 5 years
  Begin at age 12 years (or onset of puberty, if earlier)
  Begin before age 12 years (if prepubertal) only if positive family history
Type 2
  Obtain lipid profile at diagnosis and then every 2 years
Goals
  LDL < 100 mg/dL
  HDL > 35 mg/dL
  Triglycerides < 150 mg/dL
Treatment strategies
  Diet
  Maximize glycemic control
  Weight reduction, if indicated
  Medications
    Age > 10 y
    LDL 160 mg/dL or greater
    LDL 130–159 mg/dL; consider based on CVD risk profile
    Statins ± resins
    Fibric acid derivatives if triglycerides > 1000 mg/dL
Manage other CVD risk factors
  BP
  Tobacco use
  Obesity
  Inactivity

FIGURE 7-31. Ongoing laboratory evaluation and monitoring for complications after diagnosis. Health care professionals must address multiple medical and psychosocial concerns. Several interventions have proven effective in preventing diabetes complications among adults, and evaluation of these measures in children are currently under way. **A,** The current recommendations based on adult data. Systemic hypertension is defined as systolic or diastolic blood pressure (BP) greater than 95% for age. In type 2 diabetes, the BP goal is less than 90%. The diagnosis of hypertension should be confirmed on three separate occasions, and the possibility of renal and heart disease should be evaluated. If BP reduction is not achieved by lifestyle changes, then drug therapy is necessary. Angiotensin-converting enzyme (ACE) inhibitors are first-line agents because of their cardiovascular and renal benefits. Microalbuminuria is a sign of incipient diabetic nephropathy. Improved glycemic and BP control have been shown to slow down the progression of nephropathy in adults. ACE inhibitors are additional treatment modality [40]. Children with diabetes are at risk of developing hyperlipidemia, which compounds their risk for cardiovascular disease. The American Heart Association recommends that children's total cholesterol concentration is less than 170 mg/dL and low-density lipoprotein (LDL) is less than 110 mg/dL. Because of significantly higher risk of cardiovascular disease in youths with diabetes, optimal LDL level for those with diabetes is set at less than 100 mg/dL. Recent evidence indicates non–high-density lipoprotein (HDL) cholesterol is a better predictor of atherogenesis than LDL cholesterol. If a fasting measurement is not possible, HDL cholesterol is an alternative. High triglyceride levels are increasingly recognized as an additional risk factor. A lipoprotein analysis after a 12-hour fast is recommended by the American Diabetes Association to obtain triglyceride concentrations for computation of accurate LDL concentration. **B,** The most current American Diabetes Association recommendations for management of dislipidemia in children and adolescents based on a synthesis of current pediatric recommendations and recommendations for adults. CVD—cardiovascular disease. (Adapted from the American Diabetes Association [41].)

CHILDHOOD NAFLD AS CURRENTLY REPORTED: DIFFERENTIATING SIMPLE STEATOSIS FROM NASH IS POSSIBLE ONLY WITH LIVER BIOPSY DATA

Study	Children Reported, n	Gender	Age, y	Acanthosis Nigricans, %	Liver Biopsy Reported, n	Histologic Findings
Moran et al. [44]	3	2 M, 1 F	10–15	NR	3	3 SH
Kinugasa et al. [45]	11	9 M, 2 F	9–15	NR	11	5 fibrosis; 1 cirrhosis
Vajro et al. [46]	9	6 M, 3 F	4–11	NR	1	1 SH
Baldridge et al. [47]	14	10 M, 4 F	10–18	NR	14	14 SH; 13 fibrosis
Rashid and Roberts [48]	36	21 M, 15 F	4–16	30	24	24 steatosis; 21 SH; 16 fibrosis; 1 cirrhosis
Manton et al. [49]	17	11 M, 6 F	9–5	6	17	
Willner et al. [50]	4	1 M, 3 F*	14–17	NR	1	9 fibrosis; 1 evolving cirrhosis
Kocak et al. [51]	5	5 M	4–14	NR	0	1 cirrhosis
Squires (Personal communication; see [43])	39	28 M, 21 F	*	49	31	NR
						31 SH; 21 fibrosis; 2 cirrhosis
Sathya et al. [52]	27	17 M, 10 F	8–16	NR	5	3 steatosis; 2 fibrosis
Molleston et al. [53]	2	2 M	10, 14	0	2	2 cirrhosis
Totals	167	~112 M			109	8 cirrhosis

*Data incomplete.

FIGURE 7-32. Non-alcoholic fatty liver disease (NAFLD) in children is a growing problem and is frequently associated with obesity, insulin resistance, and type 2 diabetes. NAFLD is characterized by presence of macrovesicular steatosis with parenchymal inflammation. The histologic findings can range from fatty changes in liver alone to non-alcoholic steatohepatitis (NASH), cirrhosis, and liver failure. In adult studies, there is higher correlation of incidence and severity of NAFLD with insulin resistance than with body mass index. Prepubertal children can be affected. The largest pediatric series published included 36 patients ages 4 to 16 years of whom liver biopsy was performed in 24 cases. Most had weight greater than 120% of ideal body weight, and 30% had acanthosis nigricans. One 9-year-old child had cirrhosis, and 24 children had some degree of fibrosis [42]. Most affected children are asymptomatic and may be referred because of abnormal liver enzymes or an abnormal liver sonogram, consistent with fatty infiltration. Definite diagnosis, however, can be made only by liver biopsy, which remains gold standard for diagnosis and evaluation of severity, as well as for monitoring disease progression. This figure summarizes data on current reports on childhood NAFLD, including histopathology. Treatment strategies include weight loss by decreasing caloric intake and increasing exercise. A low-glycemic index diet has been proposed to lower postprandial hyperinsulinemia. Few drugs have been investigated, but they include vitamin E, metformin, and thiazolidinediones in adults. NR—not reported; SH—steatohepatitis. (*Adapted from* Roberts [43].)

References

1. American Diabetes Association: Hyperglycemic crises in patients with diabetes mellitus. *Diabetes Care* 2001, 24:1992.

2. *Clinical Practice Guidelines: Type 1 Diabetes in Children and Adolescents.* Sydney: National Diabetes Strategy Group and Australasian Paediatric Endocrine Group; 2003.

3. Franklin, SL, Geffner ME, Kaiserman KB: Outpatient management of children with diabetes. DIABETES: don't immediately admit before evaluating the entire situation. *West J Med* 2000, 172:194–196.

4. Glaser N, Barnett P, McCaslin I, et al.: Risk factors for cerebral edema in children with diabetic ketoacidosis. *N Engl J Med* 2001, 344:264–269.

5. Roe TF, Crawford TO, Huff KR, et al.: Brain infarction in children with diabetic ketoacidosis. *J Diabetes Complications* 1996, 2:100–108.

6. The International Society for Pediatric and Adolescent Diabetes (ISPAD): *Consensus Guidelines for the Management of Type 1 Diabetes Mellitus in Children and Adolescents.* The Netherlands: Medical Forum International; 2000.

7. Kaufman FR, Halvorson M: The treatment and prevention of diabetic ketoacidosis in children and adolescents with type 1 diabetes mellitus. *Pediatr Ann* 1999, 28:9.

8. Karvonen M, Viik-Kajander M, Moltchanova E, et al.: Incidence of childhood type 1 diabetes worldwide. *Diabetes Care* 2000, 23:1516–1526.

9. Kaufman FR, Epport K, Halvorson M: Neurocognitive functioning in children diagnosed with diabetes before age 10 years. *Diabetes* 1997, 46:67A.

10. Ryan CM, Becker DJ: Hypoglycemia in children with type 1 diabetes mellitus. Risk factors, cognitive functioning and management. *Endocrinol Metab Clin North Am* 1999, 28:883–900.

11. Diabetes Control and Complications Trial Research Group: Effect of intensive diabetes treatment in the development and progression of long-term complications in adolescents with insulin-dependent diabetes. *J Pediatr* 1994, 125:177–188.

12. Kaufman FR: Diabetes in children and adolescents: prevention and treatment of diabetes and its complications. *Med Clin North Am* 1998, 82:721–738.

13. White NH, Cleary PA, Dahms W, et al.: Beneficial effects of intensive therapy of diabetes during adolescence: outcomes after the conclusion of the Diabetes Control and Complications Trial (DCCT). *J Pediatr* 2001, 139:804–812.

14. Svensson M, Eriksson JW, Dahlquist G: Early glycemic control, age at onset, and development of microvascular complications in childhood-onset type 1 diabetes. *Diabetes Care* 2004, 27:955–962.

15. Buckingham BA, Bluck B, Wilson DM: Intensive diabetes management in pediatric patients. *Curr Diabetes Rep* 2001, 1:111–118.

16. Kaufman FR, Halvorson M, Carpenter S: Use of a plastic insulin dosage guide to correct blood glucose levels out of the target range and for carbohydrate counting in subjects with type 1 diabetes. *Diabetyou es Care* 1999, 22:1252–1257.

17. Chase HP, Kim LM, Owen SL, et al.: Continuous subcutaneous glucose monitoring in children with type 1 diabetes. Pediatrics 2002, 107:222–226.

18. Kaufman FR, Gibson LC, Halvorson M, et al.: A pilot study of the continuous glucose monitoring system. Diabetes Care 2001, 24:2030–2034.

19. Kaufman FR, Halvorson M, Carpenter S, et al.: Insulin pump therapy in young children with diabetes. Diabetes Spectrum 2001, 14:84–89.

20. American Diabetes Association: Care of children with diabetes in the school and day care setting. Diabetes Care 2004, 27(suppl 1):124–126.

21. Brink SJ: Limited joint mobility. In Pediatric and Adolescent Diabetes Mellitus. Edited by Brink SJ. Chicago: Year Book Medical Publishers; 1987:305–312.

22. Infante JR, Rosenbloom AL, Silverstein JH, et al.; Changes in frequency and severity of limited joint mobility in children with type 1 diabetes mellitus between 1976–1978 and 1998. J Pediatr 2001, 138:33–37.

23. The American Diabetes Association: Clinical Practice Recommendations for 2001. Diabetes Care 2001, 24:S1–S126.

24. Kaufman FR, Halvorson M: New trends in managing type 1 diabetes. Contemp Pediatr 1999, 16:112–123.

25. Schiffrin A: Psychosocial issues in pediatric diabetes. Curr Diabetes Rep 2001, 1:33–40.

26. Murphy NP, Keane SM, Ong KK, et al.: Randomized cross-over trial of insulin glargine plus lispro or NPH insulin plus regular human insulin in adolescents with type 1 diabetes on intensive insulin regimens. Diabetes Care 2003, 26:799–804.

27. Hoey H, Aanstoot HJ, Chiarelli F, et al.: Good metabolic control is associated with better quality of life in 2,101 adolescents with type 1 diabetes. Diabetes Care 2001, 24:1923–1928.

28. Kaufman FR, Halvorson M, Miller D, et al.: Insulin pump therapy in type 1 pediatric patients: now and into the year 2000. Diabetes Metab Res Rev 1999, 15:338–352.

29. Silverstein JH, Rosenbloom AL: Type 2 diabetes in children. Curr Diabetes Rep 2001, 1:19–27.

30. American Diabetes Association: Type 2 diabetes in children and adolescents. Diabetes Care 2000, 23:381–389.

31. Silverstein JH, Rosenbloom AL: Treatment of type 2 diabetes mellitus in children and adolescents. J Pediatr Endocrinol Metab 2000, 13:1402–1409.

32. Wei JN, Sung FC, Li CY, et al.: Low birth weight and high birth weight infants are at an increased risk to have type 2 diabetes among school children in Taiwan. Diabetes Care 2003, 26:343–348.

33. Hattersley AT: Maturity-onset diabetes of the young: clinical heterogeneity explained by genetic heterogeneity. Diabet Med 1998, 15:15–24.

34. Hathout EH, Thomas W, El-Shahawy, et al.: Diabetic autoimmune markers in children and adolescents with type 2 diabetes. Pediatrics 2001, 107:102–106.

35. Stuart CA, Pate CJ, Peters EJ: Prevalence of acanthosis nigricans in an unselected population. Am J Med 1989, 87:269–272.

36. CDC/National Center for Health Statistics: Prevalence of Overweight Among Children and Adolescents. Available at: http://www.cdc.gov/nchs/products/pubs/pubd/hestats/overwght99.htm

37. Cook S, Weitzman M, Awinger P, et al.: Prevalence of a metabolic syndrome phenotype in adolescents. Arch Pediatr Adolesc Med 2003, 157:821–827.

38. Jones KL, Arslanian S, Peterokova VA, et al.: Effect of metformin in pediatric patients with type 2 diabetes. Diabetes Care 2002, 25:89–94.

39. STOPP-T2D Treatment Protocol. Washington, DC: STOPP-T2 Coordinating Center, George Washington University Biostatistics Center; 2004.

40. Gahagan S, Silverstein J, and the Committee on Native American Child Health and Section of Endocrinology, American Academy of Pediatrics: Prevention and treatment of type 2 diabetes mellitus in children, with special emphasis on American Indian and Alaska Native children. Pediatrics 2003, 112:e328–347.

41. American Diabetes Association. Consensus statement. Management of dyslipidemia in children and adolescents with diabetes. Diabetes Care 3003, 26:2194–2197.

42. Rashid M, Roberts EA: Nonalcoholic steatohepatitis in children. J Pediatr Gastroenterol Nutr 2000, 30:48–53.

43. Roberts E: Nonalcoholic steatohepatitis in children. Curr Gastroenterol Rep 2003, 5:253–259.

44. Moran JR, Ghishan FK, Halter SA, Greene HL: Steatohepatitis in obese children: a cause of chronic liver dysfunction. Am J Gastroenterol 1983, 78:374–377.

45. Kinugasa A, Tsunamoto K, Furukawa N, et al.: Fatty liver and its fibrous changes found in simple obesity of children. J Pediatr Gatroenterol Nutrit 1984, 3:408–414.

46. Vajro P, Fontanella A, Perna C, et al.: Persistent hypertransaminasemia resolving after weight reduction in obese children. J Pediatr 1994, 125:239–241.

47. Baldridge AD, Perez-Atayde AR, Graeme-Cooke F, et al.: Idiopathic steatohepatitis in childhood: a multicenter retrospective study. J Pediatr 1995, 127:700–704.

48. Rashid M, Roberts EA: Nonalcoholic steatohepatitis in children. J Pediatr Gastroenterol Nutr 2000, 30:48–53.

49. Manton ND, Lipsett J, Moore DJ, et al.: Non-alcoholic steatohepatitis in children and adolescents. Med J Aust 2000, 173:476–479.

50. Willner IR, Waters B, Patil SR, et al.: Ninety patients with nonalcoholic steatohepatitis: insulin resistance, familial tendency, and severity of disease. Am J Gastroenterol 2001, 96:2957–2961.

51. Kocak N, Yuce A, Gurakan F, Ozen H: Obesity: a cause of steatohepatitis in children. Am J Gastroenterol 2000, 95:1099–1100.

52. Sathya P, Martin S, Alvarez F: Nonalcoholic fatty liver disease (NAFLD) in children. Curr Opin Pediatr 2002, 14:593–600.

53. Molleston JP, White F, Teckman J, Fitxgerald JF: Obese children with steatohepatitis can develop cirrhosis in childhood. Am J Gastroenterol 2002, 97:2460–2462.

8

PATHOGENESIS OF TYPE 2 DIABETES

John E. Gerich and Ervin Szoke

Type 2 diabetes is among the most common chronic diseases, affecting about 6% of the United States population (approximately 18 million people) [1]. Phenotypically, about 95% of people with diabetes mellitus have type 2 diabetes [2]. This disorder, however, is extremely heterogeneous (*see* Fig. 8-1). Approximately 10% of patients have late-onset type 1 diabetes; about another 5% develop diabetes as a result of rare monogenic defects in either insulin secretion or insulin action. The remaining patients have "garden variety" type 2 diabetes. The number of people with type 2 diabetes worldwide is expected to increase from 135 million to more than 300 million by 2025, with most of this increase occurring in developing countries. The prevalence of type 2 diabetes in the United States has increased rapidly over the past 50 years (*see* Fig. 8-2) and is highest in minority populations, including blacks, Hispanics, and especially Native Americans. In the Pima Indians of Arizona, 50% of adults older than age 35 years have the disease [3]. In all populations, the prevalence increases with age; in whites, the prevalence reaches 20% by age 80 years [2] (Fig. 8-3).

The pathogenesis of type 2 diabetes involves the interaction of genetic and environmental (acquired) factors that adversely affect insulin secretion (pancreatic β-cell function) and tissue responses to insulin (insulin sensitivity) (*see* Fig. 8-4). Impaired β-cell function and insulin resistance are present before the onset of type 2 diabetes and are predictive of its subsequent development [4–7]. Type 2 diabetes is a polygenic disorder [8]; the additive effects of an as yet unknown number of genetic polymorphisms (risk factors) are required for development of the disorder, although they may not be sufficient necessarily in the absence of environmental (acquired) risk factors (*see* Fig. 8-5). Although searches for candidate genes based on various proteins involved in mediating insulin action have failed to find diabetic genes in this category [8], these genetic factors will likely be elucidated as the Human Genome Project progresses. To date, three polymorphisms have been identified. The first involves an amino acid polymorphism (pro12 ala) in the peroxisome proliferator receptor gamma, which is expressed in insulin target tissues and pancreatic β cells and is involved in modulating effects of insulin [9]. The second involves the gene encoding calpain-10, a cysteine protease that modulates insulin secretion and insulin effects in muscle and adipose tissue [10]. The third involves a site linked to adiponectin, a cytokine released from adipocytes that has effects on insulin secretion and insulin sensitivity [11–14].

The importance of inheritable factors is underscored by the fact that a person with both parents or a monozygotic twin with type 2 diabetes has up to an 80% lifetime risk of developing this disorder [15]. Having a single parent or sibling with type 2 diabetes carries a risk of about 30%, which represents a two- to fourfold increase above that of the general population [16,17]. Impaired β-cell function is the earliest detectable defect in people with normal glucose tolerance who are genetically predisposed to developing type 2 diabetes [6,7,18] (*eg*, first-degree relatives of individuals with type 2 diabetes); *see* Fig. 8-9) [19]. The strongest evidence for this comes from studies of monozygotic twins in which one twin has type 2 diabetes but the other has normal glucose tolerance [20]. The twin with normal glucose tolerance has about an 80% chance of developing type 2 diabetes and thus can be considered to be a true genetically prediabetic individual. All four studies of such twin pairs have found that the twin with normal glucose tolerance had impaired β-cell function [20–23]; the only study that simultaneously assessed insulin sensitivity found it to be normal [20].

Environmental (acquired) factors, however, are also critical for developing diabetes because without these, genetic factors may be insufficient to cause type 2 diabetes. The most important factors are those that influence insulin sensitivity: obesity (especially visceral obesity), physical inactivity, high-fat/low-fiber diets, smoking, and low birth weight (*see* Fig. 8-6) [17,24–29]. Intervention trials have consistently demonstrated that the risk for developing type 2 diabetes can be reduced by up to 60% by caloric restriction, diet modification, and increased physical activity (*see* Fig. 8-7) [30–38]. Although most (> 90%) patients with classic type 2 diabetes are obese (and, therefore, insulin resistant), most insulin-resistant obese individuals are not diabetic. What distinguishes obese individuals with and without diabetes is the ability to compensate for insulin resistance with increased insulin secretion (*see* Fig. 8-8) [39].

There are numerous examples in the literature in which type 2 diabetes can occur solely as a result of impaired insulin secretion in the absence of insulin resistance [40–48]. Most of the insulin resistance found in people with type 2 diabetes can be ascribed to environmental (acquired) factors such as obesity, physical inactivity, high-fat diets, and glucose and lipid toxicity [49]. After binding to its receptor, insulin triggers a complex series of events (*see* Fig. 8-11). The insulin resistance of obesity is associated with reduced numbers of insulin receptors, reduced insulin receptor kinase activity, and reduced activation of insulin signaling proteins and glucose transport [50]. Quantitatively similar defects have been found in obese individuals with type 2 diabetes compared with obese individuals without type 2 diabetes [50]. Several factors may be involved in the insulin resistance associated with obesity: altered release from adipose tissue of free fatty acids [51], tumor necrosis factor-α [52], resistin [53], leptin [54], adipsin [55], and adiponectin [56], as well as accumulation of lipid in insulin target organs [57,58] (*see* Fig. 8-12).

People destined to develop type 2 diabetes initially have impaired glucose tolerance (IGT), a state characterized by isolated postprandial hyperglycemia in which impaired early insulin release and to some extent excessive glucagon release and insulin resistance result in increased postprandial glucose production—the key factor responsible for postprandial hyperglycemia (see Figs. 8-13, 8-15, and 8-16). In type 2 diabetes, the basic metabolic derangements are the same as in IGT except that progressive deterioration in β-cell function and a modest decrease in insulin sensitivity now result in overproduction of glucose by the liver and kidney in the postabsorptive state (ie, fasting hyperglycemia) and impaired splanchnic glucose sequestration (ie, glycogen formation) in the postprandial state [59,60]. Fasting hyperglycemia is directly related to rates of glucose production (see Fig. 8-17). Because of the mass action effect of hyperglycemia and prevailing insulin levels, glucose utilization rates are still, in an absolute sense, normal in type 2 diabetes, although the distribution of tissue uptake and metabolic fates may be altered (see Fig. 8-18) [60]. For example, in type 2 diabetes [61], overall postprandial tissue glucose uptake, glycolysis, and storage are normal but glucose oxidation is reduced; nonoxidative glycolysis is increased; glucose storage via and the direct pathway is increased, but glucose storage via the indirect pathway is reduced because gluconeogenic carbons are released into plasma as glucose rather than being stored as glycogen. As a result of increased glycogenolysis, net hepatic glucose storage is reduced (eg,. increased glycogen cycling). Thus, it appears that the mass action effects of hyperglycemia can overcome the major defect in peripheral glucose metabolism [62] but cannot overcome defects in intracellular pathways that appear to be related to oxidative processes [63].

Poorly controlled diabetes leads to microvascular complications (retinopathy, nephropathy, neuropathy) and macrovascular complications (premature atherosclerosis). Interventional clinical trials (eg, the Diabetes Control and Complications Trial, United Kingdom Prospective Diabetes Study, Kumamoto Study, and Stockholm Diabetes Intervention Study) [64–66] have shown that microvascular complications can be prevented if HbA_{1c} levels are maintained below 7.0% (upper limit of normal, 6.0%) (see Fig. 8-19), but it appears that lower HbA_{1c} levels are needed to prevent macrovascular complications [67–69]. Because IGT is associated with an approximate twofold increase in cardiovascular mortality [70] and because a clinical trial [71] has shown that reduction in postprandial hyperglycemia reduces cardiovascular events, in the future, considerable attention will be paid to reducing hyperglycemia. Currently, the American Diabetes Association recommends a target HbA_{1c} of less than 7.0; the American Association of Clinical Endocrinologists recommends a target of less than 6.5% [72]. The main difference between people with HbA_{1c} values of 7.0 and 6.5 is their postprandial glucose levels [72]. Improved insulin preparations and new oral agents that specifically target impaired insulin secretion and insulin resistance are now available that can achieve this degree of glycemic control (see Fig. 8-20). Furthermore, lifestyle changes (eg, weight loss, exercise) and drugs that reduce insulin resistance can reverse IGT and prevent its progression to type 2 diabetes. Because of the progressive deterioration in insulin secretion, most patients initially successfully managed on one oral agent will need additional drugs, and up to 50% may ultimately need some form of insulin therapy to maintain adequate glycemic control [73–84].

Epidemiology

HETEROGENEITY OF PHENOTYPIC TYPE 2 DIABETES

Subtype	Patients, %
I. Late-onset autoimmune diabetes (LADA) [85]	~10
II. Maturity onset diabetes of youth (MODY) [86]	~3
MODY 1: HNF-4α	
MODY 2: Glucokinase	
MODY 3: HNF-1α	
MODY 4: PDX-1 (IPF-1)	
MODY 5: HNF-1β	
MODY 6: Neuro D1/BETA 2	
III. Maternally inherited diabetes and deafness [87] (mutations in mitochondrial DNAtRNA)	< 1
IV. Insulin receptor defects [88]	< 1
Leprechanism	
Type A insulin resistance and acanthosis nigricans	
Rabson-Mendenhall syndrome	
V. Type 2 diabetes mellitus	~85

FIGURE 8-1. Heterogeneity of phenotypic type 2 diabetes. Patients with late-onset autoimmune diabetes (LADA) [85] experience onset of disease after age 30 years, are generally lean, have islet cell or glutamic acid decarboxylase antibodies, and usually progress to insulin dependence in less than 5 years. Patients with maturity-onset diabetes of youth (MODY) [86] generally experience onset of disease between ages 15 and 30 years, can be either obese or lean, and have a strong family history of diabetes consistent with an autosomal dominant inheritance resulting in impaired insulin release but little or no insulin resistance. Five monogenetic mutations have been identified, and more are expected. HNF—hepatic nuclear factor; IPF—insulin-promoting factor; neuro D1/BETA 2—1/b cell box transactivator 2; PDX—pancreatic development factor.

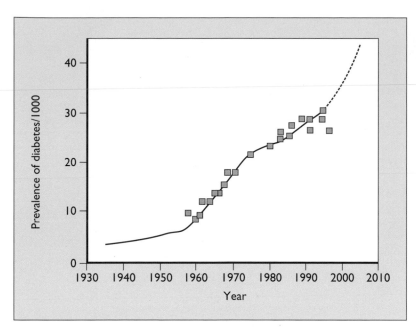

FIGURE 8-2. Increasing prevalence of diabetes in the United States. The prevalence of diagnosed diabetes in the United States has risen steadily since 1930 and is expected to continue to increase rapidly in the early part of the 21st century. About 90% of cases of diagnosed diabetes are of type 2 diabetes. It is estimated that at any given time, at least one third of persons with type 2 diabetes are undiagnosed. (*Adapted* from Diabetes in America [1].)

PERCENT OF POPULATION WITH TYPE 2 DIABETES AND IMPAIRED GLUCOSE TOLERANCE

	Diabetes		Impaired Glucose Tolerance	
Age, y	Men	Women	Men	Women
20–39	1.6	1.7	—	—
30–49	6.8	6.1	12.6	11.2
50–59	12.9	12.4	13.3	15.3
60–74	20.2	17.8	19.2	21.9
> 75	21.1	17.5	—	—

FIGURE 8-3. Prevalence of type 2 diabetes and impaired glucose tolerance (IGT). (*Data from* Harris et al. [2].)

FIGURE 8-4. Incidence of diabetes among Pima Indians. The relative impact of variations in β-cell function and insulin sensitivity on the subsequent development of diabetes among 262 Pima Indians is shown. The acute insulin secretory response to intravenous glucose and insulin action at baseline was measured in patients who initially had normal glucose tolerance. Patients were divided into tertiles of insulin secretion and insulin sensitivity and were followed for an average of 7 years. The observations, however, do not take into consideration whether the β-cell function was appropriate for the degree of insulin resistance; they merely illustrate the fact that both factors influence the risk for developing type 2 diabetes. (*Adapted from* Pratley and Weyer [7].)

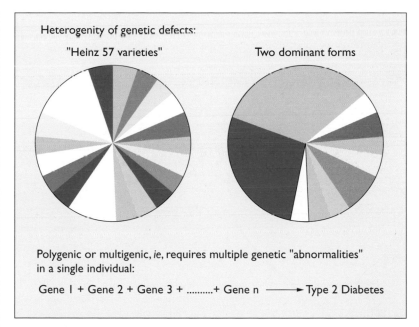

FIGURE 8-5. Two major features of the genetics of type 2 diabetes in the general population. First, this disease is a genetically heterogeneous disorder. At present, however, it is not clear how many forms of diabetes exist, whether there are one or two predominant forms, or whether each form represents only a small percentage of the total population. For most patients, the disease is polygenic: some abnormality or sequence polymorphism is present in several genes, each contributing a small amount to the overall pathogenesis. Although there is no definitive information on the number of genes involved in each form, most investigators believe that at least three genes—and perhaps as many as 10 or 20—may contribute to the final phenotype. Most likely, these are "normal" genetic variants or sequence polymorphisms, which slightly alter insulin action or insulin secretion [89].

Environmental Factors

RELATIVE RISK FOR TYPE 2 DIABETES OF THREE COMMON FACTORS

Obesity (BMI, kg/m^2)	Relative risk
< 23	1
23–25	3
25–30	8
30–35	20
> 35	40
Physical activity (exercise, h/wk)	
> 7.0	1.0
4.0–7.0	1.1
2.0–4.0	1.2
0.5–2.0	1.5
< 0.5	1.8
Healthy diet (quintiles based on fat/fiber content)	
5	1.00
4	1.15
3	1.30
2	1.50
1	2.00

FIGURE 8-6. Relative risks for developing type 2 diabetes. A physically inactive individual (< 30 min/wk of exercise) who consumes an unhealthy diet (level 1) and is modestly overweight (body mass index [BMI] of 25 to 30) would have a 30-fold increased (1.8 x 3 x 2.0 x 3 8) risk of developing type 2 diabetes compared with the general population, which would translate to a lifetime risk of nearly 100%. (*Adapted from* Choi and Shi [25].)

USE OF LIFESTYLE MODIFICATIONS AND DRUGS TO REDUCE THE DEVELOPMENT OF TYPE 2 DIABETES IN PEOPLE WITH IMPAIRED GLUCOSE TOLERANCE

Study	Patients, n	Interventions	Reduction
Eriksson, Lindgarde [34]	181	Diet and exercise in nonobese IGT	37% (11 vs 29%/6 y)
Pan et al. [33]	577	Diet and exercise in nonobese IGT	~40% (9 vs 16%/6 y)
Tuomilehto et al. [32]	522	Diet and exercise in obese IGT	~58% (11 vs 23%/6 y)
Knowler et al [31]	3234	Obese high-risk IGT	58% (14 vs 29%/4 y)
		Diet and exercise	31% (22 vs 29%/4 y)
		Metformin (500 mg BID)	
Wenying et al. [35]	321	Diet and exercise	30% (11 vs 8%/y)
		Acarbose	80%
		Metformin	64%
Chiasson et al. [36]	1348	Obese IGT	25% (32 vs 42%/4 y)
		Acarbose (100 mg TID)	
Buchanan et al. [37]	266	Postgestational diabetetic obese Hispanic women (72% IGT)	50% (6 vs 12%/2.5 y)
		Troglitazone (400 mg/d)	
Torgerson et al. [38]	794	Obese IGT	35% (19 vs 29%/4 y)
		Lifestyle vs lifestyle and orlistat	

FIGURE 8-7. Use of lifestyle modifications and drugs to reduce the development of type 2 diabetes in people with impaired glucose tolerance (IGT). People with IGT have a 20% to 40% risk of developing type 2 diabetes over a 5-year period. Numerous clinical trials [31–38] have demonstrated that lifestyle modifications (eg, diet and exercise) or drugs that reduce insulin resistance (metformin, troglitazone) or obesity (orlistat) can decrease the development of type 2 diabetes in individuals with IGT.

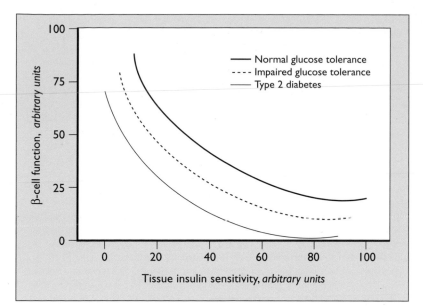

FIGURE 8-8. Reciprocal relationship between β-cell function and tissue insulin sensitivity. A hyperbolic function relates β-cell function to tissue insulin sensitivity such that when insulin decreases, β-cell function increases to maintain normal glucose homeostasis. Patients who develop impaired glucose tolerance (IGT) or type 2 diabetes have an inadequate β-cell compensation for insulin resistance in that for any degree of reduced tissue insulin sensitivity, the β-cell response is below normal [5–7,90].

Genetic Factors

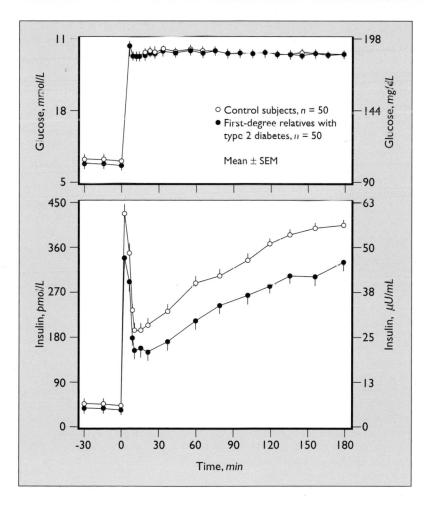

FIGURE 8-9. Plasma glucose (*top*) and insulin (*bottom*) concentrations in hyperglycemic clamp experiments. In response to an acute elevation of blood glucose concentrations, insulin is secreted in a biphasic manner; a first phase lasting approximately 10 minutes followed by a gradually increasing second phase. The first phase of insulin release has been linked to insulin granules located near the β-cell membrane (rapidly releasable pool). Second-phase insulin release depends partly on mobilizing insulin granules from a storage pool to the rapidly releasable pool as well as increased synthesis of insulin. In this study [19], subjects with normal glucose tolerance but a first-degree relative with type 2 diabetes were studied using a hyperglycemic clamp to assess their β-cell function and insulin sensitivity relative to a group of subjects with normal glucose tolerance but no family history of diabetes. Subjects were matched for age, gender, and obesity to exclude environmental (acquired) risk factors. It was demonstrated that individuals with a first-degree relative with type 2 diabetes had reduced early (first-phase) and late (second-phase) insulin release and were not insulin resistant. (*Adapted from* Pimenta *et al.* [19].)

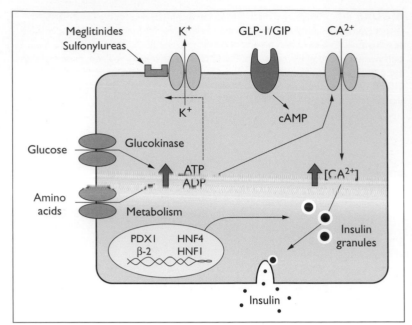

FIGURE 8-10. Nutrient sensing and insulin secretion by the pancreatic β cell. The β cell takes up glucose and amino acids via specific transporters on the cell membrane, such as the GLUT2 glucose transporter. This isoform of transporter is expressed only by the β cell and the liver and has a Km in the physiologic range. After it is inside the cell, glucose is phosphorylated by a specialized form of hexokinase called glucokinase. The subsequent metabolism of glucose results in a change in the ratio of adenosine triphosphate (ATP) to adenosine diphosphate (ADP) in the cell, which in turn causes activation of the ATP-sensitive potassium channel. This results in depolarization of the cell, an influx of calcium, and subsequent release of insulin from secretory granules. The sulfonylurea receptor can also activate the ATP-sensitive potassium channel, mimicking the effect of glucose. Other secretagogues, such as glucagon-like peptide-I (GLP-I), bypass this system by changing cellular cyclic adenosine monophosphate (cAMP) levels. The level of expression of the several molecules involved in glucose sensing, including the GLUT2 glucose transporter and the development of the β cell, are controlled by several nuclear transcription factors. The best studied of these are hepatocyte nuclear factor (HNF)-Iα, HNF-Iβ, HNF-4α, and pancreatic duodenal homeobox-I (PDX-I; insulin promoting factor-I [IPF-I]). Maturity-onset diabetes of youth can result from genetic defects in any of these transcription factors or a genetic defect in glucokinase. In type 2 diabetes, the exact site of the defect in glucose sensing is unknown, but studies in animal models of disease have suggested that this may be the result of a downregulation of the GLUT2 glucose transporter [91].

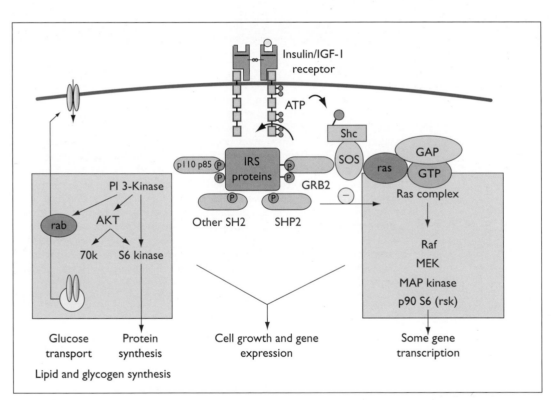

FIGURE 8-11. The insulin signaling network. The full network is complex and can be divided into five levels: 1) activation of the insulin receptor tyrosine kinase and closely linked events; 2) phosphorylation of a family of substrate proteins; 3) interaction of the receptor and its substrates with several intermediate signaling molecules via SH2 (src homology 2) and other recognition domains; 4) activation of serine and lipid kinases, resulting in a broad range of phosphorylation–dephosphorylation events; and 5) regulation of the final biological effectors of insulin action, such as glucose transport, lipid synthesis, gene expression, and mitogenesis. The SH2 proteins link the insulin receptor substrate (IRS) proteins to a series of cascading reactions involving serine/threonine kinases and phosphatases such as the mitogen-activated protein (MAP) kinases, S6 kinases, and protein phosphatase-IA. These serine kinases act on enzymes such as glycogen synthase, transcription factors, and other proteins to produce many of the final biologic effects of the hormone. In adipose tissue and muscle, insulin stimulation also increases glucose uptake by promoting translocation of an intracellular pool of glucose transporters to the plasma membrane. Exactly how this action is linked to the phosphorylation cascade is unknown, but several studies suggest that this important action of insulin, as well as most metabolic effects, is downstream of the enzyme phosphatidylinositol 3-kinase (PI 3-kinase). Other effects of insulin, such as stimulation of glycogen and lipid synthesis, occur through additional intracellular effects to stimulate the enzymes involved in these reactions. ATP—adenosine triphosphate; GAP—GTPase-activating protein; GRB2—growth-factor receptor binding protein 2; GTP—guanosine triphosphate; IGF—insulin-like growth factor; MEK—MAP-Erk kinase; SOS—son-of-sevenless.

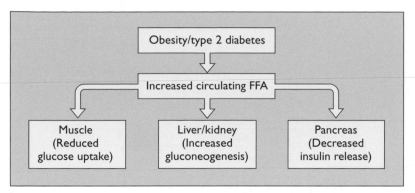

FIGURE 8-12. Insulin resistance and obesity. The insulin resistance associated with type 2 diabetes can be largely explained by obesity because comparably obese individuals with and without type 2 diabetes have quantitatively similar reductions in insulin-receptor binding, insulin-receptor tyrosine kinase activity, and muscle glucose transport [50,92]. Most of these abnormalities in patients with type 2 diabetes can be normalized by weight loss [93]. Current evidence indicates that the most important factor involved in the insulin resistance of obesity in humans is the increased circulating levels of plasma free fatty acids (FFAs) [51]. Experimental elevation of FFAs in normal humans decreases muscle glucose uptake and increases endogenous glucose production; in animal models, this elevation impairs insulin secretion [94,95]. All of these actions would promote hyperglycemia by altering rates of the balance between entry and removal of glucose from the circulation. The mechanisms for the effects of FFAs are twofold: substrate competition [96] and impaired insulin signaling [97]. Acetylated products of FFA metabolism decrease glucose oxidation via inhibition of pyruvate dehydrogenase and activate serine/threonine kinases, possibly through increases in protein kinase C (theta), leading to reduced activity of insulin receptor substrate (IRS) proteins. The main effect of the latter appears to be a reduction in glucose transport [98–100].

STAGES IN THE DEVELOPMENT OF TYPE 2 DIABETES MELLITUS

	Impaired β cell function	Insulin Resistance	Glucose Tolerance
Stage 1	Demonstrable on testing (+)	Absent	Normal
Stage 2	Demonstrable on testing (++)	Present (variable)	Normal
Stage 3	Clearly abnormal (+++)	Worse than above	IGT*
Stage 4	More abnormal (++++)	Worse than above	IGT + IFG†
Stage 5	Markedly abnormal (+++++)	Worse than above	Type 2 diabetes mellitus‡

*Fasting plasma glucose generally normal < 110 mg/dL (6.1 mM), but 2-hour postprandial > 140 mg/dL (7.8 mM) < 200 mg/dL (11.1 mM).
† Fasting plasma glucose > 110 mg/dL (6.1 mM) but less than 126 mg/dL (7.0 mM), and 2-hour postprandial.
‡ Fasting plasma glucose > 126 mg/dL (7.0 mM) or 2-hour postprandial > 200 mg/dL (11.1 mM).

FIGURE 8-13. Stages in development of type 2 diabetes. Longitudinal and cross-sectional studies indicate that individuals destined to develop type 2 diabetes pass through five stages. The first stage begins at birth, when glucose homeostasis is normal but individuals are at risk for type 2 diabetes because of genetic polymorphisms predisposing them to become obese and limiting the ability of their pancreatic β cells to compensate for insulin resistance. During stage 2, decreases in insulin sensitivity emerge as a result of a genetic predisposition and unhealthy lifestyle, which is initially compensated for by an increase in β-cell function so that glucose tolerance remains normal. During stage 3, β-cell function and insulin sensitivity both deteriorate so that when challenged, as during a glucose tolerance test or a standardized meal, postprandial glucose tolerance becomes abnormal. At this point, β-cell function is clearly abnormal but sufficient to maintain normal fasting plasma glucose concentrations. In stage 4, as a result of further deterioration in β-cell functioning and worsening of insulin sensitivity (probably a result of postprandial hyperglycemia), fasting plasma glucose concentrations increase because of an increase in basal endogenous glucose production. Finally, in stage 5, as a result of further deterioration in β-cell function (because of genetic and environmental factors such as glucose and lipotoxicity), both fasting and postprandial glucose levels reach diabetic levels. IFG—impaired fasting glucose; IGT—impaired glucose tolerance.

β-CELL MASS IN TYPE 2 DIABETES MELLITUS

Study	Reduction
Butler et al. [101]	Reduced
Yoon et al. [102]	Reduced
Guiot et al. [103]	Reduced
Stefan et al. [104]	Reduced
Sakuraba et al. [105]	Reduced
Clark et al. [106]	Reduced
Kloppel et al. [107]	Reduced
Gepts et al. [108]	Reduced
Saito et al. [109]	Reduced
Maclean et al. 110]	Reduced
Westermark et al. [111]	Reduced
Rahier et al. [112]	Normal
Deng et al. [113]	Reduced

FIGURE 8-14. Twelve of 13 studies have reported β-cell mass to be reduced in patients with type 2 diabetes [101–113], and one has found β-cell mass to be reduced in people with impaired glucose tolerance [101]. Islet cells from patients with type 2 diabetes have increased rates of apoptosis but normal rates of replication and regeneration [101]. To what extent this decrease in β-cell mass is acquired or genetically programmed is unclear. Various factors have been implicated: intrauterine malnutrition [114,115], glucose toxicity [116–121], lipotoxicity [94,122–124], cytokines [125–127], and accumulation of amyloid within islet cells [128,129]. In addition to a reduced β-cell mass, isolated islet cells from patients with type 2 diabetes secrete less insulin than islet cells from nondiabetic individuals [113], indicating that functional as well as structural abnormalities exist.

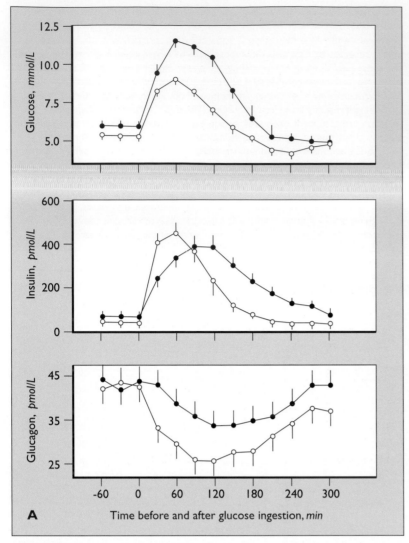

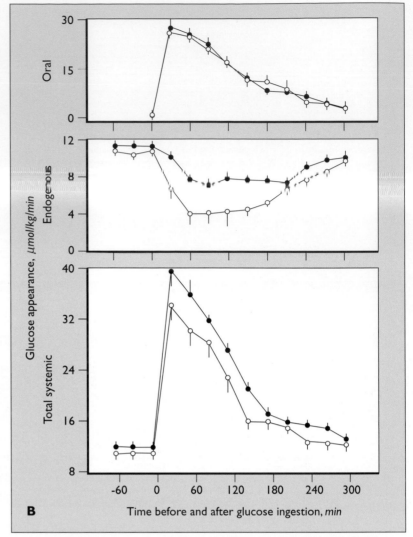

FIGURE 8-15. Comparison of changes in hormones (insulin and glucagon) and rates of glucose production and utilization after glucose ingestion in patients with impaired glucose tolerance (*closed circles*) and in healthy patients (*open circles*). Patients with impaired glucose tolerance (IGT) have normal fasting plasma glucose, insulin, and glucagon levels and normal fasting rates of glucose production and utilization. However, after an oral glucose challenge or a meal, they have a reduced early release of insulin during the initial 30 to 60 minutes accompanied by a reduced decrease in plasma glucagon levels (**A**). These hormonal abnormalities lead to a reduction in the suppression of endogenous glucose production with preservation of normal splanchnic sequestration of the ingested glucose. Consequently, more than a normal amount of glucose enters the systemic circulation (**B**). This exceeds the rates of glucose removal from the circulation during the first

1 to 2 hours so that plasma glucose levels increase more than normal. The hyperglycemia eventually leads to delayed and greater-than-normal plasma insulin levels that, along with the hyperglycemia, cause glucose utilization to exceed glucose production so that plasma glucose eventually returns to normal fasting levels [130,131]. During the 4- to 6-hour postprandial period, a greater-than-normal amount of glucose enters the circulation, and plasma glucose levels start at a normal level and return to a normal level; therefore, it is obvious that a greater-than-normal amount of glucose has been removed from circulation. Although tissue glucose utilization is not reduced in patients with IGT) it is less than would have been found in patients with normal glucose tolerance whose plasma glucose and insulin levels match those of patients with IGT, indicating that patients with IGT are insulin resistant [132]. (*Adapted from* Mitrakou *et al.* [130].)

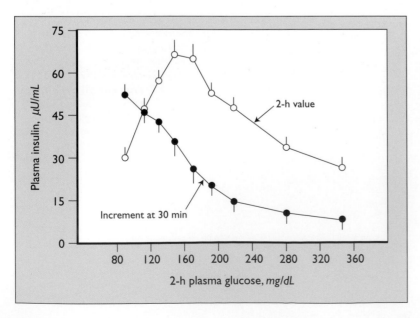

FIGURE 8-16. Comparison of early and late plasma insulin responses during oral glucose tolerance tests. The decrease in early (30 min) postprandial insulin secretion has been correlated with the reduced suppression of endogenous glucose production [130] and decreases progressively as glucose tolerance deteriorates [132]. In contrast, 2-hour insulin levels increase initially and only decrease after 2-hour plasma glucose levels reach diabetic values [18]. The latter phenomenon had been erroneously interpreted to imply that insulin resistance occurs earlier than impaired insulin secretion in the evolution of type 2 diabetes [133], but it is now evident that this results from the hyperglycemia caused by delayed early insulin release [6,7,18,134].

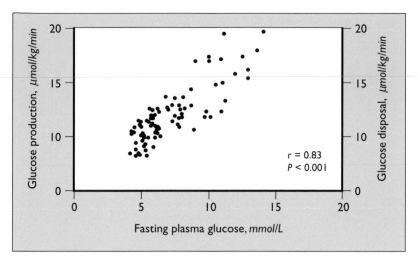

FIGURE 8-17. Glucose production and disposal in the postabsorptive state. With further deterioration in β-cell function, plasma glucose levels in the fasting state increase as a result of impaired suppression of hepatic and renal glucose release by insulin [60]. This is largely due to increased gluconeogenesis [135–138]. As shown in this figure, glucose removal from the circulation also increases as fasting blood glucose levels increase, illustrating that the primary cause of fasting hyperglycemia is overproduction of glucose, not reduced glucose utilization. The increased glucose production results from impaired β-cell function as well as insulin resistance, mediated in part indirectly by increased plasma free fatty acids, increased availability of gluconeogenic substrates, and lack of appropriate suppression of glucagon secretion. (*Adapted from* Dinneen *et al.* [60].)

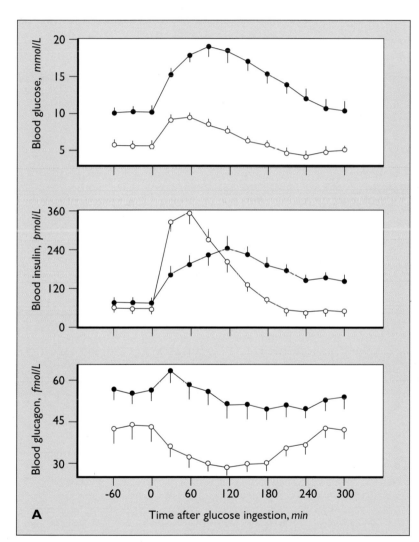

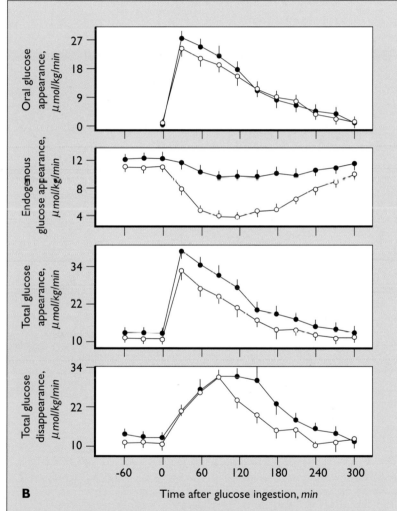

FIGURE 8-18. Comparison of postprandial changes in plasma insulin and glucagon levels (**A**) and rates of glucose appearance and removal from plasma (**B**) in patients with type 2 diabetes and healthy patients. The postprandial abnormalities in patients with type 2 diabetes (*closed circles*) are quite similar to those of people with impaired glucose tolerance (*open circles*), except that they are more exaggerated. The only major difference is that with excessive glycosuria, uptake of glucose in liver is diminished [59,60,139,140]. (*Adapted from* Mitrakou *et al.* [59].)

Control, Complications, and Treatment

UKPDS: EFFECTS OF INTENSIVE TREATMENT OF TYPE 2 DIABETES

Reduced HbA_{1c} by 11% with intensive therapy (7.9% vs 7.0%)

This leads to

12% decrease in any diabetes-related endpoint

25% decrease in microvascular endpoints

21% decrease in retinopathy at 12 years

33% decrease in microalbuminuria at 12 years

25% decrease in cataract

16% decrease in myocardial infarction (ns)

5% decrease in stroke (ns)

FIGURE 8-19. Effects of intensive treatment of type 2 diabetes. Results of the United Kingdom Prospective Diabetes Study (UKPDS) showed an unequivocal effect of intensive insulin therapy on long-term complications of diabetes and mortality [141,142]. HbA_{1c}—glycated hemoglobin.

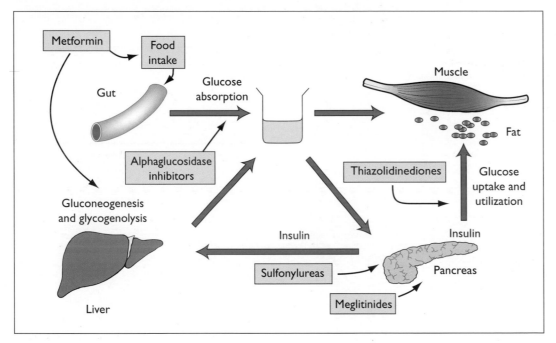

FIGURE 8-20. Sites of action of drugs used to treat type 2 diabetes. Various oral agents are now available for the treatment of type 2 diabetes. These agents differ in their modes of action, efficacy, pharmacokinetics, and side effects. Sulfonylureas and meglitinides are insulin secretagogues that act directly on the pancreatic β cells via inhibiting adenosine triphosphate (ATP)-sensitive potassium channels [73]. Metformin, a biguanide, and the thiazolidinediones (TZDs) are classified as insulin sensitizers [77,143]. Metformin appears to act preferentially to inhibit glucose production and to reduce appetite [144], and the TZDs are thought to work primarily on adipose tissue and muscle to reduce free fatty acid (FFA) release and increase glucose uptake, respectively [78]. The exact mechanism of action of these agents on a molecular level is still poorly understood. Metformin may act on gluconeogenic and mitochondrial enzymes, and the TZDs acting on peroxisome proliferator gamma receptors may alter adipose tissue metabolism (eg, decreased FFAs, tumor necrosis factor-α and resistin release), which then has secondary effects on muscle and liver metabolism [145,146]. In contrast, the mechanism of action of the alphaglucosidase inhibitors is well established [147]. By inhibiting the digestion of dietary starches, they slow the postprandial absorption of glucose. Recently, so-called designer insulins produced by modification of their molecular structure have led to preparations with improved pharmacokinetics. Lispro and aspart insulins are absorbed more rapidly than regular insulin and have a shorter half-life, so that injection of these agents immediately before meal ingestion more closely mimics the normal physiologic profile than that of regular human insulin, which, for optimal benefit, must be injected 30 minutes before meal ingestion [80,148–150]. Glargine insulin is a peakless insulin preparation that lasts an average of 24 hours and has distinct advantages over neutral protamine Hagedorn (NPH) insulin, which peaks at 6 to 8 hours and lasts only 14 hours [80,81,151,152].

References

1. *Diabetes in America*. Bethesda, MD: National Institutes of Health; 1995.

2. Harris M, Flegal K, Cowie C, et al.: Prevalence of diabetes, impaired fasting glucose, and impaired glucose tolerance in U.S. adults. The Third National Health and Nutrition Examination Survey, 1988–1994. *Diabetes Care* 1998, 21:518–524.

3. Bogardus C, Lillioja S, Bennett P: Pathogenesis of NIDDM in Pima Indians. *Diabetes Care* 1991, 14:685–690.

4. Weyer C, Tataranni PA, Bogardus C, Pratley R: Insulin resistance and insulin secretory dysfunction are independent predictors of worsening of glucose tolerance during each stage of type 2 diabetes development. *Diabetes Care* 2000, 24:89–94.

5. Weyer C, Bogardus C, Mott D, Pratley R: The natural history of insulin secretory dysfunction and insulin resistance in the pathogenesis of type 2 diabetes mellitus. *J Clin Invest* 1999, 104:787–794.

6. Kahn S: The importance of β-cell failure in the development and progression of type 2 diabetes. *J Clin Endocrinol Metab* 2001, 86:4047–4058.

7. Pratley R, Weyer C: The role of impaired early insulin secretion in the pathogenesis of type II diabetes mellitus. *Diabetologia* 2001, 44:929–945.

8. Hamman R: Genetic and environmental determinants of noninsulin dependent diabetes mellitus (NIDDM). *Diabetes Metab Rev* 1992, 8:287–338.

9. Stefan N, Fritsche A, Haring H, Stumvoll M: Effect of experimental elevation of free fatty acids on insulin secretion and insulin sensitivity in healthy carriers of the Pro12Ala polymorphism of the peroxisome proliferator-activated receptor-gamma2 gene. *Diabetes* 2001, 50:1143–1148.

10. Horikawa Y, Oda N, Cox N, et al.: Genetic variation in the gene encoding calpain-10 is associated with type 2 diabetes mellitus. *Nat Genet* 2000, 26:163–175.

11. Chandran M, Phillips SA, Ciaraldi T, Henry RR: Adiponectin: more than just another fat cell hormone? *Diabetes Care* 2003, 26:2442–2450.

12. Vasseur F, Lepretre F, Lacquemant C, Froguel P: The genetics of adiponectin. *Curr Diab Rep* 2003, 3:151–158.

13. Havel PJ: Update on adipocyte hormones: regulation of energy balance and carbohydrate/lipid metabolism. *Diabetes* 2004, 53(suppl 1):S143–S151.

14. Yamauchi T, Hara K, Kubota N, et al.: Dual roles of adiponectin/Acrp30 in vivo as an anti-diabetic and anti-atherogenic adipokine. *Curr Drug Targets Immune Endocr Metabol Disord* 2003, 3:243–254.

15. Gloyn A: The genetics of diabetes: a progress report. *Practical Diabetes Int* 2001, 18:246–250.

16. Shaw J, Purdie D, Neil H, et al.: The relative risks of hyperglycemia, obesity and dyslipidemia in relatives of patients with type II diabetes mellitus. *Diabetologia* 1999, 42:24–27.

17. Shatten B, Smith G, Kuller L, Neation J: Risk factors for the development of type 2 diabetes among men enrolled in the usual care group of the multiple risk factor intervention trial. *Diabetes* 1993, 16:1331–1338.

18. Gerich J, Van Haeften T: Insulin resistance versus impaired insulin secretion as the genetic basis for type 2 diabetes. *Curr Opin Endocrinol Diab* 1998, 5:144–148.

19. Pimenta W, Kortytkowski M, Mitrakou A, et al.: Pancreatic beta-cell dysfunction as the primary genetic lesion in NIDDM. *JAMA* 1995, 273:1855–1861.

20. Vaag A, Alford F, Beck-Nielsen H: Intracellular glucose and fat metabolism in identical twins discordant for non-insulin-dependent diabetes mellitus (NIDDM): acquired versus genetic metabolic defects. *Diabetic Med* 1996, 13:806–815.

21. Cerasi E, Luft R: Insulin response to glucose infusion in diabetic and nondiabetic monozygotic twin pairs: genetic control of insulin response. *Acta Endocrinol* 1967, 55:330–345.

22. Barnett A, Spiliopoulos A, Pyke D, et al.: Metabolic studies in unaffected co-twins of noninsulin dependent diabetics. *Br Med J* 1981, 282:1656–1658.

23. Pyke D, Taylor K: Glucose tolerance and serum insulin in unaffected identical twins of diabetics. *Br Med J* 1967, 4:21–22.

24. Hu F, Manson J, Stampfer M, et al.: Diet, lifestyle, and the risk of type 2 diabetes mellitus in women. *N Engl J Med* 2001, 345:790–797.

25. Choi B, Shi F: Risk factors for diabetes mellitus by age and sex: results of the national population health survey. *Diabetologia* 2001, 44:1221–1231.

26. Marshall J, Hoag S, Shetterly S, Hammon R: Dietary fat predicts conversion of impaired glucose tolerance to NIDDM. *Diabetes Care* 1994, 17:50–56.

27. Wei M, Schweitner H, Blair S: The association between physical activity, physical fitness and type 2 diabetes mellitus. *Compr Ther* 2000, 26:176–182.

28. Wannamethee S, Shaper A, Perry I: Smoking as a modifiable risk factor for type 2 diabetes in middle aged men. *Diabetes Care* 2001, 24:1590–1595.

29. Rich-Edwards J, Colditz G, Stampfer M, et al.: Birthweight and the risk for type 2 diabetes mellitus in adult women. *Ann Intern Med* 1999, 130:278–284.

30. Eriksson J, Lindstrom J, Tuomilehto J: Potential for prevention of type 2 diabetes. *Br Med Bull* 2001, 60:183–199.

31. Knowler W, Barrett-Connor E, Fowler S, et al. and the Diabetes Prevention Program Research Group: Reduction in the incidence of type 2 diabetes with lifestyle intervention or metformin. *N Engl J Med* 2002, 346:393–403.

32. Tuomilehto J, Lindstrom J, Eriksson J, et al.: Prevention of type 2 diabetes mellitus by changes in lifestyle among subjects with impaired glucose tolerance. *N Engl J Med* 2001, 344:1343–1350.

33. Pan X-R, Li G-W, Hu Y-H, et al.: Effects of diet and exercise in preventing NIDDM in people with impaired glucose tolerance: The Da Qing IGT and Diabetes Study. *Diabetes Care* 1997, 20:537–544.

34. Erikkson K, Lindgarde F: Prevention of type 2 (noninsulin dependent) diabetes mellitus by diet and exercise. *Diabetologia* 1991, 34:891–898.

35. Wenying Y, Lixiang L, Jinwu Q, et al.: The preventive effect of acarbose and metformin on the progression to diabetes mellitus in the IGT population: a 3-year multicenter prospective study. *Clin J Endocrinol Metab* 2001, 17:131–136.

36. Chiasson J, Josse R, Gomis R, et al.: Acarbose for prevention of type 2 diabetes mellitus: the STOP-NIDDM randomised trial. *Lancet* 2002, 359:2072–2077.

37. Buchanan TA, Xiang AH, Peters RK, et al.: Preservation of pancreatic beta-cell function and prevention of type 2 diabetes by pharmacological treatment of insulin resistance in high-risk hispanic women. *Diabetes* 2002, 51:2796–2803.

38. Torgerson JS, Hauptman J, Boldrin MN, Sjostrom L: XENical in the prevention of diabetes in obese subjects (XENDOS) study: a randomized study of orlistat as an adjunct to lifestyle changes for the prevention of type 2 diabetes in obese patients. *Diabetes Care* 2004, 27:155–161.

39. Porte D, Jr., Kahn S: Beta-cell dysfunction and failure in type 2 diabetes: potential mechanisms. *Diabetes* 2001, 50(suppl 1):S160–S163.

40. Carey D, Jenkins A, Campbell L, et al.: Abdominal fat and insulin resistance in normal and overweight women: direct measurements reveal a strong relationship in subjects at both low and high risk of NIDDM. *Diabetes* 1996, 45:633–638.

41. Banerji M, Chaiken R, Gordon D, et al.: Does intra-abdominal adipose tissue in black men determine whether NIDDM is insulin-resistant or insulin-sensitive? *Diabetes* 1995, 44:141–146.

42. Byrne M, Sturgis J, Sobel R, Polonsky K: Elevated plasma glucose 2h postchallenge predicts defects in B-cell function. *Am J Physiol* 1996, 270:E572–E579.

43. Nesher R, Casa Della L, Litvin Y, et al.: Insulin deficiency and insulin resistance in type II (noninsulin dependent) diabetes: quantitative contributions of pancreatic and peripheral responses to glucose homeostasis. Eur J Clin Invest 1987, 17:266–274.

44. Campbell P, Mandarino L, Gerich J: Quantification of the relative impairment in actions of insulin on hepatic glucose production and peripheral glucose uptake in non-insulin-dependent diabetes mellitus. Metabolism 1988, 37:15–21.

45. Kalant N, Leibovici D, Fukushima N, et al.: Insulin responsiveness of superficial forearm tissues in type 2 (noninsulin-dependent) diabetes. Diabetologia 1982, 22:239–244.

46. Bonora E, Bonadonna R, DelPrato S, et al.: In vivo glucose metabolism in obese and type II diabetic subjects with or without hypertension. Diabetes 1993, 42:764–772.

47. Nosadini R, Solini A, Velussi M, et al.: Impaired insulin-induced glucose uptake by extrahepatic tissue is hallmark of NIDDM patients who have or will develop hypertension and microalbuminuria. Diabetes 1994, 43:491–499.

48. Groop L, Ekstrand A, Forsblom C, et al.: Insulin resistance, hypertension and microalbuminuria in patients with type 2 (non-insulin-dependent) diabetes mellitus. Diabetologia 1993, 36:642–647.

49. Gerich J: The genetic basis of type 2 diabetes mellitus: impaired insulin secretion versus impaired insulin sensitivity. Endocr Rev 1998, 19:491–503.

50. Dohm GL, Tapscott E, Pories W, et al.: An in vitro human muscle preparation suitable for metabolic studies. Decreased insulin stimulation of glucose transport in muscle from morbidly obese and diabetic subjects. J Clin Invest 1988, 82:486–494.

51. Boden G: Role of fatty acids in the pathogenesis of insulin resistance and NIDDM. Diabetes 1997, 46:3–10.

52. Hotamisligil G, Spiegelman B: Tumor necrosis factor a: a key component of the obesity-diabetes link. Diabetes 1994, 43:1271–1278.

53. Steppan C, Bailey S, Bhat S, et al.: The hormone resistin links obesity to diabetes. Nature 2001, 409:307–312.

54. Ahima R, Flier J: Leptin. Annu Rev Physiol 2000, 62:413–437.

55. Ahima R, Flier J: Adipose tissue as an endocrine organ. Trends Endocrinol Metab 2000, 11:327–332.

56. Saltiel A, Kahn C: Insulin signalling and the regulation of glucose and lipid metabolism. Nature 2001, 414:799–806.

57. Kelley D, Goodposter B: Skeletal muscle triglyceride: an aspect of regional adiposity and insulin resistance. Diabetes Care 2001, 24:933–941.

58. Virkamaki A, Korsheninnikova E, Seppala-Lindroos A, et al.: Intramyocellular lipid is associated with resistance to in vivo insulin actions on glucose uptake, antilipolysis, and early insulin signaling pathways in human skeletal muscle. Diabetes 2001, 50:2337–2343.

59. Mitrakou A, Kelley D, Veneman T, et al.: Contribution of abnormal muscle and liver glucose metabolism in postprandial hyperglycemia in noninsulin-dependent diabetes mellitus. Diabetes 1990, 39:1381–1390.

60. Dinneen S, Gerich J, Rizza R: Carbohydrate metabolism in noninsulin-dependent diabetes mellitus. N Engl J Med 1992, 327:707–713.

61. Woerle HJ., Szoke E, Gosmanov N, et al.: Abnormal postprandial splanchnic and peripheral glucose disposal in type 2 diabetes [abstract]. Diabetes 2004, 53(suppl 2):A374.

62. Perseghin G, Petersen K, Shulman GI: Cellular mechanism of insulin resistance: potential links with inflammation. Int J Obes Relat Metab Disord 2003, 27(suppl 3):S6–S11.

63. Petersen KF, Dufour S, Befroy D, et al.: Impaired mitochondrial activity in the insulin-resistant offspring of patients with type 2 diabetes. N Engl J Med 2004, 350:664–671.

64. DCCT Research Group: The effect of intensive treatment of diabetes on the development and progression of long-term complications in insulin dependent diabetes mellitus. N Engl J Med 1993, 329:977–986.

65. UK Prospective Diabetes Study (UKPDS) Group: Effect of intensive blood-glucose control with metformin on complications in overweight patients with type 2 diabetes (UKPDS 34). Lancet 1998, 352:854–865.

66. Reichard P, Pihl M, Rosenqvist U, Sule J: Complications in IDDM are caused by elevated blood glucose level: The Stockholm Diabetes Intervention Study (SDIS) at 10-year follow up. Diabetologia 1996, 39:1483–1488.

67. Stratton I, Adler A, Neil HA, et al.: Association of glycaemia with macrovascular and microvascular complications of type 2 diabetes (UKPDS 35): prospective observational study. Br Med J 2000, 321:405–412.

68. Gerstein H, Pais P, Pogue J, Yusuf S: Relationship of glucose and insulin levels to the risk of myocardial infarction: a case-control study. J Am Coll Cardiol 1999, 33:612–619.

69. Khaw K-T, Wareham N, Luben R, et al.: Glycated haemoglobin, diabetes, and mortality in men in Norfolk cohort of European Prospective Investigation of Cancer and Nutrition (EPIC-Norfolk). Br Med J 2001 322:15–18.

70. Gerich JE: Clinical significance, pathogenesis, and management of postprandial hyperglycemia. Arch Intern Med 2003, 163:1306–1316.

71. Chiasson JL, Josse RG, Gomis R, et al.: Acarbose treatment and the risk of cardiovascular disease and hypertension in patients with impaired glucose tolerance: the STOP-NIDDM trial. JAMA 2003, 290:486–494.

72. Woerle HJ, Pimenta W, Meyer C, et al.: Diagnostic and therapeutic implications of relationships between fasting, 2 hour postchallenge plasma glucose and HbA$_{1c}$ values. Arch Intern Med 2004, 164:1627–1632.

73. Lebovitz H: Insulin secretagogues: old and new. Diab Rev 1999, 7:139–153.

74. Langtry H, Balfour J: Glimepiride. A review of its use in the management of type 2 diabetes mellitus. Drugs 1998, 55:563–584.

75. Dunn C, Faulds D: Nateglinide. Drugs 2000, 60:607–615.

76. Lee Y, Hirose H, Ohneda M, et al.: Beta-cell lipotoxicity in the pathogenesis of non-insulin-dependent diabetes mellitus of obese rats: impairment in adipocyte-beta-cell relationships. Proc Natl Acad Sci U S A 1994, 91:10878–10882.

77. Mudaliar S, Henry R: New oral therapies for type 2 diabetes mellitus: the glitazones or insulin sensitizers. Annu Rev Med 2001, 52:239–257.

78. Inzucchi S, Maggs D, Spollett G, et al.: Efficacy and metabolic effects of metformin and troglitazone in type II diabetes mellitus. N Engl J Med 1998, 338:867–872.

79. Campbell L, Baker D, Campbell RK: Miglitol: assessment of its role in the treatment of patients with diabetes mellitus. Ann Pharmacother 2000, 34:1291–1301.

80. Bolli G, Di Marchi R, Park G, et al.: Insulin analogues and their potential in the management of diabetes mellitus. Diabetologia 1999, 42:1151–1167.

81. Lepore M, Pampanelli S, Fanelli C, et al.: Pharmacokinetics and pharmacodynamics of subcutaneous injection of long-acting human insulin analog glargine, NPH insulin, and ultralente human insulin and continuous subcutaneous infusion of insulin lispro. Diabetes 2000, 49:2142–2148.

82. Abraira C, Henderson W, Colwell J, et al. and the VA CSDM Group: Response to intensive therapy steps and glipizide dose in combination with insulin in type 2 diabetes. Diabetes Care 1998, 21:574–579.

83. Turner R, Cull C, Frighi V, Holman R: Glycemic control with diet, sulfonylurea, metformin, or insulin in patients with type 2 diabetes mellitus. Progressive requirement for multiple therapies (UKPDS 49). JAMA 1999, 281:2005–2012.

84. Siegel E, Mayer G, Nauck M, Creutzfeldt W: Factitious hypoglycemia caused by taking a sulfonylurea drug [German]. Dtsch Med Wochenschr 1987, 112:1575–1579.

85. Wroblewski M, Gottsater A, Lindgarde F, et al.: Gender, autoantibodies, and obesity in newly diagnosed diabetic patients aged 40–75 years. Diabetes Care 1998, 21:250–255.

86. Bell G, Polonsky K: Diabetes mellitus and genetically programmed defects in b-cell function. Nature 2001, 414:788–791.

87. Maassen J, Kadowaki T: Maternally inherited diabetes and deafness: a new diabetes subtype. Diabetologia 1996, 39:375–382.

88. Taylor S, Cama S, Accili D, et al.: Mutations in the insulin receptor gene. Endocr Rev 1992, 13:566–595.

89. Kahn C: Insulin action, diabetogenes, and the cause of type II diabetes. *Diabetes* 1994, 43:1066–1084.

90. Kahn S: The importance of the β-cell in the pathogenesis of type 2 diabetes mellitus. *Am J Med* 2000, 108(suppl 6A):2S–8S.

91. Thorens B, Wu Y, Leahy J, Weir G: The loss of GLUT2 expression by glucose-unresponsive beta cells of db/db mice is reversible and is induced by the diabetic environment. *J Clin Invest* 1992, 90:77–85.

92. Caro J, Sinha M, Raju SM, et al.: Insulin receptor kinase in human skeletal muscle from obese subjects with and without noninsulin dependent diabetes. *J Clin Invest* 1987, 79:1330–1337.

93. Bak J, Moller N, Schmitz O, et al.: In vivo action and muscle glycogen synthase activity in type II (noninsulin dependent) diabetes mellitus: effects of diet treatment. *Diabetologia* 1992, 35:777–784.

94. McGarry J, Dobbins R: Fatty acids, lipotoxicity and insulin secretion. *Diabetologia* 1999, 42:128–138.

95. Unger R, Zhou Y: Lipotoxicity of beta-cells in obesity and in other causes of fatty acid spillover. *Diabetes* 2001, 50(suppl 1):S118–S121.

96. Randle P, Priestman D, Mistry S, Halsall A: Glucose fatty acid interactions and the regulation of glucose disposal. *J Cell Biochem* 1994, 55S:1–11.

97. Shulman G: Cellular mechanisms of insulin resistance. *J Clin Invest* 2000, 106:171–176.

98. Garvey W, Huecksteadt T, Matthaei S, Olefsky J: Role of glucose trans-porters in the cellular insulin resistance of type II noninsulin-dependent diabetes mellitus. *J Clin Invest* 1988, 81:1528–1536.

99. Kelley D, Mintun M, Watkins S, et al.: The effect of non-insulin-dependent diabetes mellitus and obesity on glucose transport and phosphorylation in skeletal muscle. *J Clin Invest* 1996, 97:2705–2713.

100. Cline G, Petersen K, Krssak M, et al.: Impaired glucose transport as a cause of decreased insulin-stimulated muscle glycogen synthesis in type 2 diabetes. *N Engl J Med* 1999, 341:240–246.

101. Butler AE, Janson J, Bonner-Weir S, et al.: Beta-cell deficit and increased beta-cell apoptosis in humans with type 2 diabetes. *Diabetes* 2003, 52:102–110.

102. Yoon KH, Ko SH, Cho JH, et al.: Selective beta-cell loss and alpha-cell expansion in patients with type 2 diabetes mellitus in Korea. *J Clin Endocrinol Metab* 2003, 88:2300–2308.

103. Guiot Y, Sempoux C, Moulin P, Rahier J: No decrease of the beta-cell mass in type 2 diabetic patients. *Diabetes* 2001, 50(suppl 1):S188.

104. Stefan Y, Orci L, Malaisse-Lagae F, et al.: Quantitation of endocrine cell content in the pancreas of nondiabetic and diabetic humans. *Diabetes* 1982, 31:694–700.

105. Sakuraba H, Mizukami H, Yagihashi N, et al.: Reduced beta-cell mass and expression of oxidative stress-related DNA damage in the islet of Japanese Type II diabetic patients. *Diabetologia* 2002, 45:85–96.

106. Clark A, Wells C, Buley I, et al.: Islet amyloid, increased alpha-cells, reduced beta-cells and exocrine fibrosis: quantitative changes in the pancreas in type 2 diabetes. *Diabetes Res* 1988, 9:151–159.

107. Kloppel G, Lohr M, Habich K, et al.: Islet pathology and the pathogenesis of type 1 and type 2 diabetes mellitus revisited. *Surv Synth Pathol Res* 1985, 4:110–125.

108. Gepts W: Contribution to the morphological study of the islands of Langerhans in diabetes; study of the quantitative variations of the different insular constituents. *Ann Soc R Sci Med Nat Brux* 1957, 10:5–108.

109. Saito K, Yaginuma N, Takahashi T: Differential volumetry of A, B, and D cells in the pancreatic islets of diabetic and nondiabetic subjects. *Tohoku J Exp Med* 1979, 129:273–283.

110. Maclean N, Ogilvie RF: Quantitative estimation of the pancreatic islet tissue in diabetic subjects. *Diabetes* 1955, 4:367–376.

111. Westermark P, Wilander E: The influence of amyloid deposits on the islet volume in maturity onset diabetes mellitus. *Diabetologia* 1978, 15:417–421.

112. Rahier J, Goebbels R, Henquin J: Cellular composition of the human diabetic pancreas. *Diabetologia* 1983, 24:366–371.

113. Deng S, Vatamaniuk M, Huang X, et al.: Structural and functional abnor-malities in the islets isolated from type 2 diabetic subjects. *Diabetes* 2004, 53:624–632.

114. Hales C, Barker D, Clark P, et al.: Fetal and infant growth and impaired glucose tolerance at age 64. *Br Med J* 1991, 303:1019–1022.

115. Dahri S, Snoeck A, Reusens-Billen B, et al.: Islet function in offspring of mothers on low-protein diet during gestation. *Diabetes* 1991, 40(suppl 2):115–120.

116. Moran A, Zhang HJ, Olson LK, et al.: Differentiation of glucose toxicity from beta cell exhaustion during the evolution of defective insulin gene expression in the pancreatic islet cell line, HIT-T15. *J Clin Invest* 1997, 99:534–539.

117. Olson LK, Redmon JB, Towle HC, Robertson RP: Chronic exposure of HIT cells to high glucose concentrations paradoxically decreases insulin gene transcription and alters binding of insulin gene regulatory protein. *J Clin Invest* 1993, 92:514–519.

118. Lu M, Seufert J, Habener JF: Pancreatic beta-cell-specific repression of insulin gene transcription by CCAAT/enhancer-binding protein beta. Inhibitory interactions with basic helix-loop-helix transcription factor E47. *J Biol Chem* 1997, 272:28349–28359.

119. Jonas JC, Sharma A, Hasenkamp W, et al.: Chronic hyperglycemia triggers loss of pancreatic beta cell differentiation in an animal model of diabetes. *J Biol Chem* 1999, 274:14112–14121.

120. Tanaka Y, Gleason CE, Tran PO, et al.: Prevention of glucose toxicity in HIT-T15 cells and Zucker diabetic fatty rats by antioxidants. *Proc Natl Acad Sci U S A* 1999, 96:10857–10862.

121. Tajiri Y, Moller C, Grill V: Long-term effects of aminoguanidine on insulin release and biosynthesis: evidence that the formation of advanced glyco-sylation end products inhibits B cell function. *Endocrinology* 1997, 138:273–280.

122. Cnop M, Hannaert JC, Hoorens A, et al.: Inverse relationship between cytotoxicity of free fatty acids in pancreatic islet cells and cellular triglyceride accumulation. *Diabetes* 2001, 50:1771–1777.

123. Maedler K, Spinas GA, Dyntar D, et al.: Distinct effects of saturated and monounsaturated fatty acids on beta-cell turnover and function. *Diabetes* 2001, 50:69–76.

124. Gremlich S, Bonny C, Waeber G, Thorens B: Fatty acids decrease IDX-1 expression in rat pancreatic islets and reduce GLUT2, glucokinase, insulin, and somatostatin levels. *J Biol Chem* 1997, 272:30261–30269.

125. Farney AC, Xenos E, Sutherland DE, et al.: Inhibition of pancreatic islet beta cell function by tumor necrosis factor is blocked by a soluble tumor necrosis factor receptor. *Transplant Proc* 1993, 25:865–866.

126. Bolaffi JL, Rodd GG, Wang J, Grodsky GM: Interrelationship of changes in islet nicotine adeninedinucleotide, insulin secretion, and cell viability induced by interleukin-1 beta. *Endocrinology* 1994, 134:537–542.

127. Campbell IL, Oxbrow L, Harrison LC: Interferon-gamma: pleiotropic effects on a rat pancreatic beta cell line. *Mol Cell Endocrinol* 1987, 52:161–167.

128. Janson J, Ashley R, Harrison D, et al.: The mechanism of islet amyloid polypeptide toxicity is membrane disruption by intermediate-sized toxic amyloid particles. *Diabetes* 1999, 48:491–498.

129. Clark A, Nilsson MR: Islet amyloid: a complication of islet dysfunction or an aetiological factor in Type 2 diabetes? *Diabetologia* 2004, 47:157–169.

130. Mitrakou A, Kelley D, Mokan M, et al.: Role of reduced suppression of glucose production and diminished early insulin release in impaired glucose tolerance. *N Engl J Med* 1992, 326:22–29.

131. Gerich J: Metabolic abnormalities in impaired glucose tolerance. *Metabolism* 1997, 46(suppl 1):40–43.

132. Van Haeften T, Pimenta W, Mitrakou A, et al.: Relative contributions of b-cell function and tissue insulin sensitivity to fasting and post-glucose-load glycemia. *Metabolism* 2000, 49:1318–1325.

133. DeFronzo R: The triumvirate: B-cell, muscle, and liver: a collusion responsible for NIDDM. *Diabetes* 1988, 37:667–687.

134. Calles-Escandon J, Robbins D: Loss of early phase of insulin release in humans impairs glucose tolerance and blunts thermic effect of glucose. *Diabetes* 1987, 36:1167–1172.

135. Meyer C, Stumvoll M, Nadkarni V, et al.: Abnormal renal and hepatic glucose metabolism in type 2 diabetes mellitus. *J Clin Invest* 1998, 102:619–624.

136. Consoli A, Nurjhan N, Capani F, Gerich J: Predominant role of gluconeogenesis in increased hepatic glucose production in NIDDM. *Diabetes* 1989, 38:550–561.

137. Magnusson I, Rothman D, Katz L, *et al.*: Increased rate of gluconeogenesis in type II diabetes. A 13C nuclear magnetic resonance study. *J Clin Invest* 1992, 90:1323–1327.

138. Nurjhan N, Consoli A, Gerich J: Increased lipolysis and its consequences on gluconeogenesis in noninsulin-dependent diabetes mellitus. *J Clin Invest* 1992, 89:169–175.

139. Kelley D, Mokan M, Veneman T: Impaired postprandial glucose utilization in non-insulin-dependent diabetes mellitus. *Metabolism* 1994, 43:1549–1557.

140. Roden M, Petersen K, Shulman G: Nuclear magnetic resonance studies of hepatic glucose metabolism in humans. *Recent Prog Horm Res* 2001, 56:219–237.

141. UK Prospective Diabetes Study (UKPDS) Group: Intensive blood-glucose control with sulphonylureas or insulin compared with conventional treatment and risk of complications in patients with type 2 diabetes (UKPDS 33). *Lancet* 1998, 352:837–853.

142. Turner R: The U.K. Prospective Diabetes Study. A review. *Diabetes Care* 1998, 21(suppl 3):C35–C38.

143. Cusi K, DeFronzo R: Metformin: a review of its metabolic effects. *Diab Rev* 1998, 6:89–131.

144. Stumvoll M, Nurjhan N, Perriello G, *et al.*: Metabolic effects of metformin in non-insulin-dependent diabetes mellitus. *N Engl J Med* 1995, 333:550–554.

145. Gerich J: Oral hypoglycemic agents. *N Engl J Med* 1989, 321:1231–1245.

146. Inzucchi S: Oral antihyperglycemic therapy for type 2 diabetes: scientific review. *JAMA* 2002, 287:360–372.

147. Goke B, Herrmann-Rinke C: The evolving role of alpha-glucosidase inhibitors. *Diabetes Metab Rev* 1998, 14:S31–S38.

148. Mudaliar S, Lindberg F, Joyce M, *et al.*: Insulin aspart (B28 Asp-Insulin): a fast-acting analog of human insulin. Absorption kinetics and action profile compared with regular human insulin in healthy nondiabetic subjects. *Diabetes Care* 1999, 22:1501–1506.

149. Dimitriadis G, Gerich J: Importance of timing preprandial subcutaneous insulin administration in the management of diabetes mellitus. *Diabetes Care* 1983, 6:374–377.

150. Hedman C, Lindstrom T, Arnqvist H: Direct comparison of insulin lispro and aspart shows small differences in plasma insulin profiles after subcutaneous injection in type 1 diabetes. *Diabetes Care* 2001, 24:1120–1121.

151. Ratner R, Hirsch I, Neifing J, *et al.*: Less hypoglycemia with insulin glargine in intensive insulin therapy for type 1 diabetes. *Diabetes Care* 2000, 23:639–643.

152. Rosenstock J, Schwartz S, Clark C, *et al.*: Basal insulin therapy in type 2 diabetes. *Diabetes Care* 2001, 24:631–636.

MANAGEMENT OF TYPE 2 DIABETES MELLITUS

Jennifer B. Marks

9

Diabetes and its complications are a significant cause of morbidity and mortality in the United States. The prevalence of diabetes has been steadily increasing in the US population, based on national household interview surveys conducted during the past 40 years [1–3]. Undiagnosed diabetes and abnormal glucose tolerance are considered to have substantial clinical importance (*see* Fig. 9-1) [1,2].

Approximately 90% to 95% of people with diabetes have type 2 diabetes [1]. The pathogenesis of type 2 diabetes involves inadequate insulin secretion from pancreatic β cells and inadequate insulin action in target tissues (insulin resistance) (*see* Figs. 9-2 and 9-3). When these tissues become insulin resistant, hepatic glucose production increases, glucose uptake is decreased, and lipolysis is enhanced. Increased free fatty acids (FFAs) from lipolysis stimulate cellular uptake of FFAs and lipid oxidation. In muscle, the increased FFA availability accelerates fat oxidation, resulting in decreased insulin-mediated glucose uptake and disposal. In the liver, elevated FFAs stimulate gluconeogenesis and increase hepatic glucose output. When β-cell dysfunction is also present, insulin resistance in the target tissues leads to hyperglycemia, elevated plasma FFA levels, and the development of type 2 diabetes(*see* Figs. 9-2 and 9-3) [4–8].

Insulin resistance is present before the onset of clinical disease and is a predictor of its development [9–11]. In the natural history of progression to diabetes, β cells increase insulin secretion in response to insulin resistance and for a period of time are able to effectively maintain glucose levels below the diabetic range. However, when β-cell function begins to decline, insulin production is insufficient to overcome the insulin resistance, and blood glucose levels increase. The increase in glycemia is paralleled by the decline in β-cell function. After it is established, insulin resistance remains relatively stable over time. Therefore, progression of diabetes is a result of worsening β-cell function with preexisting established insulin resistance. (*see* Fig. 9-4).

Environmental factors, particularly abdominal obesity and a sedentary lifestyle, are important contributors to the development of diabetes, largely because of their effects on insulin sensitivity (*see* Fig. 9-5) [3,12–16]. Specific population subgroups have a higher prevalence of diabetes than the population as a whole (*see* Fig. 9-6) [16]. The greater the number of risk factors present in an individual, the greater the chance that that individual will develop diabetes. The risk of developing diabetes increases with increasing age (> 45 years), obesity (body mass index > 25 kg/m^2), and lack of physical activity. Type 2 diabetes is more common in individuals with a family history of the disease and in members of certain racial or ethnic groups (*eg*, African Americans, Hispanic Americans, Native Americans, Asian Americans, and Pacific Islanders). It occurs frequently in women with a history of gestational diabetes or polycystic ovarian syndrome and in individuals with hypertension, dyslipidemia (high-density lipoprotein cholesterol < 35 mg/dL or triglyceride level > 250 mg/dL), vascular disease, impaired glucose tolerance (IGT), or impaired fasting glucose (IFG). Routine screening for diabetes is recommended for those age 45 or older; however, individuals who fall into any of these higher risk categories should be screened earlier.

The diagnostic criteria for diabetes and the two high-risk states of abnormal glucose metabolism, IFG, and IGT are defined [17]. IFG is a fasting plasma glucose level of 100 mg/dL or greater but less than 126 mg/dL. IGT is a plasma glucose level of greater than or equal to 140 mg/dL but less than 200 mg/dL 2 hours after a 75-g oral glucose load. If symptoms are present, a casual plasma glucose of greater than 200 mg/dL is diagnostic of diabetes. In the absence of unequivocal hyperglycemia, the diagnosis of diabetes must be confirmed on a subsequent day by the measurement of fasting plasma glucose or 2 hours after an oral glucose load (*see* Fig. 9-7).

Chronic poor glucose control is associated with development of diabetic vascular complications. These include microvascular (retinopathy, neuropathy, and nephropathy) and macrovascular (premature cardiovascular disease [CVD]) complications. CVDs (coronary and cerebrovascular) account for 65% of deaths in patients with type 2 diabetes (*see* Fig. 9-8) [18]. Epidemiologic studies have shown the risk of a myocardial infarction (MI) or CVD death in a diabetic individual with no history of CVD is similar to that of an individual who has had a previous CVD event (*see* Figs. 9-9 and 9-10) [19,20]. Glycemic levels in the high-normal but nondiabetic range may even be associated with increased CVD risk (*see* Fig. 9-11) [21].

In addition to hyperglycemia, individuals with type 2 diabetes often have a myriad of other metabolic abnormalities that increase their cardiovascular risk, including dyslipidemia, hypertension, and abnormalities of fibrinolysis and coagulation (*see* Fig. 9-12) [22–29]. The Multiple Risk Factor Intervention Trial (MRFIT), which studied 347,978 men aged 35 to 57 years, demonstrated the absolute risk of CVD death to be approximately three times higher for men with diabetes than for those without diabetes, regardless of age, ethnic background, and risk factor level (*see* Fig. 9-13). With progressively less favorable baseline risk factor status, the CVD mortality rate increased much more steeply for men with diabetes than for their nondiabetic counterparts [30]. In the United Kingdom Prospective Diabetes Study (UKPDS), coronary heart disease (CHD) risk factors were evaluated by inclusion in a Cox proportional hazards model [31]. In order, and all statistically significant, the variables were low-density lipoprotein cholesterol, high-density lipoprotein cholesterol, hemoglobin A_{1C}, and systolic blood pressure (*see* Fig. 9-14).

A number of interventional trials (the Diabetes Control and Complications Trial, UKPDS, Kumamoto Study, Stockholm Diabetes Intervention Study) have demonstrated that microvascular complications can be delayed or prevented by maintaining excellent glycemic control (*see* Figs. 9-15 and 9-16) [32–38]. In several studies in the setting of acute illness, intensive insulin therapy with improved glycemic control has been shown in to improve outcomes in people with and without diabetes (*see* Fig. 9-17) [39,40].

Direct evidence of the impact of improved glycemic control on macrovascular complications is lacking. In the UKPDS, a 16% reduction in the risk of MI, including nonfatal and fatal MI and sudden death, was observed in the cohort of type 2 diabetic patients randomized to tight blood glucose control, just missing the level for statistical significance [36]. A secondary multivariate observational analysis of the 10-year follow-up data of the original UKPDS cohort was performed to evaluate the relationship between exposure to hyperglycemia and the development of vascular complications [41]. The results showed that for every 1% reduction in A_{1C}, there was a 14% decrease in fatal and nonfatal MI (*see* Fig. 9-18). Similar risk reduction was shown in a secondary multivariate observational analysis of systolic blood pressure [42]. Based on results from clinical trials of glycemic control and impact on diabetic microvascular complications, recommendations for targets of glycemic control have been put forth (*see* Fig. 9-19) [43].

Other interventions have been demonstrated to be effective in reducing CVD in type 2 diabetes. The Micro-Hope Study included 3577 with types 1 and 2 diabetes, with and without hypertension, and compared the cardiovascular event rates with the angiotensin-converting enzyme (ACE) inhibitor ramipril versus placebo [44]. The results demonstrated that treatment with ramipril lowered the risk of the combined primary outcome of combined MI, stroke, or CVD mortality by 25%, MI by 22%, stroke by 33%, and cardiovascular death by 37% (*see* Fig. 9-20). Lowering of serum cholesterol has been demonstrated in many studies to be effective at reducing CVD risks as primary and secondary prevention. Recent studies have questioned whether more aggressive low-density lipoprotein cholesterol lowering in high-risk individuals should be the appropriate target of such treatment (*see* Figs. 9-21 and 9-22) [45,46].

The many antidiabetic agents for the treatment of type 2 diabetes target different mechanisms in the underlying pathogenesis of the disease [47,48]. Sulfonylureas and the glitinides (repaglinide, nateglinide) are insulin secretagogues that stimulate release of insulin from the pancreas. Metformin improves insulin sensitivity primarily by reducing insulin resistance in the liver, thereby decreasing hepatic glucose production. The thiazolidinediones (rosiglitazone, pioglitazone) improve insulin sensitivity primarily in the muscle, thereby increasing peripheral uptake and utilization of glucose. The α-glucosidase inhibitors (acarbose, precose) prevent the breakdown of carbohydrates to glucose in the gut by inhibiting the enzymes that catalyze this process, delaying carbohydrate absorption. Insulin and insulin analogues increase insulin levels in the presence of declining β-cell function and diminished endogenous insulin secretion (*see* Fig. 9-23). The efficacy of the different classes of antidiabetic drugs are similar when used as monotherapy. In addition to taking antihyperglycemic agents, all patients with type 2 diabetes should be encouraged to maintain a healthy lifestyle by exercising and following an appropriate diet (*see* Fig. 9-24) [48,49]. A variety of insulins and insulin analogues complete the armamentarium of treatment options for therapy of type 2 diabetes (*see* Fig. 9-25) [50–55].

Recently, a national sample of 733 adults with type 2 diabetes was studied from 1991 to 1994 in the Third National Health and Nutrition Examination Survey (NHANES III) [56]. Of the patients with hypertension, 83% were diagnosed and treated with antihypertensive agents and only 17% were undiagnosed or untreated; most of the patients known to have dyslipidemia were treated with medication or diet (89%). Health status and outcomes were less than optimal: 58% had hemoglobin A_{1c} (HbA$_{1c}$) greater than 7.0, 45% had a body mass index above 30, 28% had microalbuminuria, and 8% had clinical proteinuria. Of patients known to have hypertension and dyslipidemia, 60% were not controlled to accepted levels. In addition, 22% of patients smoked cigarettes, 26% had to be hospitalized during the previous year, and 42% assessed their health status as fair or poor (*see* Fig. 9-26).

Risk determinants of CVD in addition to low-density lipoprotein (LDL) cholesterol include the presence or absence of CHD, other clinical forms of atherosclerotic disease, and the major risk factors other than LDL (cigarette smoking, hypertension, low high-density lipoprotein cholesterol, family history of premature CHD, and older age [men > 45 years, women > 55 years]). Based on these other risk determinants, the Expert Panel on Detection, Evaluation, and Treatment of High Blood Cholesterol in Adults (Adult Treatment Panel III) identified three categories of risk that modify the goals and modalities of LDL-lowering therapy (*see* Fig. 9-27) [57].

In the NHANES III 1999–2000, and NHANES III, US adults aged 20 years and older with previously diagnosed diabetes were surveyed [58]. Only 37% of the NHANES 1999–2000 participants achieved the target goal of HbA$_{1c}$ below 7%, and only 35.8% achieved the target systolic blood pressure of less than 130 mm Hg and diastolic blood pressure of less than 80 mm Hg. More than 50% the participants had total cholesterol levels of greater than 200 mg/dL, and only 7.3% of adults with diabetes had overall "good control" (*ie*, attained target goals for all vascular risk factors) (*see* Fig. 9-28).

An important recent study used a focused, multifactorial intervention with continued patient education and motivation and strict targets and individualized risk assessment in patients with type 2 diabetes and microalbuminuria who are at increased risk for macrovascular and microvascular complications. Such patients may represent about one third of the population of patients with type 2 diabetes. The data suggest that a long-term, targeted, intensive intervention involving multiple risk factors reduces the risk of cardiovascular and microvascular events by about 50% among these patients. The advantages of a multifactorial approach to the reduction of cardiovascular risk are clear. The challenge remains to ensure that this approach can be widely adopted [59].

Using a focused, multifaceted approach in individuals at risk has demonstrated that the onset of clinical type 2 diabetes can be delayed or prevented [60,61]. The Diabetes Prevention Program was a 27-center, randomized, controlled trial. It included 3234 people with impaired glucose tolerance, randomized to placebo, metformin (850 mg twice daily), or a lifestyle modification program with the goals of at least a 7% weight loss and at least 150 minutes of physical activity per week. The participants were followed for an average of 2.8 years. After 4 years of follow-up, the results demonstrated a 58% reduction in the incidence of diabetes development in the intensive lifestyle group, compared with a 31% reduction in the incidence of diabetes development in the metformin group, both highly statistically significant compared with the placebo group (*see* Fig. 9-29).

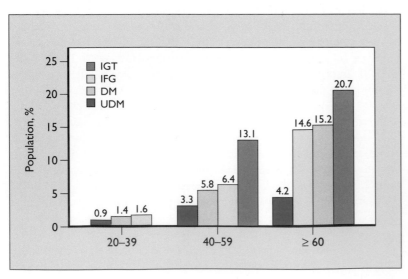

FIGURE 9-1. Prevalence of diagnosed diabetes (DM), undiagnosed diabetes (UDM), and impaired fasting glucose (IFG), 1999–2000, and impaired glucose tolerance (IGT), 1988–1994, National Health and Nutrition Examination Survey (NHANES) III and NHANES 1999–2000 in the US adult population [1,2].

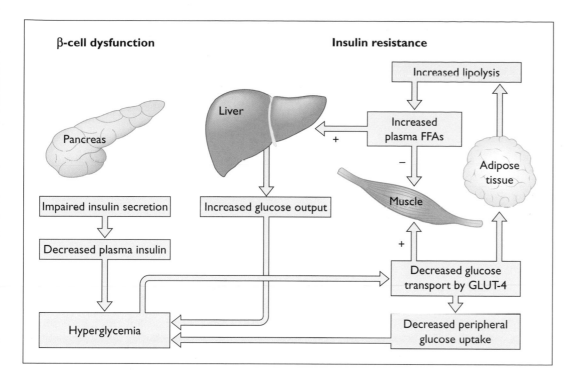

β-cell dysfunction

Insulin resistance

FIGURE 9-2. Defects in the pancreas and target tissues for insulin action in type 2 diabetes. In nondiabetic individuals, insulin suppresses hepatic glucose production, stimulates glucose uptake into muscle and adipose tissue, and suppresses lipolysis in adipose tissue. When these tissues become insulin resistant, hepatic glucose production increases, glucose uptake is decreased, and lipolysis is enhanced. Increased free fatty acids (FFAs) from lipolysis stimulate cellular uptake of FFAs and lipid oxidation. In muscle, the increased FFA availability accelerates fat oxidation, resulting in decreased insulin-mediated glucose uptake and disposal. In the liver, elevated FFAs stimulate gluconeogenesis and increase hepatic glucose output. When β-cell dysfunction is also present, insulin resistance in the target tissues leads to hyperglycemia and the development of type 2 diabetes [4]. GLUT—glucose transporter.

FIGURE 9-3. Defects in metabolism in type 2 diabetes as a result of insulin resistance and deficient insulin secretion. Insulin resistance in the liver results in increased gluconeogenesis, decreased glycogen synthesis and glucose oxidation, and increased free fatty acid (FFA) oxidation. The net result is increased hepatic glucose production. In muscle and adipose tissue, glucose transport and oxidation are decreased. In muscle, glycogen synthesis is decreased and FFA oxidation is increased. In adipose tissue, lipolysis is increased. The net result is hyperglycemia and elevated plasma FFA levels [4–8]. GLUT—glucose transporter.

SUMMARY OF DEFECTS IN INSULIN ACTION IN TYPE 2 DIABETES

	Liver	Muscle	Apidose
Gluconeogenesis	Y	—	—
GLUT-4 translocation	—	Y	Y
Glucose transport	—	Y	Y
Glycogen synthesis	Y	Y	—
Glucose oxidation	Y	Y	Y
FFA oxidation	Y	Y	—
Lipolysis	—	—	Y

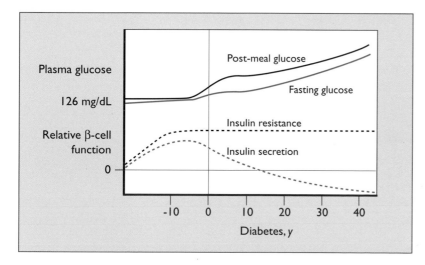

FIGURE 9-4. Natural history of type 2 diabetes. In the natural history of the development of type 2 diabetes, insulin resistance is present before the onset of clinical disease. β cells increase insulin secretion in response to insulin resistance and for a period of time are able to effectively overcome it and maintain glucose levels below the diabetic range. However, when β-cell function begins to decline, insulin production is insufficient to overcome the insulin resistance, and blood glucose levels increase. As illustrated, the increase in glycemia is paralleled by the decline in β-cell function. Note that once it is established, insulin resistance remains relatively stable over time. Therefore, progression of diabetes is a result of worsening β-cell function with preexisting established insulin resistance. Note also that the increase in postmeal glucose in this graph occurs before the increase in fasting glucose, a commonly seen occurrence in the prediabetic phase [9–11]. (*Adapted from* International Diabetes Center, Minneapolis, MN.)

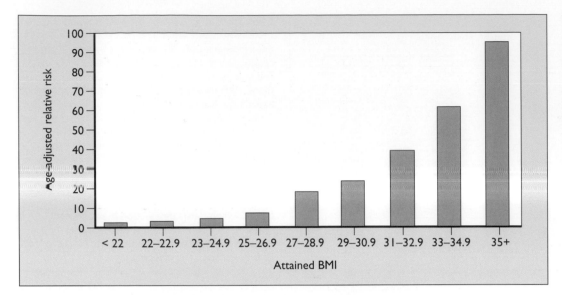

FIGURE 9-5. Relative risk of the development of type 2 diabetes based on body mass index (BMI) in women. Body weight is one of the strongest environmental predictors of the development of type 2 diabetes. Studies such as the Nurses Health Study, which followed 114,281 women age 30 to 55 years for 14 years, found that BMI was the dominant predictor of risk for diabetes mellitus, and the age-adjusted relative risk for diabetes development began to increase at a BMI of 24 mg/kg^2 and increased dramatically as BMI increased beyond that level [12].

RISKS FOR TYPE 2 DIABETES

Age 45 years or older
Overweight or obesity (BMI 25 kg/m^2 or greater)
Family history of type 2 diabetes
Habitual physical inactivity
Race/ethnicity
IGT or IFG
History of gestational diabetes or delivery of a baby > 9 pounds
Hypertension
HDL cholesterol 35 mg/dL or less and/or triglyceride level 250 mg/dL or greater
Polycystic ovarian syndrome
History of vascular disease

FIGURE 9-6. Populations at increased risk for type 2 diabetes. Specific population subgroups have a much higher prevalence of diabetes than the population as a whole. The greater the number of risk factors present in an individual, the greater the chance of that individual developing diabetes. The risk of developing diabetes increases with increasing age, obesity, and lack of physical activity. Type 2 diabetes is more common in individuals with a family history of the disease and in members of certain racial or ethnic groups (eg, African Americans, Hispanic Americans, Native Americans, Asian Americans, and Pacific Islanders). It occurs with great frequency in women with prior gestational diabetes or polycystic ovarian syndrome and in individuals with hypertension, dyslipidemia, impaired glucose tolerance (IGT), or impaired fasting glucose (IFG) [16]. BMI—body mass index; HDL—high-density lipoprotein.

CRITERIA FOR THE DIAGNOSIS OF DIABETES

Normal	IFG or IGT	Diabetes
FPG < 100 mg/dL	FPG 100 or greater and < 126 mg/dL	FPG 126 mg/dL or greater
2-h PG < 140 mg/dL	2-h PG 140 or greater and < 200 mg/dL	2-h PG 200 mg/dL or greater
		Symptoms of diabetes and CPG 200 mg/dL or greater

FIGURE 9-7. The diagnostic criteria for diabetes and the classification of impaired fasting glucose (IFG) and impaired glucose tolerance (IGT). In the absence of unequivocal hyperglycemia, a diagnosis of diabetes must be confirmed on a subsequent day by measurement of fasting plasma glucose (FPG) or 2-hour FPG (2-hour post 75 g glucose load). A casual plasma glucose (CPG) above 200 mg/dL, is diagnostic if symptoms are present [16].

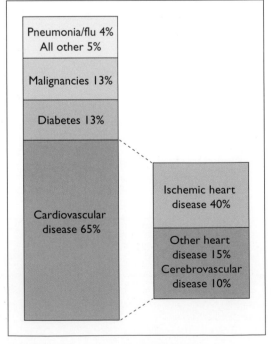

FIGURE 9-8. Causes of death in diabetic individuals. Cardiovascular diseases (coronary and cerebrovascular) account for 65% of deaths in patients with diabetes. (Adapted from Geiss et al. [18].)

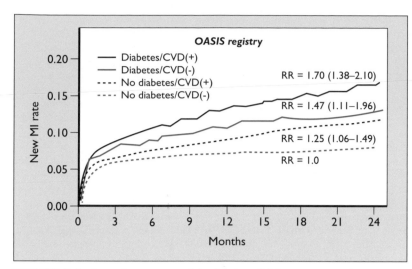

FIGURE 9-9. Rate of new myocardial infarctions (MIs) in patients with and without diabetes and with and without cardiovascular disease (CVD). The OASIS (Organization to Assess Strategies for Ischemic Syndromes) registry was a multicenter European registry of individuals with and without diabetes and risk for new coronary events. The data demonstrated that across this population, those with diabetes and a history of previous CVD had the highest risk for a subsequent event over the follow-up period of 2 years. Those without diabetes or CVD had the lowest risk. Most significantly, the data demonstrated that the risk of a MI in diabetic individuals with no history of CVD was very similar to that of individuals who had already had a previous CVD event [19]. RR—relative risk.

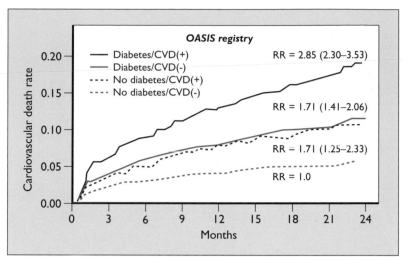

FIGURE 9-10. Cardiovascular disease (CVD) death rates for patients with and without diabetes. The OASIS (Organization to Assess Strategies for Ischemic Syndromes) registry demonstrated that the risk of cardiac death in a diabetic individual with no history of CVD was exactly the same as that of an individual who had already had CVD [19]. RR—relative risk.

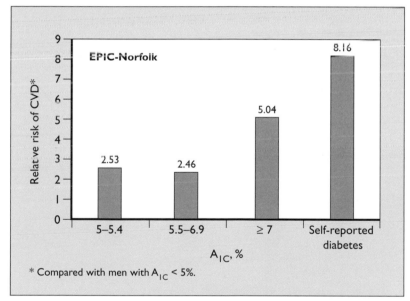

* Compared with men with A_{1C} < 5%.

FIGURE 9-11. Risk of cardiovascular disease (CVD) mortality correlated with hemoglobin A_{1C} (HbA$_{1C}$). Khaw et al. [21] studied the relation between A_{1C} concentrations, diabetes, and subsequent mortality in 4662 men age 45 to 79 years from the Norfolk cohort of the European Prospective Investigation into Cancer and Nutrition (EPIC—Norfolk). They found that A_{1C} (to values < 5%) was *continuously* related to subsequent all-cause, cardiovascular, and ischemic heart disease mortality with no evidence of a threshold. An increase of 1% in A_{1C} was associated with a 28% (P < 0.002) increase in the risk of death independent of age, blood pressure, serum cholesterol, basal metabolic index, and cigarette smoking.

Furthermore, the small increased risk of CVD (per person) in persons without diabetes but with relatively high normal A1C levels (5% to 6.9%), who accounted for approximately 70% of the total population, contributed more to the total population mortality than did the larger increased risk of CVD in patients with diabetes, who accounted for only approximately 5% of the total population. The total contribution to excess mortality from CVD in nondiabetic persons with glycemia was 82%. In contrast, the total contribution from CVD in patients with self-reported diabetes was only 18%.

Thus, in addition to the use of treatments for controlling glycemia in patients with diabetes, some consideration should perhaps be given to the introduction of strategies for reducing glycemia in nondiabetic persons with elevated A_{1C} levels. Lowering their CVD risk would decrease the total population mortality. Based on data from the men in this cohort with A_{1C} of 5% or above, a reduction of only 0.1% or 0.2% would reduce the total population mortality by 5% or 10%, respectively [21].

POTENTIAL FACTORS IN DEVELOPMENT OF DIABETIC VASCULAR COMPLICATIONS

Abnormalities in apoproteins and lipoproteins

Hemodynamic stress

Glycosylation and advanced glycosylation end-products; altered protein structure and function

Glycoxidation and oxidative stress

Decreased NO production and increased vascular permeability

Increased growth factors and extracellular matrix overproduction

Endothelial dysfunction, prothrombotic, proinflammatory state

Insulin resistance

FIGURE 9-12. Potential factors contributing to diabetic vascular complications. Microvascular disease is a leading cause of blindness, kidney failure, and nerve damage in individuals with diabetes. Accelerated atherosclerosis and macrovascular disease in diabetes leads to increased risk of myocardial infarctions, strokes, and nontraumatic lower extremity amputations [22–29]. AGEs—advanced glycation endproducts; NO—nitric oxide.

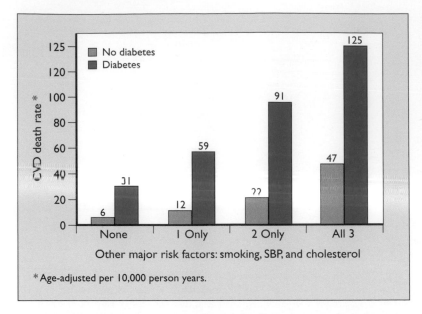

*Age-adjusted per 10,000 person years.

FIGURE 9-13. The interaction of diabetes with other risk factors on the risk of cardiovascular disease (CVD) death as shown in the Multiple Risk Factor Intervention Trial (MRFIT). The MRFIT, with 347,978 men age 35 to 57 years who were followed for 12 years, demonstrated that the absolute risk of CVD death was about three times higher for men with diabetes than for those without diabetes, regardless of age, ethnic background, or risk factor level. The significant predictors in both groups of men were serum cholesterol level, systolic blood pressure (SBP), and cigarette smoking.

With progressively less favorable baseline risk factor status, the CVD mortality rate increased much more steeply for men with diabetes than for their nondiabetic counterparts. Therefore, the absolute excess risk of CVD death became progressively greater for diabetic than for nondiabetic men, and men with diabetes and poorer baseline risk factors had worse prognoses.

This graph shows that the men with diabetes in this trial had a fivefold increased risk of CVD mortality during an average 12-year interval, even in the absence of the three other major CVD risk factors (ie, cholesterol level > 200 mg/dL, SBP > 120 mm Hg, and cigarette smoking). In addition, diabetes was associated with a much higher risk of CVD death in the presence of any one, two, or three of these other factors (with relative risks: 4.82, 4.05, and 2.64, respectively) [30].

RISK FACTORS IN THE UKPDS EVALUATED BY COX PROPORTIONAL HAZARDS MODEL

Coronary Artery Disease (n = 280)

Position in Model	Variable	P Value*
First	LDL cholesterol	< 0.0001
Second	HDL cholesterol	0.0001
Third	HbA$_{1c}$	0.0022
Fourth	Systolic blood pressure	0.0065
Fifth	Smoking	0.056

*Adjusted for age and gender.

FIGURE 9-14. Stepwise selection of risk factors in 2693 white patients with type 2 diabetes with dependent variable as time to first event. In the United Kingdom Prospective Diabetes Study (UKPDS), coronary heart disease (CHD) risk factors were evaluated by their inclusion in a Cox proportional hazards model. In order, the variables included in the model were low-density lipoprotein (LDL) cholesterol, high-density lipoprotein (HDL) cholesterol, hemoglobin A$_{1c}$ (HbA$_{1c}$), systolic blood pressure, and smoking. Although HbA$_{1c}$ was highly statistically significant, so were conventional cardiovascular risk factors, the most important of which seem to be LDL and HDL. Triglyceride level did not enter the multivariate analysis and was not a powerful predictor, even when HDL was not included in the model [31].

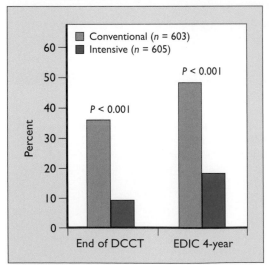

FIGURE 9-15. Progression of retinopathy for the Epidemiology of Diabetes Interventions and Complications (EDIC) participants. The post-Diabetes Control and Complications Trial (DCCT) long-term follow-up study, known as the EDIC trial, is following a cohort of subjects from the DCCT. Those who had been treated with intensive insulin therapy during the DCCT had a 76% reduction in the risk of progression of retinopathy compared with the conventional treatment cohort at the end of the DCCT. At the completion of the 4-year EDIC follow-up, participants who had been in the intensive treatment arm of the DCCT demonstrated a continued 75% reduction in the risk of progression of retinopathy despite maintaining the same level of glycemic control over these 4 years as the conventional treatment group [32,33].

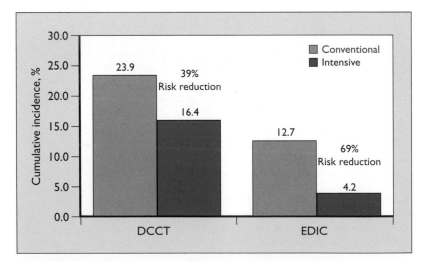

FIGURE 9-16. Progression of microalbuminuria for the Epidemiology of Diabetes Interventions and Complications (EDIC) participants. At the completion of the 4-year EDIC follow-up, participants who had been in the intensive treatment arm of the Diabetes Control and Complications Trial (DCCT) also demonstrated a continued 69% reduction in the risk of progression of microalbuminuria despite maintaining the same level of glycemic control over these 4 years as the conventional treatment group [34,35].

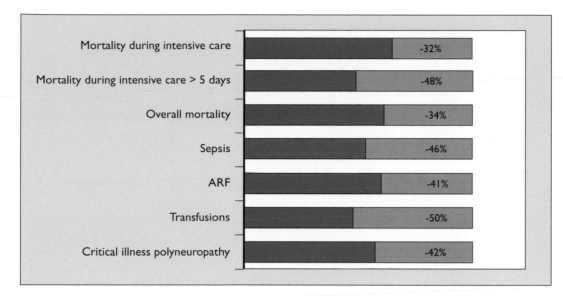

FIGURE 9-17. Benefits of intensive insulin therapy in critically ill patients with and without diabetes. A total of 1548 adults patients admitted to a surgical intensive care unit who were receiving mechanical ventilation were randomly assigned to receive intensive insulin therapy (maintenance of blood glucose at a level between 80 and 110 mg/dL) or conventional treatment (infusion of insulin only if the blood glucose level exceeded 215 mg/dL and maintenance of glucose at a level between 180 and 200 mg/dL).

The authors found that intensive insulin therapy reduced mortality during intensive care from 8.0% with conventional treatment to 4.6% (*P* < 0.04, with adjustment for sequential analyses). The benefit of intensive insulin therapy was attributable to its effect on mortality among patients who remained in the intensive care unit for more than 5 days (20.2% with conventional treatment compared with 10.6% with intensive insulin therapy; *P* = 0.005). The greatest reduction in mortality involved deaths attributable to multiple-organ failure with a proven septic focus. Intensive insulin therapy also reduced overall in-hospital mortality by 34%, bloodstream infections by 46%, acute renal failure (ARF) requiring dialysis or hemofiltration by 41%, the median number of red blood cell transfusions by 50%, and critical illness polyneuropathy by 44%. Additionally, patients receiving intensive therapy were less likely to require prolonged mechanical ventilation and intensive care [40].

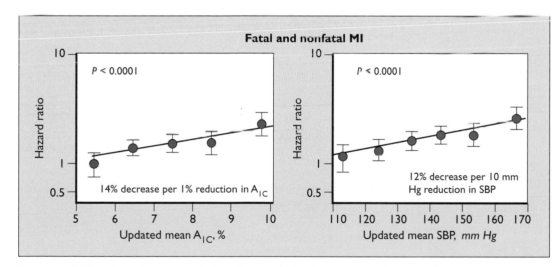

FIGURE 9-18. Glycemia- and systolic blood pressure (SBP)-associated risk reduction for myocardial infarction (MI) in the United Kingdom Prospective Diabetes Study (UKPDS). In the UKPDS, a 16% reduction (*P* = 0.052) in the risk of MI, including nonfatal and fatal MI and sudden death, was observed in the cohort of type 2 diabetic patients randomized to tight blood glucose control, just missing the level for statistical significance. The cohort assigned to tight blood pressure control had a nonsignificant 21% reduction in risk of MI (*P* = 0.13).

These graphs illustrate the results of secondary multivariate observational analyses of the 10-year follow-up data of the original UKPDS cohort performed to evaluate the relationships between exposure to hyperglycemia and hypertension over time and the development of vascular complications. Exposure to glycemia was measured as the updated mean of annual measurements of hemoglobin A_{1c} (HbA$_{1c}$) concentration and exposure to hypertension, the updated mean of annual SBP measurements. Shown are the hazard ratios of fatal and nonfatal MI as log linear plots of the estimated association between categories of the updated mean HbA$_{1c}$ (*left panel*) and the updated mean SBP (*right panel*). The reference categories (hazard ratio = 1.0) were HbA$_{1c}$ less than 6.0% and SBP less than 120 mm Hg, respectively. The P values reflected a contribution of glycemia and SBP, respectively, to the multivariate model. Reduction in the risks of fatal and nonfatal MI for each 1.0% reduction in updated HbA$_{1c}$, 14% (8% to 21%, *P* < 0.0001), and for each 10–mm Hg reduction in updated mean SBP, 12% (7% to 16%, *P* < 0.0001), were similar [41,42].

GLYCEMIC GOALS

	ADA	AACE
HbA$_{1c}$	< 7.0%	< 6.5%
FPG, *mg/dL*	80–120	< 110
2-h BG, *mg/dL*	< 180	< 140
HS BG, *mg/dL*	100–140	100–140

FIGURE 9-19. Glycemic goals (whole blood values) as recommended by the American Diabetes Association (ADA) and the American Association of Clinical Endocrinologists (AACE) [43]. BG—blood glucose; FPG—fasting plasma glucose; HbA$_{1c}$—hemoglobin A$_{1c}$; HS BG—bedtime blood glucose.

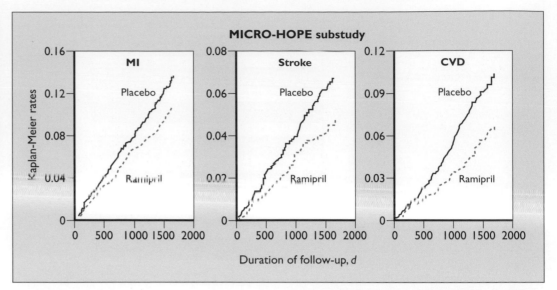

FIGURE 9-20. Angiotensin-converting enzyme (ACE) inhibitor effects on cardiovascular disease (CVD). The MICRO-HOPE (Heart Outcomes Prevention Evaluation) study included 9297 high-risk patients, 3577 with types 1 and 2 diabetes, with and without hypertension, and compared the cardiovascular event rates with the ACE inhibitor ramipril versus placebo. The primary endpoint was combined myocardial infarction (MI), stroke, or CVD mortality.

The results demonstrated that treatment with ramipril lowered the risk of the combined primary outcome by 25% (95% confidence interval [CI], 12–36; P = 0.0004), MI by 22% (CI, 6–36), stroke by 33% (CI, 10–50), cardiovascular death by 37% (CI 21–51), total mortality by 24% (CI, 8–37), revascularization by 17% (CI, 2–30), and overt nephropathy by 24% (CI, 3–40; P =0.027). After adjustment for the changes in systolic (2.4 mm Hg) and diastolic (1.0 mm Hg) blood pressures, ramipril still lowered the risk of the combined primary outcome by 25% (CI, 12–36; P =0.0004) [44].

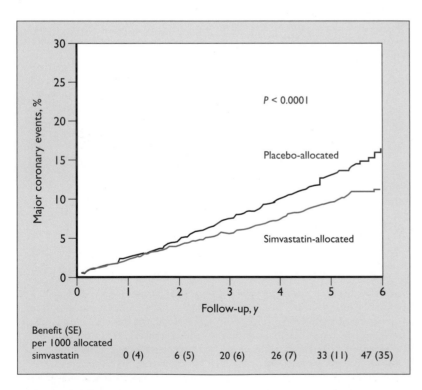

FIGURE 9-21. Heart Protection Study: effect of cholesterol lowering on vascular events in diabetic subjects. A total of 5963 adults with diabetes and 14,573 with occlusive arterial disease age 40 to 80 years were randomized to simvastatin 40 mg/day or placebo and followed for 5 years. The average difference in total cholesterol between the two groups was 39 mg/dL. The results of the study for individuals with diabetes showed that lowering low-density lipoprotein cholesterol by 1 mmol/L (40 mg/dL) reduces the risk of major vascular events by about 25% during 5 years of treatment, and continued statin treatment prevents not only first but also subsequent major vascular events. [45].

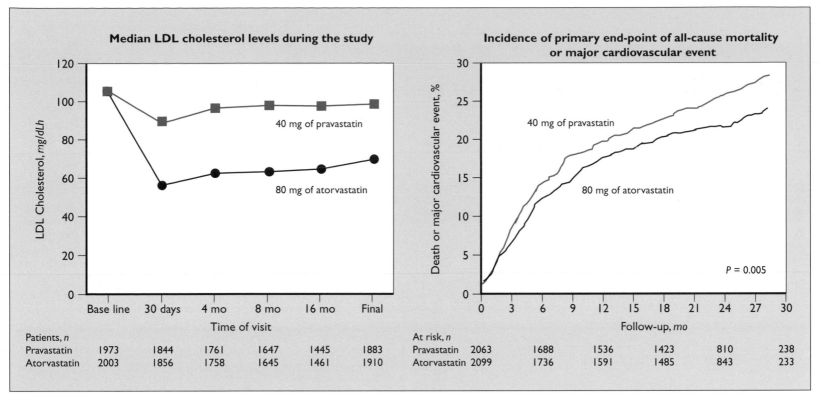

Median LDL cholesterol levels during the study

Incidence of primary end-point of all-cause mortality or major cardiovascular event

Patients, n	Base line	30 days	4 mo	8 mo	16 mo	Final
Pravastatin	1973	1844	1761	1647	1445	1883
Atorvastatin	2003	1856	1758	1645	1461	1910

At risk, n						
Pravastatin	2063	1688	1536	1423	810	238
Atorvastatin	2099	1736	1591	1485	843	233

FIGURE 9-22. Pravastatin or Atorvastatin Evaluation and Infection Therapy Thrombolysis in Myocardial Infarction (PROVE-IT TIMI 22): effect of cholesterol lowering in patients with acute coronary events. A total of 4162 patients who had been hospitalized for an acute coronary syndrome within the preceding 10 days, age 40 to 80 years, were randomized to pravastatin 40 mg/day or atorvastatin 80 mg/day and followed for 18 to 36 months. Approximately 17.5% of each group had diabetes. The primary endpoint was a composite of death, myocardial infarction (MI), unstable angina, revascularization, or stroke. Median levels of low-density lipoprotein (LDL) cholesterol in the two groups were 95 and 62 mg/dL, respectively.

Kaplan-Meier estimates of the rates of the primary endpoint at 2 years were 26.3% in the pravastatin group and 22.4% in the atorvastatin group, reflecting a 16% reduction in the hazard ratio in favor of the group with the lower LDL levels (P = 0.005; 95%, 5% to 26%) [46].

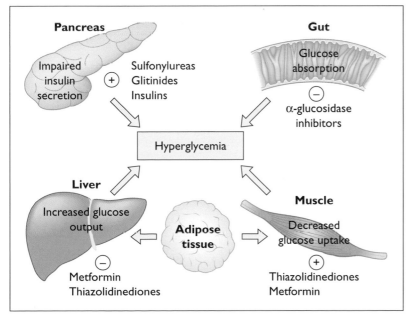

FIGURE 9-23. Antidiabetic agents and their mechanisms of action. The many antidiabetic agents used in the treatment of patients with type 2 diabetes target different mechanisms in the underlying pathogenesis of the disease. Sulfonylureas and the glitinides (repaglinide, nateglinide) are insulin secretagogues that stimulate release of insulin from the pancreas. Metformin improves insulin sensitivity primarily by reducing insulin resistance in the liver, thereby decreasing hepatic glucose production. The thiazolidinediones (rosiglitazone, pioglitazone) improve insulin sensitivity primarily in the muscle, thereby increasing peripheral uptake and utilization of glucose. The α-glucosidase inhibitors (acarbose, precose) prevent the breakdown of carbohydrates to glucose in the gut by inhibiting the enzymes that catalyze this process, delaying carbohydrate absorption. Insulin and insulin analogues increase insulin levels in the presence of declining β-cell function and diminished endogenous insulin secretion [47,48].

EFFICACY OF MONOTHERAPY WITH ORAL DIABETES AGENTS

Drug	Fasting Plasma Glucose Reduction, mg/dL	A_1c Reduction, %
Thiazolidinedione	35–40	0.5–1.0
Sulfonylurea	60–70	1.0–2.0
Biguanide	60–70	1.0–2.0
Glitinide	60–70	1.0–2.0
α-Glucosidase inhibitor	20–30	0.5–1.0

FIGURE 9-24. Fasting glucose and glycohemoglobin responses to pharmacologic treatment in patients with type 2 diabetes. A number of antihyperglycemic agents are available for patients with type 2 diabetes. Treatment decisions must take into consideration patient conditions that may contraindicate the use of the drug, any adverse effects as well as any beneficial effects such as weight loss, and patient and physician preferences. In addition to taking antihyperglycemic agents, all patients with type 2 diabetes should be encouraged to maintain a healthy lifestyle by exercising and following an appropriate diet [43,48,49].

COMPARISON OF HUMAN INSULINS AND ANALOGS

Insulin Preparations	Onset of Action	Peak, h	Duration of action, h
Lispro/aspart	5–15 min	1–2	4–6
Regular human	30–60 min	2–4	6–10
Human NPH/Lente	1–2 h	4–8	10–20
Human Ultralente	2–4 h	10–16	16–20
Glargine	1–2 h	Flat	~24
Detimir	~2–3 h	4–8	10–20

FIGURE 9-25. Comparison of human insulins and analogs. Genetically engineered human insulin preparations generally show a rapid onset of action and durations of action ranging from 4 to 6 hours to approximately 1 full day. The absorption of insulin glargine is prolonged and usually without unwanted peaks; thus, it fulfills the basal insulin requirements without the disadvantages of other currently used insulin preparations. It is recommended for once-daily dosing. Insulin detemir is also a long-acting, twice-a-day insulin analogue that binds to albumin and may provide more predictable fasting blood glucose with lower intrasubject variation and reduced risk of hypoglycemia compared with neutral protamine Hagedorn (NPH). Insulin glargine and human NPH insulin demonstrate an onset of action within 1 to 2 hours after subcutaneous administration. Insulin detemir has a slower onset of action and a milder peak than NPH. Insulin glargine has approximately twice the duration of action of NPH [50–55].

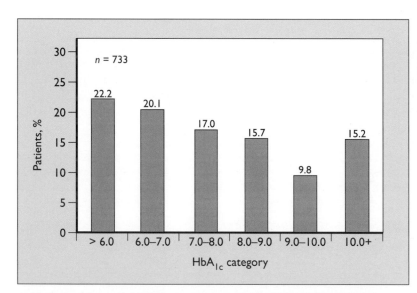

FIGURE 9-26. Health status of US adults: distribution of hemoglobin A_{1c} (HbA$_{1c}$) values in type 2 diabetic patients. A national sample of 733 adults with type 2 diabetes was studied from 1991 to 1994 in the Third National Health and Nutrition Examination Survey (NHANES). Structured questionnaires and clinical and laboratory assessments were used to determine the frequencies of physician visits; health insurance coverage; screening for diabetes complications; treatment for hyperglycemia, hypertension, and dyslipidemia; and the proportion of patients who met their treatment goals. The study established criteria for health outcome measures, including hyperglycemia, albuminuria, obesity, hypertension, and dyslipidemia. Almost all (95%) patients had one source of primary care, two or more physician visits during the past year (88%), and health insurance coverage (91%). Most (76%) were treated with insulin or oral agents for their diabetes, and 45% of patients taking insulin monitored their blood glucose at least once a day. The patients were frequently screened for retinopathy (52%), hypertension (88%), and dyslipidemia (84%). Of patients with hypertension, 83% were diagnosed and treated with antihypertensive agents, and only 17% were undiagnosed or untreated; most of the patients known to have dyslipidemia were treated with medication or diet (89%). Health status and outcomes were less than optimal: 58% had HbA$_{1c}$ levels greater than 7.0, 45% had a body mass index above 30, 28% had microalbuminuria, and 8% had clinical proteinuria. Of patients known to have hypertension and dyslipidemia, 60% were not controlled to accepted levels. In addition, 22% of patients smoked cigarettes, 26% had to be hospitalized during the previous year, and 42% assessed their health status as fair or poor [56].

NCEP ATP III: LDL GOALS AND THERAPY

CHD or CHD equivalent (10 y risk > 20%) TLC at 100 mg/dL or greater	Goal < 100 mg/dL Drug Rx at 130 mg/dL or greater
2+ risk factors (10 y risk 20% or less) TLC at 130 mg/dL or greater	Goal < 130 mg/dL Drug Rx at 130–160 mg/dL or greater
0–1 risk factor TLC at 160 mg/dL or greater	Goal < 160 mg/dL Drug Rx at 190 mg/dL or greater

FIGURE 9-27. National Cholesterol Education Program (NCEP) Adult Treatment Panel III (ATP III): low-density lipoprotein (LDL) goals and therapy according to risk category. Risk determinants in addition to LDL cholesterol include the presence or absence of coronary heart disease (CHD), other clinical forms of atherosclerotic disease, and the major risk factors other than LDL (ie, cigarette smoking, hypertension, low high-density lipoprotein (HDL), family history of premature CHD, and age [men 45 y and older, women 55 y and older]). Based on these other risk determinants, the ATP III identifies three categories of risk that modify the goals and modalities of LDL-lowering therapy [57]. TLC—therapeutic lifestyle change.

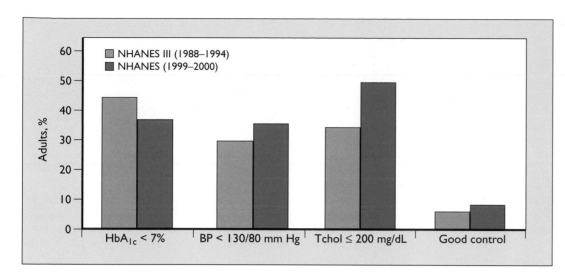

FIGURE 9-28. US adults with recommended levels of vascular disease risk factors. In the National Health and Nutrition Examination Survey (NHANES) 1999–2000 and NHANES III, US adults age 20 years and older with previously diagnosed diabetes were surveyed. In NHANES 1999–2000, participants were diagnosed at an earlier age, had greater body mass indexes, and were more likely to use insulin in combination with oral agents. Only 37% of the NHANES 1999–2000 participants achieved the target goal of hemoglobin A_{1c} (HbA_{1c}) below 7%, and only 35.8% achieved the target systolic blood pressure of less than 130 mm Hg and diastolic blood pressure of less than 80 mm Hg. More than half of the participants had total cholesterol levels of greater than 200 mg/dL. Additionally, only 7.3% of adults with diabetes had overall "good control" (*ie*, attained target goals for all vascular risk factors) [58]. BP—blood pressure; Tchol—total cholesterol.

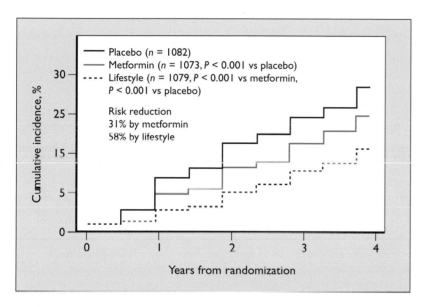

FIGURE 9-29. Prevention of type 2 diabetes: Diabetes Prevention Program (DPP). The DPP was a 27-center, randomized, controlled trial that included 3234 people with impaired glucose tolerance, age 25 to 85 years, with a mean body mass index of 34 mg/kg^2. The subjects were randomized to one of three groups: placebo, metformin (850 mg twice daily), or a lifestyle modification program with the goals of at least a 7% weight loss and at least 150 minutes of physical activity per week. The participants were followed for an average of 2.8 years. The results demonstrated a 58% reduction in the incidence of diabetes development in the intensive lifestyle group compared with a 31% reduction in the incidence of diabetes development in the metformin group; both are highly statistically significant compared with the placebo group [60].

References

1. Harris MI, Flegal KM, Cowie CC, *et al*.: Prevalence of diabetes, impaired fasting glucose, and impaired glucose tolerance in US adults. The Third National Health and Nutrition Examination Survey, 1988–1994. *Diabetes Care* 1998, 21:518–524.

2. Cowie CC, Rust KF, Byrd-Holt D, *et al*.: Prevalence of diabetes and impaired fasting glucose in adults, United States, 1999-2000. *MMWR Morb Mortal Wkly Rep* 2003, 52:833–837.

3. Mokdad AH, Ford ES, Bowman BA, et. al.: Diabetes trends in the US: 1990–1998. *Diabetes Care* 2000, 23:1278–1283.

4. DeFronzo RA: Lilly lecture 1987. The triumvirate: beta-cell, muscle, liver. A collusion responsible for NIDDM. *Diabetes* 1988, 37:667–687.

5. Boden G, Chen X: Effects of fat on glucose uptake and utilization in patients with non-insulin-dependent diabetes. *J Clin Invest* 1995, 96:1261–1268.

6. Groop LC, Bonadonna RC, DelPrato S, *et al*.: Glucose and free fatty acid metabolism in non-insulin-dependent diabetes mellitus. Evidence for multiple sites of insulin resistance. *J Clin Invest* 1989, 84:205–213.

7. Lewis GF, Carpentier A, Vranic M, Giacca A: Resistance to insulin's acute direct hepatic effect in suppressing steady-state glucose production in individuals with type 2 diabetes *Diabetes* 1999, 48:570–576.

8. Shepard PR, Kahn BB. Mechanisms of Disease: glucose transporters and insulin action — implications for insulin resistance and diabetes mellitus. *N Engl J Med* 1999, 341:248–257.

9. Weyer C, Tataranni PA, Bogardus C, *et al*.: Insulin resistance and insulin secretory dysfunction are independent predictors of worsening of glucose tolerance during each stage of type 2 diabetes development. *Diabetes Care* 2000, 24:89–94.

10. Kahn S: The importance of β-cell failure in the development and progression of type 2 diabetes. *J Clin Endocrinol Metab* 2001, 86:4047–4058.

11. Weyer C, Bogardus C, Mott D, *et al*.: The natural history of insulin secretory dysfunction and insulin resistance in the pathogenesis of type 2 diabetes mellitus. *J Clin Invest* 1999, 104:787–794.

12. Colditz GA, Willett WC, Rotnitzky A, Manson JE: Weight gain as a risk factor for clinical diabetes mellitus in women. *Ann Intern Med* 1995, 122:481–486.

13. Choi B, Shi F: Risk factors for diabetes mellitus by age and sex: results of the national population health survey. *Diabetologia* 2001, 44:1221–1231.

14. Hu F, Manson J, Stamfer M, *et al*.: Diet, lifestyle, and the risk of type 2 diabetes in women. *N Engl J Med* 2001, 345:790–797.

15. Wei M, Schweitner H, Blair S: The association between physical activity, physical fitness, and type 2 diabetes mellitus. *Compr Ther* 2000, 26:176–182.

16. American Diabetes Association: Position statement. Screening for type 2 diabetes. *Diabetes Care* 2004, 27(suppl 1):S11–S14.

17. American Diabetes Association: Position statement. Standards of medical care for diabetes. *Diabetes Care* 2004 27: S15–S35.

18. Geiss LS, Herman WH, Smith PJ: Mortality in non-insulin dependent diabetes. In *Diabetes in America*, edn 2. National Diabetes Data Group, National Institutes of Health, NIDDK. NIH pub no. 95-1468; 1995:233–257.

19. Malmberg K, Yusuf S, Gerstein HC, *et al.*: Impact of diabetes on long-term prognosis in patients with unstable angina and non-Q-wave myocardial infarction: results of the OASIS (Organization to Assess Strategies for Ischemic Syndromes) registry. *Circulation* 2000, 102:1014–1019.

20. Haffner SM, Lehto S, R÷nnemaa T, *et al.*: Mortality from coronary heart disease in subjects with type 2 diabetes and in nondiabetic subjects with and without prior myocardial infarction. *N Engl J Med* 1998, 339:229–234.

21. Khaw K-T, Wareham N, Luben R, *et al.*: Glycated hemoglobin, diabetes, and mortality in men in Norfolk cohort of European Prospective Investigation of Cancer and nutrition (EPIC-Norfolk). *Br Med J* 2001, 322:15–18.

22. Bierman EL: George Lyman Duff Memorial Lecture. Atherogenesis in diabetes. *Arterioscler Thromb* 1992, 12:647–656.

23. Ginsberg HN: Insulin resistance and cardiovascular disease. *J Clin Invest* 2000, 106:453–458.

24. Hsueh WA, Law RE: Cardiovascular risk continuum: implications of insulin resistance and diabetes. *Am J Med* 1998, 105:4S–14S.

25. Williams SB, Goldfine AB, Timimi FK, *et al.*: Acute hyperglycemia attenuates endothelium-dependent vasodilation in humans in vivo. *Circulation* 1998, 97:1695–1701.

26. Adler AI, Stratton IM, Neil HA, *et al.*: Association of systolic blood pressure with macrovascular complications of type 2 diabetes (UKPDS: 36). *Br Med J* 2000, 321:412–419.

27. Meigs JB, Mittleman MSA, Nathan DM, *et al.*: Hyperinsulinemia, hyperglycemia and impaired homeostasis. The Framingham Offspring Study. *JAMA* 2000, 283:221–228.

28. Cooper ME, Bonnet F, Oldfield M, Jandeleit-Dahm K: Mechanisms of diabetic vasculopathy: an overview. *Am J Hypertens* 2001, 14:475–486.

29. Brownlee M: Biochemistry and molecular cell biology of diabetic complications. *Nature* 2001, 414:813–820.

30. Stamler J, Vaccaro O, Neaton JD, Wentworth D: Diabetes, other risk factors, and 12-yr cardiovascular mortality for men screened in the Multiple Risk Factor Intervention Trial. *Diabetes Care* 1993, 16:434–444.

31. Turner RC, Millns H, Neil HA, *et al.*: Risk factors for coronary artery disease in non-insulin dependent diabetes mellitus: United Kingdom Prospective Diabetes Study (UKPDS: 23). *BMJ* 1998, 316:823–828.

32. The Diabetes Control and Complications Trial Research Group: The effect of intensive treatment of diabetes on the development and progression of long-term complications in insulin-dependent diabetes mellitus. *N Engl J Med* 1993, 329:977–986.

33. The Diabetes Complications and Control/Epidemiology of Diabetes Interventions and Complications Research Group: Retinopathy and nephropathy in patients with type 1 diabetes four years after a trial of intensive therapy. *N Engl J Med* 2000, 342:381–389.

34. The Diabetes Control and Complications (DCCT) Research Group: Effect of intensive therapy on the development and progression of diabetic nephropathy in the Diabetes Control and Complications Trial. *Kidney Int* 1995 47:1703–1720.

35. Steffes MW, Molitch M, Chavers BM, *et al.* and the DCCT/EDIC Study Group: Sustained reduction in albuminuria six years after the Diabetes Control and Complications Trial. *Diabetes* 2001, 50(suppl):A63.

36. United Kingdom Prospective Diabetes Study Group: Effect of intensive blood glucose control with sulfonylurea or insulin compared with conventional treatment and risk of complications in patients with type 2 diabetes. *Lancet* 1998, 352:837–853.

37. Ohkubo Y, Kishikawa H, Araki E, *et al.*: Intensive insulin therapy prevents the progression of diabetic microvascular complications in Japanese patients with non-insulin-dependent diabetes mellitus: a randomized prospective 6-year study. *Diabetes Res Clin Pract* 1995, 28:103–117.

38. Reichard P, Pihl M, Rosenqvist U, Sule J: Complications in IDDM are caused by elevated blood glucose level: the Stockholm Diabetes Intervention Study (SDIS) at 10-year follow up. *Diabetologia* 1996, 39:1483–1488.

39. Malmberg K, Ryden L, Efendic S, *et al.*: Randomized trial of insulin-glucose infusion followed by subcutaneous insulin treatment in diabetic patients with acute myocardial infarction (DIGAMI Study): effects on mortality at 1 year. *J Am Coll Cardiol* 1995, 26:57–65.

40. Van den Berghe G, Wouters P, Weekers F, *et al.*: Intensive insulin therapy in critically ill patients. *N Engl J Med* 2001, 345:1359–1367.

41. Stratton IM, Adler AI, Neil HAW, *et al.* for the UK Prospective Diabetes Study Group. Association of glycemia with macrovascular and microvascular complications of type 2 diabetes (UKPDS 35): prospective observational study. *BMJ* 2000, 321:405–412.

42. Adler AI, Stratton IM, Neil HA, *et al.*: Association of systolic blood pressure with macrovascular and microvascular complications of type 2 diabetes (UKPDS 36): prospective observational study. *Br Med J* 2000, 321:412–419.

43. American Diabetes Association: Position statement. Standards of medical care for patients with diabetes mellitus. *Diabetes Care* 2002, 25:213–229.

44. Heart Outcomes Prevention Evaluation Study Investigators: Effects of ramipril on cardiovascular and microvascular outcomes in people with diabetes mellitus: results of the HOPE study and MICRO-HOPE substudy. *Lancet* 2000, 355:253–259.

45. Collins R, Armitage J, Parish S, *et al.* and the Heart Protection Study Collaborative Group: MRC/BHF Heart Protection Study of cholesterol-lowering with simvastatin in 5963 people with diabetes: a randomised placebo-controlled trial. *Lancet* 2003, 361:2005–2016.

46. Cannon C P, Braunwald E, McCabe CH, *et al.*: Intensive versus moderate lipid lowering with statins after acute coronary syndromes. *N Engl J Med* 2004, 350:1495–1504.

47. White JR, Campbell K: Recent developments in the pharmacological reduction of blood glucose in patients with type 2 diabetes *Clin Diab* 2001, 19:153–159.

48. DeFronzo RA: Pharmacologic therapy for type 2 diabetes. *Ann Intern Med* 1999, 131:281–303.

49. Nathan DM: Initial management of glycemia in type 2 diabetes mellitus. *N Engl J Med* 2002, 347:1342–1349.

50. Bolli GB, Di Marchi RD, Park GD, *et al.*: Insulin analogues and their potential in the management of diabetes mellitus. *Diabetologia* 1999, 42:1151–1167.

51. Edelman SV, Henry RR: Insulin therapy for normalizing glycosylated hemoglobin in type II diabetes. Application, benefits, and risks. *Diabetes Rev* 1995, 3:308–334.

52. Skyler JS: Insulin therapy in type 2 diabetes mellitus. In *Current Therapy of Diabetes Mellitus*. Edited by DeFronzo RA. St Louis: Mosby-Year Book; 1998:108–116.

53. Herbst KL, Hirsch IB: Insulin strategies for primary care providers. *Clin Diab* 2002, 20:11–17.

54. Heinemann L, Sinha K, Weyer C, *et al.*: Time-action profile of the soluble, fatty acid acylated, long-acting insulin analogue NN304. *Diabetes Med* 1999, 16:332–338.

55. Home P, Bartley P, Russell-Jones D, *et al.*: Insulin detemir offers improved glycemic control compared with NPH insulin in people with type 1 diabetes: a randomized clinical trial. *Diabetes Care* 2004, 27:1081–1087.

56. Harris MI: Health care and health status and outcomes for patients with type 2 diabetes. *Diabetes Care* 2000, 23:754–758.

57. Expert Panel on Detection, Evaluation, and Treatment of High Blood Cholesterol in Adults (Adult Treatment Panel III): Executive summary of the third report of the National Cholesterol Education Program Expert Panel on detection, evaluation, and treatment of high blood cholesterol in adults. *JAMA* 2001, 285:2486–2497.

59. Saydah SH, Fradkin J, Cowie, CC: Poor control of risk factors for vascular disease among adults with previously diagnosed diabetes. *JAMA* 2004, 291:335–342.

59. Gaede P, Vedel P, Larsen N, *et al.*: Multifactorial intervention and cardiovascular disease in patients with type 2 diabetes. *N Engl J Med* 2003, 348:383–393.

60. The Diabetes Prevention Program Research Group: Reduction in the incidence of type 2 diabetes with lifestyle intervention or metformin. *N Engl J Med* 2002, 346:393–403.

61. Tuomilehto J, Lindstrom J, Eriksson JG, *et al.* and the Finnish Diabetes Prevention Study Group: Prevention of type 2 diabetes mellitus by changes in lifestyle among Subjects with impaired glucose tolerance. *N Engl J Med* 2001, 344:1343–1350.

DIABETES AND PREGNANCY

Lois Jovanovic

10

Hyperglycemia during pregnancy is the most common metabolic problem of pregnancy today [1]. The prevalence of hyperglycemia during pregnancy may be as high as 13% [2] (0.1% of the pregnant population per year have type 1 diabetes, 2% to 3% have type 2 diabetes, and up to 12% of the population have gestational diabetes mellitus [GDM]). Although all types of diabetes increase the risk of complications to the mother and the fetus, it is most important to distinguish among the types because each has a different impact on the course of pregnancy and the development of the fetus. Pregestational diabetes mellitus (type 1 or type 2) is more serious because it is present before pregnancy; thus, its effect begins at fertilization and implantation and continues throughout pregnancy and thereafter. In particular, organogenesis may be disrupted, leading to a high risk of early abortion [3], severe congenital defects [4], and retarded growth [5]. Maternal manifestations are also more serious, especially in the presence of vascular complications such as retinopathy or nephropathy [6]. GDM usually appears in the second half of pregnancy and affects mainly fetal growth rate [7]. The offspring of mothers with GDM have a higher risk of subsequent obesity and slower systemic and psychosocial development and probably other long-term metabolic effects [8,9].

Historically, few women with pregestational diabetes lived to childbearing age before the advent of insulin therapy. Until insulin became commercially available in 1924, less than 100 pregnancies were reported in diabetic women, and most likely these women had type 2, and not type 1, diabetes. Even with this assumption, these cases of diabetes and pregnancy were associated with a greater than 90% infant mortality rate and a 30% maternal mortality rate [10]. As late as 1980, some physicians were still counseling diabetic women to avoid pregnancy [11]. This philosophy was justified because of the poor obstetric history in 30% to 50% of diabetic women. Infant mortality rates finally began to improve after 1980, when treatment strategies stressed better control of maternal plasma glucose levels and after self-monitoring of blood glucose and hemoglobin A_{1c} became available to enable better metabolic control in persons with diabetes [12]. As the pathophysiology of pregnancy complicated by diabetes has been elucidated and as management programs have achieved and maintained near normoglycemia throughout pregnancy complicated by types 1 and 2 diabetes and GDM, perinatal mortality rates have become comparable with those of the general population [13]. The Pedersen [14] hypothesis links maternal hyperglycemia-induced fetal hyperinsulinemia to morbidity of the infant. Fetal hyperinsulinemia may cause increased fetal body mass (macrosomia) and, subsequently, a difficult delivery, or cause inhibition of pulmonary maturation of surfactant and, therefore, respiratory distress of the neonate. The fetus may also have decreased serum potassium levels caused by the elevated insulin and

glucose levels that may induce fatal cardiac arrhythmias. Neonatal hypoglycemia may cause permanent neurologic damage.

The literature since the advent of insulin has documented that programs of near-normal glycemia are associated with improved outcome [15]. Therefore, treatment strategies have been developed to minimize the fetal exposure to either sustained or intermittent periods of hyperglycemia [16]. The maternal postprandial glucose level has been shown to be the most important variable to affect the subsequent risk of neonatal macrosomia [17]. When the postprandial glucose levels are blunted 1 hour after beginning a meal, the risk of macrosomia is minimized [18].

There is an increased prevalence of congenital anomalies and spontaneous abortions in women with types 1 and 2 diabetes who are in poor glycemic control during the period of fetal organogenesis, which is nearly complete by 7 weeks postconception [19]. It has also been reported that some women with GDM are also at risk for bearing a malformed infant because they most probably had undiagnosed (and thus untreated) type 2 diabetes during the time of organogenesis. Because women may not know they are pregnant during the critical time period for organ formation, prepregnancy counseling and planning are essential for all pregestational diabetic women of childbearing age [20,21].

For the past 30 years, the classification, diagnosis, and treatment of GDM have been based on the recommendations of the International Workshop—Conference on Gestational Diabetes Mellitus [22]. As of 1997, four such international meetings had been held, and their recommendations were adopted by major medical institutions in Europe and America (American College of Obstetrics and Gynecology, American Diabetes Association, European Association for the Study of Diabetes, World Health Organization). Despite decades of debate on the optimal screening and diagnostic criteria, there still remains divided opinion as to the best means to diagnose GDM. At present there is an ongoing multinational trial (Hyperglycemia and Adverse Outcome in Pregnancy) that has as its objective to elucidate the optimal diagnostic criteria for gestational diabetes. The Hyperglycemia and Adverse Outcome in Pregnancy trial will be completed in 2006, and it is hoped that the results will recommend the best method to diagnose hyperglycemia during pregnancy.

Since 1980, the inception of "tight glycemia control" achieved by "intensive conventional therapy," including self-monitoring of blood glucose, has become an integral part of the treatment program for pregnancies complicated by hyperglycemia. As early as 1954, Pedersen [10] observed that "the common maternal, fetal, and neonatal complications of a diabetic pregnancy could be diminished by carefully supervised regulation of maternal metabolism." There is now a wealth of literature and experience to justify intensive approaches toward achieving normoglycemia in pregnancy. It is time to invest energy to simplify and disseminate these systems.

Pregestational Diabetes

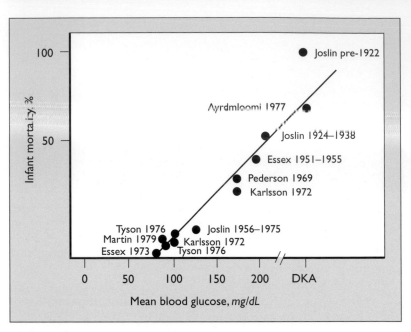

FIGURE 10-1. Literature review of the relationship between mean maternal glucose concentrations and infant mortality. Before the advent of insulin, an infant of a diabetic mother rarely survived. Before 1922, the fewer than 100 reported cases of survival are probably the offspring of type 2 rather than type 1 diabetic women [10]. A review of the major studies over the years since insulin became commercially available and when intensive glucose control systems were developed reveals that as the mean maternal blood glucose concentrations decrease, the percent infant mortality decreases [23]. A linear regression line drawn through the points on this graph indicates that at a mean maternal glucose level of 84 mg/dL, there would be no increased risk of infant mortality over the risk in the general population. (*Adapted from* Jovanovic and Peterson. [24].)

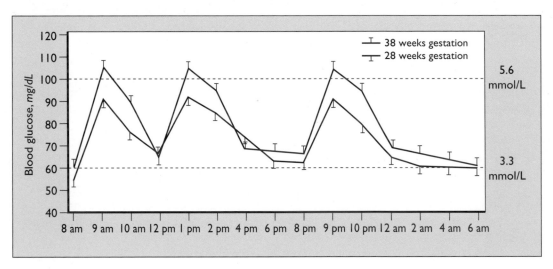

FIGURE 10-2. The report by Parretti *et al.* [25] on the blood glucose levels in normal, healthy pregnant women shows that the overall daily mean fasting glucose level is 56 mg/dL and the peak postprandial response occurs at 1 hour after the meal. This peak level never exceeds 105.2 mg/dL. The calculated mean glucose concentration in their population was 85 mg/dL, close to the projected mean glucose concentration derived from the literature review [24].

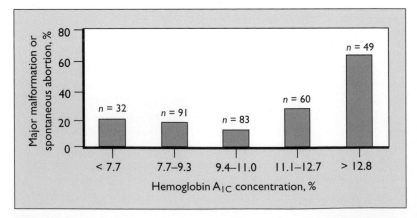

FIGURE 10-3. Combined prevalence of major malformation and spontaneous abortion according to the glycosylated hemoglobin (A_{1C}) concentration during the first trimester of pregnancy. In women with preexisting diabetes (pregestational diabetes), pregnancy should be deferred until the patient is under good glycemic control and has been thoroughly evaluated for complications of diabetes. Prepregnancy counseling should begin at the onset of puberty, with the need for abstinence or effective contraception clearly explained and understood [20]. A_{1C} values provide the best assessment of the degree of chronic glycemic control, reflecting the average blood glucose concentration during the preceding 6 to 8 weeks. As a result, measurement of A_{1C} can, in early preg-

nancy, estimate the level of glycemic control during the period of fetal organogenesis [21,23,26]. There are two important consequences in this regard: 1) A_{1C} values early in pregnancy are correlated with the rates of spontaneous abortion and major congenital malformations and 2) normalizing blood glucose concentrations before and early in pregnancy can reduce the risks of spontaneous abortion and congenital malformations nearly to that of the general population [5,21,27]. One report compared 110 women who were already 6 to 30 weeks pregnant at the time of referral with 84 women recruited before conception and then put on a daily glucose-monitoring regimen [21]. The mean blood glucose concentration was between 60 and 140 mg/dL (3.3 and 7.8 mmol/L) in 50% of the latter women. The incidence of anomalies was 1.2% in the women recruited before conception versus 10.9% in those first seen during pregnancy. Very similar findings were noted in another study: 1.4% versus 10.4% incidence of congenital abnormalities [27]. Major congenital malformations (specifically, caudal regression, 252 times more common in infants of diabetic mothers; situs inversus, 84 times common than in the normal population; and renal and cardiac defects, six and four times more common, respectively, than in the infants of diabetic mothers compared with the normal population), which either require surgical correction or significantly affect the health of the child, are more common in infants of mothers with poorly controlled diabetes [19]. There is also a substantial increase in spontaneous abortions in women who enter pregnancy in poor metabolic control as reflected by an elevated hemoglobin A_{1C} level [3]. The teratogenicity of glucose appears to be the major factor before the seventh gestational week [19].

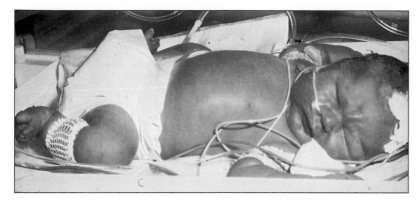

FIGURE 10-4. Diabetic fetopathy. The most common and significant neonatal complication clearly associated with diabetes in pregnancy is macrosomia: an oversized baby with a birth weight greater than the 90th percentile for gestational age and gender or a birth weight greater than 2 standard deviations (SD) above the normal mean birth weight. This infant was macrosomic, weighed 4583 g, was delivered 1 month prematurely, had all of the signs of an infant of a diabetic mother (hypoglycemia, hypocalcemia, hyperbilirubinemia), and died of respiratory distress 2 days after this photograph was taken.

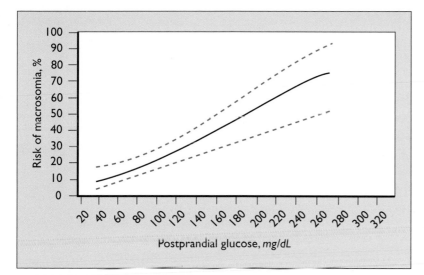

FIGURE 10-5. The relationship between the peak postprandial glucose concentration and the risk of macrosomia. Although controversial, the rate of complications in pregnancies complicated by diabetes has been tied to metabolic control of maternal glucose [5,15,17,21,23,26]. Perhaps the debate remains because many of the reports claim that neonatal complications occur despite excellent metabolic control, but these reports fail to measure postprandial glucose levels [17]. Postprandial glucose control has been suggested as key to neonatal outcome for pregnant women with either type 1 or gestational diabetes [17,28]. The Diabetes in Early Pregnancy (DIEP) study was a multicenter trial of type 1 diabetic pregnant women who were compared with control women throughout pregnancy. This group studied the relationship of maternal glucose levels and risk of macrosomia [17]. The DIEP study reported that the 1-hour postprandial glucose levels predicted 28.5% of the macrosomic infants born to diabetic mothers. This figure shows that the risk of macrosomia is a continuum. Any postprandial peak increases the risk of macrosomia above that seen in the normal population (10% risk). In addition, when the peak postprandial response is greater than 120 mg/dL, then the risk of macrosomia rises rapidly. (*Adapted from* Jovanovic *et al.* [17].)

STEPWISE LOGISTIC REGRESSION OF MATERNAL METABOLIC FACTORS AND ESTIMATES OF NEONATAL BODY COMPOSITION*

	r^2	$*\Delta*r^2$
Birthweight		
Insulin sensitivity index[†]	0.28	—
Maternal weight gain	0.48	0.20
Fat-free mass		
Insulin sensitivity index[†]	0.33	—
Maternal weight gain	0.53	0.20
Fat mass		
Insulin sensitivity[‡]	0.15	—
Parity	0.29	0.14
Neonatal sex	0.39	0.10
Insulin sensitivity index[†]	0.46	0.07

*In 16 neonates of women with normal glucose tolerance (n = 6) or gestational diabetes (n = 10).
[†]Late pregnancy.
[‡]Pregravid.

FIGURE 10-6. Stepwise logistic regression of maternal metabolic factors and estimates of neonatal body composition. Catalano *et al.* [7] evaluated the relationship of various aspects of maternal carbohydrate metabolism and estimates of neonatal body composition. They evaluated 16 infants of women who participated in a long-term study of alterations in glucose metabolism. The results of a stepwise logistic regression of maternal carbohydrate metabolism factors showed that maternal weight gain played the most significant role. (*Adapted from* Catalano *et al.* [7].)

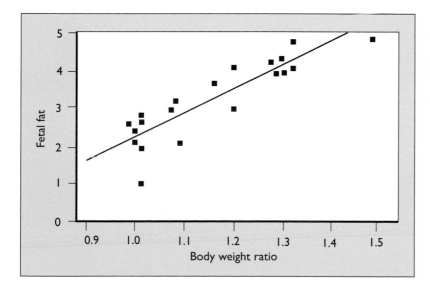

FIGURE 10-7. Relationship between fetal fat and subsequent birth weight, as measured by ponderal index or body weight ratio. Using magnetic resonance imaging (MRI), Jovanovic *et al.* [29] also found that the mother's adiposity was a predictor of the baby's birth weight. The relationship of fetal fat, as determined by the mean of two points of maximal thickness of the fetal abdominal wall subcutaneous fat on the MRI taken at 36 weeks of gestation compared with the infant birth weight ratio was highly significant ($P < 0.001$; $r = 0.88$). (*Adapted from* Jovanovic *et al.* [29].)

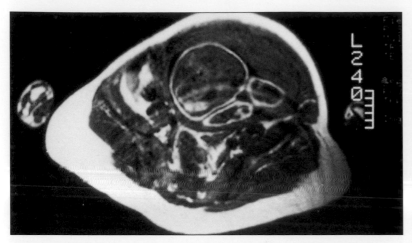

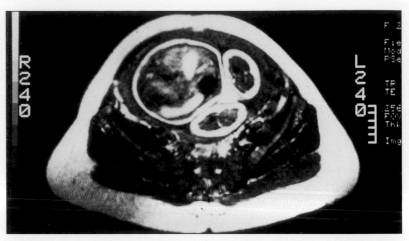

FIGURE 10-8. Magnetic resonance image of the fetus of a diabetic woman in excellent glucose control. This image was taken at the level of the maternal umbilicus at 38 weeks of gestation [29]. The mother had gestational diabetes mellitus and maintained excellent glucose control with preprandial glucose concentrations of 70 to 90 mg/dL; all of her blood glucose levels at 1 hour after the meal were less than 120 mg/dL. This infant weighed 3300 g at birth and was normal for percent body fat. (*From* Jovanovic *et al.* [29]; with permission).

FIGURE 10-9. Magnetic resonance image of the fetus of a diabetic woman in poor glucose control. This image was taken at the level of the maternal umbilicus at 38 weeks of gestational age. As can be seen, this fetus not only has increased subcutaneous fat but also already has accrual of visceral fat [29]. This mother had no antenatal care and presented to the emergency room with a urinary tract infection. She was found to have severe hyperglycemia. Her glucose concentration on admission was 396 mg/dL, probably indicative that she had undiagnosed type 2 diabetes. This fetus weighed 4340 g at birth, had 50% of its neonatal weight composed of fat, and had all of the signs of an infant of a diabetic mother. (*From* Jovanovic *et al.* [29]; with permission.)

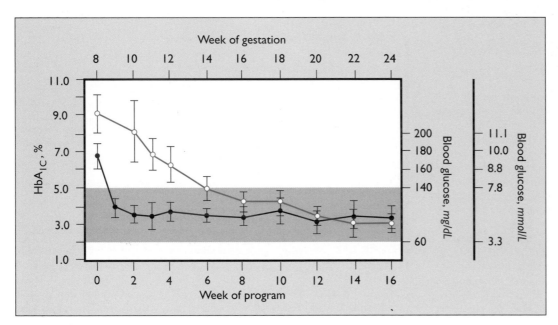

FIGURE 10-10. The time course for normalization of maternal glycosylated hemoglobin level in relationship to the normalization of maternal glucose concentrations. One of the first reports of a significant improvement in the outcome of type 1 diabetic pregnancies was published by Jovanovic *et al.* [26] in 1980. This report showed that when maternal blood glucose levels were normalized by the eighth gestational week, the birth weights of the infants were also normalized. This figure shows the time course for the normalization of glycosylated hemoglobin (HbA$_{1C}$) and blood glucose for 10 pregnant women with type 1 diabetes. The *open circles* represent the mean HbA$_{1C}$, and the *closed circles* represent mean blood glucose concentrations of (each time point is based on eight to 10 glucose determinations obtained from all 10 patients over 2-week intervals). The *shaded area* is the normal range for both HbA$_{1C}$ and blood glucose concentrations in the third trimester. All 10 women had normal infants at term. (*Adapted from* Jovanovic *et al.* [26].)

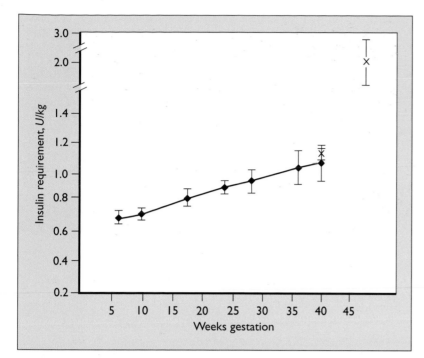

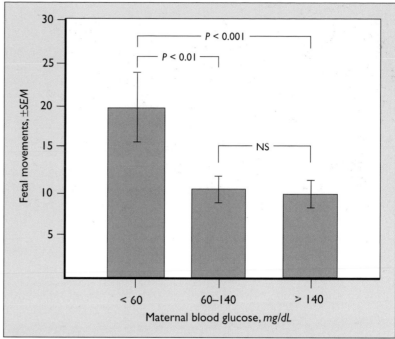

FIGURE 10-11. The insulin requirement throughout pregnancy in type 1 diabetic women. In a larger study of type 1 diabetic women who were maintained with normoglycemia from the sixth gestational week onward, there was a smooth increase in the insulin requirement throughout pregnancy. Fifty-three infants born to 52 type 1 diabetic women were all normal at birth. The insulin requirement of the woman who delivered twins was double that of the other 51 women. This increased need for insulin was manifested from the sixth gestational week onward. The x shows the mean daily dosage of insulin during weeks 34 to 37 of gestation. (*Adapted from* Jovanovic *et al.* [15].)

FIGURE 10-12. The relationship between fetal movements and maternal glucose concentrations. In this same population of diabetic women whose glucose control was documented in the study shown in Figure 10-11, the assessment of fetal well being using the parameter of fetal movements associated with heart rate (HR) acceleration is shown here. The *bars* show comparison of fetal movements with accelerations with maternal blood glucose concentrations less than 60 mg/dL, with maternal blood glucose concentrations of 60 to 140 mg/dL, and with maternal blood glucose concentrations greater than 140 mg/dL. It can be seen that the fetuses had significantly more movements with HR acceleration when the blood glucose concentrations were low. It appears, therefore, that transient, mild hypoglycemia is well tolerated by fetuses and may actually be preferred by them. NS— not significant; SEM— standard error of the mean. (*Adapted from* Holden *et al.* [30].)

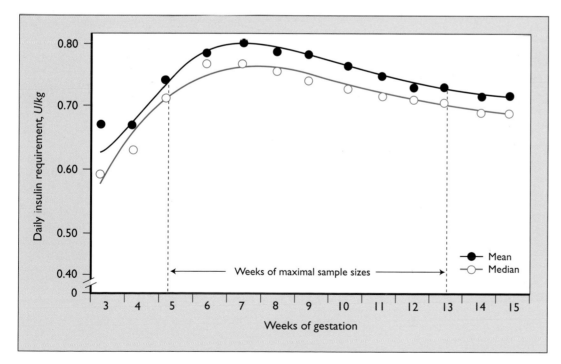

FIGURE 10-13. The declining insulin requirement in the first trimester of type 1 diabetic pregnant women. In the Diabetes in Early Pregnancy Study, the insulin requirement in the first trimester was studied. The daily insulin dosage (expressed as either a weekly mean or median in units per kg from weeks 3 to 8) increased, but there was an insulin dosage decrease in the late first trimester. The *open circles* represent the mean dosage of 346 type 1 diabetic women who had healthy infants. The *closed circles* represent the median dosage of these same patients. (*Adapted from* Jovanovic *et al.* [31].)

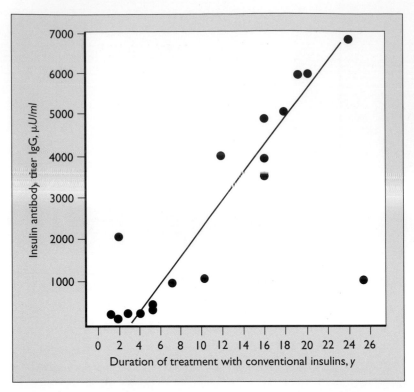

FIGURE 10-14. The relationship between anti-insulin antibody levels and duration of treatment with animal insulin. Although maternal glucose is the most likely causal agent of neonatal macrosomia, some have suggested that neonatal morbidity is secondary to the variability of maternal serum glucose and presence of antibodies to insulin. Placental transfer of insulin bound to immunoglobulin G (IgG) has also been associated with fetal macrosomia in mothers with near-normal glycemic control during gestation. Menon *et al.* [32] reported that antibody-bound insulin transferred to the fetus was proportional to the concentration of antibody-bound insulin measured in the mother. Also, the amount of antibody-bound insulin transferred to the fetus correlated directly with macrosomia in the infant and was independent of maternal blood glucose levels. In contrast, researchers found that only improved glucose control, as evidenced by lower postprandial glucose excursions but not lower insulin antibody levels, correlated with lower fetal weight [33]. They showed that insulin antibodies to exogenous insulin do not influence infant birth weight or insulin dosage. They did report, however, that there is a relationship between duration of treatment with conventional insulin and IgG antibody titer, as shown here. (*Adapted from* Jovanovic *et al.* [34].)

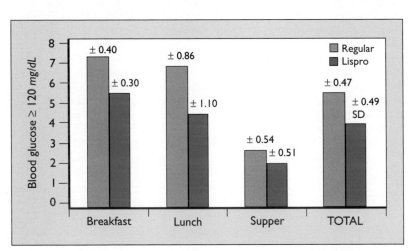

FIGURE 10-15. The postprandial glucose concentrations of diabetic women treated with insulin lispro compared with the postprandial glucose concentrations of diabetic women treated with human insulin during pregnancy. Our group reported that insulin lispro, an analog of human insulin with a peak insulin action achieved within 1 hour after injection, significantly improves the postprandial glucose concentrations in pregnant diabetic patients. Jovanovic *et al.* [35] showed that the postprandial glucose level is significantly lower ($P < 0.01$) throughout pregnancy in insulin-requiring gestational diabetic women treated with lispro insulin compared with gestational diabetic women treated with human insulin. SD—standard deviation. (*Adapted from* Jovanovic *et al.* [35].)

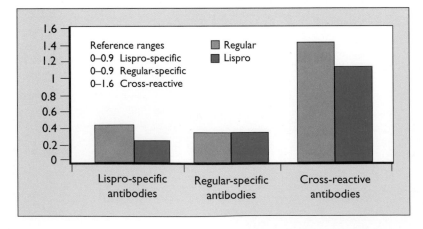

FIGURE 10-16. Insulin antibody findings. The antibody levels were no different in the women treated with lispro insulin compared with human insulin. In addition, lispro was not detected in the cord blood of the infants whose mothers were treated with lispro. A clinical trial [36] has shown the safety and efficacy of insulin aspart for the treatment of gestational diabetes. In this study, similar to the lispro study, insulin aspart proved to lower the postprandial glucose concentrations better than the concentrations achieved with human regular insulin, and the insulin appeared not to be immunogenic. Because of the importance of blunting the postprandial peak glucose concentration and the lack of immunogenicity of rapid-acting insulin analogues, the treatment of choice in pregnancy is now to suggest that these insulins be used in pregnancies complicated by diabetes. (*Adapted from* Jovanovic *et al.* [35].)

Insulin dosage regimen for diabetic pregnancy

"BIG I"	Date & Time	☐ 1. Pregnancy NPH plus regular insulin schedule Patient weight in kg = _____ . Nursing will calculate and administer the starting dose of insulin as outlined below: "Big I" = total daily units of insulin. Date: Circle one: Gestational weeks = 0–12 | 13–28 | 29–34 | 35–40 | OTHER Units of insulin = 0.7 | 0.8 | 0.9 | 1.0 | Calculate desired units of insulin from above line. "Big I" = _____ (units X weight KG/24 hours) divide so that 4/9 of "Big I" is NPH given before breakfast, and 1/6 of "Big I" is NPH given before bedtime. Regular insulin is given before breakfast as 2/9 of "Big I", and before dinner as 1/6 of "Big I". The regular insulin is titrated based on the blood glucose.

BREAKFAST	Do not feed the patient until the blood sugar is below 120 mg/dL.	0730 Pre-breakfast: NPH = 4/9 "Big I" = _____ .
		  Check yesterday's pre-dinner BS:
		       If yesterday's pre-dinner BS is < 60, then decrease today's AM NPH by 2 units.
		       If yesterday's pre-dinner BS is 60–90, no change in today's AM NPH.
		       If yesterday's pre-dinner BS is > 90, then increase today's AM NPH by 2 units.
		Regular or aspart or lispro = 2/9 Insulin "Big I" = _____ to be adjusted according to the following scale:
		       BS < 60 = _____ = (2/9 "Big I" dose) - 3% of the "Big I".
		       60–90 = _____ = 2/9 "Big I" dose.
		       90–120 = _____ = (2/9 "Big I" dose) + 3% of "Big I".
		       >121 = _____ = (2/9 "Big I" dose) + 6% of "Big I".
		If today's BS 1 hour after breakfast is < 110, then decrease tomorrow's pre-breakfast regular insulin by 2 units.
		If today's BS 1 hour after breakfast is 110–120, no change in tomorrow's pre-breakfast regular insulin.
		If today's BS 1 hour after breakfast is > 120, then increase tomorrow's pre-breakfast regular insulin by 2 units.

LUNCH	Do not feed the patient until the blood sugar is below 120 mg/dL.	1130 Pre-lunch: Regular or aspart or lispro insulin is given based on the following scale:
		  BS < 90 = 0 insulin.
		
		       91–120 = (1/18 "Big I") = _____ .
		
		   121–140 = (1/18 "Big I") + 2 units = _____ .
		
		       > 141 = (1/18 "Big I") + 4 units = _____ .

DINNER	Do not feed the patient until the blood sugar is below 120 mg/dL.	1700 Pre-dinner: Regular or aspart or lispro insulin is 1/6 "Big I" = _____ and is based on the following scale.
		       BS < 60 = _____ = (1/6 "Big I" dose) - 3% of "Big I".
		       60–90 = _____ = 1/6 "Big I" dose.
		       91–120 = _____ = (1/6 "Big I" dose) + 3% of "Big I".
		       > 121 = _____ = (1/6 "Big I" dose) + 6% of "Big I".
		If today's BS 1 hour after dinner is < 110, then decrease tomorrow's dinner regular insulin by 2 units.
		If today's BS 1 hour after dinner is 110–120, no change in tomorrow's dinner regular insulin.
		If today's BS 1 hour after dinner is > 120, then increase tomorrow's dinner regular insulin by 2 units.

BEDTIME		2330 Bedtime NPH: Give 1/6 "Big I" = _____ .
		  If today's pre-breakfast BS is < 60, then decrease today's bedtime NPH by 2 units.
		  If today's pre-breakfast BS is 60–90, no change in today's bedtime NPH.
		  If today's pre-breakfast BS is > 90, then check the 3 AM BS and, if it is < 70 (regardless of today's pre-breakfast BS), decrease today's bedtime NPH by 2 units.
		  If today's pre-breakfast BS is > 90, and the 3 AM BS > 70, increase today's bedtime NPH by 2 units.
		  Also, if the 3 AM BS is > 90, then call the doctor for 3 AM regular insulin scale equal to the pre-lunch regular insulin scale.

FIGURE 10-17. Insulin dosage regimen for diabetic pregnancy. This treatment algorithm has proven to achieve normal glycemia in pregestational diabetic women. The insulin doses are divided into frequent injections to provide the basal and the meal-related insulin needs. The smooth increase in the total daily insulin requirement throughout pregnancy is calculated based on gestational week and maternal pregnant weight. The insulin requirement at 0 to 12 weeks of gestation is 0.7 U/kg/d (with careful monitoring of the blood glucose levels to prevent hypoglycemia from occurring if there is a decline in dosage during weeks 9 to 12). During weeks 13 to 28 of gestation, the dosage is 0.8 U/kg/d; during weeks 29 to 34, the insulin requirement is 0.9 U/kg/d. At term, the insulin requirement is 1.0 U/kg/d [15]. BS—blood sugar, NPH— neutral protamine Hagedorn. (*Adapted from* Jovanovic and Peterson [37].)

IMPORTANT TESTS FOR MONITORING CONCOMITANT DISEASES AND GLUCOSE DURING PREGNANCIES COMPLICATED BY TYPE I DIABETES

Test	Frequency
Eye examination	Prior to conception and then once each trimester
Fundus photography and/or dilated examination by an ophthalmologist	Prior to conception and once each trimester
Kidney function	Prior to conception and once each trimester
Creatinine clearance with total microalbumin	Prior to conception and once a month
Thyroid function	Premeals and 1-h postmeals
Free T$_4$ and TS-II	Target: capillary whole blood glucose:
HbA$_{1c}$	Premeal <90 mg/dL
Self–blood glucose monitoring	Postmeal <120 mg/dL
Blood pressure and weight	Prior to conception and at each visit

FIGURE 10-18. Recommended testing protocol for women with pregestational diabetes. Ideally, a diabetic woman would plan her pregnancy so that there is time to create an individualized algorithm of care. When a diabetic woman presents in her first few weeks of pregnancy, there is no time for individualization, and rather rigid protocols must be urgently instituted to provide optimal control within 24 to 48 hours and to maintain control thereafter [20,21]. The table lists the important tests for monitoring concomitant diseases and the maternal vascular status during pregnancy [28]. HbA$_{1c}$—hemoglobin A$_{1c}$; T4—thyroxine.

A. WHITE CLASSIFICATION OF PREGESTATIONAL DIABETES

Group	Age at Onset, y	Duration of Disease, y	Vascular Complication
B	> 20	< 10	None
C	< 10	< 10–19	None
D	< 10	> 20	Retinopathy-background type
F	All ages	Any duration	Nephropathy
R	All ages	Any duration	Retinopathy-proliferative
H	All ages	Any duration	Cardiac disease
T	All ages	Any duration	After organ transplantation

FIGURE 10-19. Two classifications of pregestational diabetes. Classifications of pregestational diabetes have been formulated to help physicians predict the outcome of pregnancy for both the mother and child [38,39]. **A,** The White [38] classification categorized diabetic women based on the mode of therapy, duration, age at onset of diabetes, and degree of vascular compromise of each patient at the beginning of the pregnancy. White class A referred to gestational diabetes, but many of these women probably had undiagnosed type 2 diabetes. The White classification also led to confusion because the "B" determination was given to both the pregnancy-related diabetes (gestational diabetes), which necessitated insulin, and to the pregestational woman with fewer than 10 years of insulin therapy. Treatment for all groups consisted of diet and insulin. **B,** Revised classification. As evidence mounts that maternal normoglycemia is beneficial at the time of conception, during fetal organogenesis, and throughout gestation, a newer classification that places more emphasis on maternal plasma glucose concentrations is an acceptable alternative to the White classification. This new classification is based on vascular status and type of complication, with an emphasis on glycemic control [38]. ASCVD—atherosclerotic cardiovascular disease.

B. CLASSIFICATION OF RISK ASSOCIATED WITH PREGESTATIONAL DIABETES (TYPES I AND 2) DURING PREGNANCY BASED ON GLYCEMIC CONTROL, VASCULAR DISEASE, AND TYPE OF DISEASE

Condition			Risk Classification
Optimal glucose control*	No vascular disease		Low
	Vascular disease	Retinopathy	Minimal
		Neuropathy	Minimal
		Nephropathy	Moderate
		ASCVD	
Less than optimal glucose control†	No vascular disease		High
	Vascular disease	Retinopathy	High
		Neuropathy	High
		Nephropathy	High
		ASCVD	High

*Optimal glucose control is defined as fasting blood glucose (BG) concentrations of 55–65 mg/dL, average BG level of 84 mg/dL, and 1-h postprandial BG value of <120 mg/dL [5].

†Less than optimal glucose control status is diagnosed when optimal control fails to occur.

Gestational Diabetes Mellitus

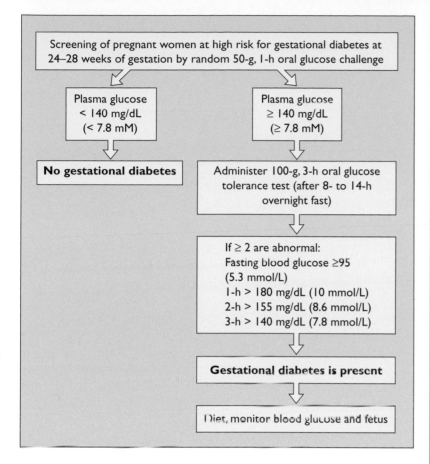

Screening of pregnant women at high risk for gestational diabetes at 24–28 weeks of gestation by random 50-g, 1-h oral glucose challenge

Plasma glucose < 140 mg/dL (< 7.8 mM)

Plasma glucose ≥ 140 mg/dL (≥ 7.8 mM)

No gestational diabetes

Administer 100-g, 3-h oral glucose tolerance test (after 8- to 14-h overnight fast)

If ≥ 2 are abnormal:
Fasting blood glucose ≥95 (5.3 mmol/L)
1-h > 180 mg/dL (10 mmol/L)
2-h > 155 mg/dL (8.6 mmol/L)
3-h > 140 mg/dL (7.8 mmol/L)

Gestational diabetes is present

Diet, monitor blood glucose and fetus

FIGURE 10-20. Treatment protocol for the screening and diagnosis of gestational diabetes (GDM). GDM is defined as glucose tolerance of variable severity with onset or first recognition during pregnancy. The prevalence of GDM is dependent on ethnic background and degree of adiposity, and thus varies from 0.1% to 12.0% [13]. Most medical centers today use the two-stage diagnostic procedure suggested at the Third International Workshop-Conference on Gestational Diabetes held in Chicago in 1991, namely, glucose challenge screen with confirmation, if necessary, by oral glucose tolerance test (OGTT). The current position paper, presented in 1997 at the Fourth International Workshop-Conference on Gestational Diabetes Mellitus in Chicago, summarizes the most recent recommendations [22]. The glucose challenge test (GCT) is performed in weeks 24 to 28 of gestation for patients at moderate risk and in early pregnancy for patients at high risk, regardless of the time of the last meal. The test involves the oral intake of 50 g of glucose within 2 minutes and measurement of plasma glucose level after 1 hour. Patients with a glucose level of more than 140 mg/dL on the GCT (14% to 18% of all pregnant women) must then undergo the OGTT for confirmation of GDM. This subgroup accounts for about 80% of all women with GDM. Some medical centers use a cutoff of 130 mg/dL on the GCT, which identifies more than 90% of all affected patients, but it increases the subgroup that requires an OGTT to 20% to 25% of all pregnant women. The OGTT identifies patients with diabetes by glucose loading. Before testing, patients ingest a 3-day diet of more than 150 g carbohydrate with regular physical activity followed by a fast of at least 8 hours (but not more than 14 hours). The test is performed in the morning of the fourth day. For diagnosis, the values of two of the four criteria listed in this figure must surpass the predetermined cutoff value, as indicated. According to the most recent recommendations [22], clinicians can use a 75- or 100-g glucose load and cutoff values equal to both tests. It is important to emphasize that capillary fingerstick glucose values are not accepted for diagnosis. The diagnosis of GDM must be based solely on plasma glucose levels on an OGTT.

DIAGNOSIS OF GESTATIONAL DIABETES MELLITUS BY RISK ASSESSMENT

A. Low risk of developing GDM*

GCT is not necessary if all of the following criteria are met:

Absence of diabetes in first-degree relatives

Age <25 y

Normal prepregnancy weight

No history of poor carbohydrate metabolism

No history of adverse pregnancy outcome

B. Average risk of developing GDM

GCT should be performed in weeks 24 to 28 of pregnancy. One of the following options may be chosen:

Two-stage testing

Stage 1: GCT; if results on GCT are abnormal, go to stage 2

Stage 2: OGTT; diagnosis is based on values listed in Figure 16-5

One-stage testing

OGTT for all suspected cases; diagnosis is based on values listed in Figure 16-20

C. High risk of developing GDM

Pregnant women who are obese or who have a family history of diabetes mellitus type 2, GDM in a past pregnancy, or known carbohydrate intolerance or high urine glucose level should undergo the GCT and/or OGTT according to the accepted criteria for diagnosis of GDM. Testing should be done as soon as feasible during pregnancy and immediately after the first visit (early first trimester). If GDM is not detected at this stage, the GCT and/or OGTT should be repeated in weeks 24 to 28 or at the first suspicious signs of diabetes.

*Because few women will meet all the criteria for low risk, we recommend that all patients be classified in groups B and C.

FIGURE 10-21. Risk assessment guide for women who need to be screened for gestational diabetes mellitus (GDM). The risk of GDM is stratified into low, average, and high [22]. Risk assessment should be undertaken at the first prenatal visit. Women with clinical characteristics consistent with a high risk (obesity, history of GDM, glycosuria, or strong family history of diabetes) must be tested as soon as feasible. Women at average risk should be tested in weeks 24 to 28 of gestation, and women at low risk need not be tested at all. However, there are many who favor universal screening for all pregnant women because there is no way to guarantee that a woman with no risks does not have GDM [39]. An 8- to 14-hour fasting glucose level above 126 mg/dL or a casual plasma glucose level above 200 mg/dL are diagnostic of diabetes; thus, no further tests are needed. Evaluation should be done as early during pregnancy as possible. New guidelines may be expected on completion of the 4-year multinational Hyperglycemia and Adverse Pregnancy Outcome (HAPO) study, which is being conducted under the aegis of the National Institutes of Health in 16 leading medical centers, including two in Israel. The study seeks to set criteria for the 75-g glucose load, which is already accepted in several European countries, to standardize the diagnosis of GDM with the diagnosis of diabetes in the nonpregnant state. GCT—glucose tolerance test; OGTT—oral glucose tolerance test.

A. COMPARISON OF NEONATAL OUTCOME WHEN WOMEN ARE MANAGED WITH ULTRASONOGRAPHY VERSUS SELF–BLOOD GLUCOSE MONITORING

Patients, n	Standard Group	Ultrasound Group	P Value
	100	99	
Gestational age at delivery, wks	39.3 ± 1.3	39.0 ± 1.9	0.2
Induction, %	23.0	23.2	0.5
Cesarean delivery, %	15.0	18.2	0.5
Birth weight, g	3271.2 ± 500	3306.1 ± 558	0.4
SGA, %	13.0	12.1	0.5
LGA, %	10.0	12.1	0.4
Neonatal BMI, kg/m^2	13.1 ± 1.2	12.8 ± 1.5	0.2
Sum of skinfolds, mm*	13.2 ± 3.2	14.1 ± 3.4	0.07
Hypoglycemia (< 40 mg/dL), %	16.0	17.0	0.5
Intravenous glucose, %	11	9.1	0.4
Cord blood insulin, $\mu U/mL^\dagger$	9.1 ± 6.2	8.8 ± 6.82	0.8
Transfer to NICU, %	15.0	14.1	0.5

*Sum of skinfold measured at four locations on the body (subscalpular, iliac crest, triceps, and thigh).
†Missing in four infants of women who did not complete the study.

B. PREGNANCY OUTCOMES OF GESTATIONAL DIABETES TREATED WITH INSULIN OR GLYBURIDE

Outcome	Glyburide (n = 201)	Insulin (n = 203)	P Value
Neonatal features			
Large size for gestational age, n (%)	24 (12)	26 (13)	0.76
Birth weight, g	3256 ± 543	3194 ± 598	0.28
Ponderal index > 2.85, n (%)*	18 (9)	24 (12)	0.33
Macrosomia, n (%)	14 (7)	9 (4)	0.26
Metabolic outcomes			
Cord serum insulin, $\mu U/mL^\dagger$	15 ± 13	15 ± 21	0.84
Intravenous glucose therapy, n (%)	28 (14)	22 (11)	0.36
Hypoglycemia, n (%)	18 (9)	12 (6)	0.25
Hypocalcemia, n (%)	2 (1)	2 (1)	0.99
Hyerpbilirubinemia, n (%)	12 (6)	8 (4)	0.36
Erythrocytosis, n (%)	4 (2)	6 (3)	0.52
Lung complications, n (%)	16 (8)	12 (6)	0.43
Respiratory support, n (%)	4 (2)	6 (3)	0.52
Admission for neonatal intensive care unit, n (%)	12 (6)	14 (7)	0.68
Congenital anomaly	5 (2)	4 (2)	0.74
Prerinatal mortality, n (%)‡			
Stillbirth	1 (0.5)	1 (0.5)	0.99
Neonatal death	1 (0.5)	1 (0.5)	0.99

Plus-minus values are mean ± SD.
*The ponderal index was calculated as 100 times the weight in grams divided by the cube of the length in centimeters.
†To convert the values for insulin to picomoles per liter, multiply by 6.0.
‡Numbers include infants with congenital abnormalities.

FIGURE 10-22. **A,** Guidelines for management of pregnancies complicated by gestational diabetes (GDM) generally call for normalization of maternal glucose concentrations. This strategy requires frequent glucose monitoring with initiation of insulin therapy if the blood glucose concentrations increase above the target levels. Management of women with GDM with the use of fetal ultrasonography has been shown to safe and can identify those who are at risk of delivering neonates who are large for gestational age if insulin therapy is withheld. Two trials testing the fetal growth–based approach in a predominately Latino population [40,41] demonstrated low rates of macrosomic infants when the fetus' abdominal circumference on ultrasonography remained below the 75th percentile during pregnancy. Recently, a third study [42] reported the management of women with GDM based predominantly on monthly fetal growth ultrasound examinations with an approach based solely on maternal glycemia. Women with GDM who attained fasting capillary glucose (FCG) below 120 mg/dL and 2-hour postprandial capillary glucose (2h-CG) below 200 mg/dL after 1 week of diet were randomized to management based on maternal glycemia alone (standard) or glycemia plus ultrasound. In the standard group, insulin was initiated if FCG was repeatedly above 90 mg/dL or 2h-CG was above 120 mg/dL. In the ultrasound group, thresholds were 120 and 200 mg/dL, respectively, or a fetal abdominal circumference above the 75th percentile (AC > p75). Outcome criteria were rates of cesarean section, small-for-gestational-age (SGA) or large-for-gestational-age (LGA) infants, neonatal hypoglycemia (< 40 mg/dL), and neonatal care admission. As seen here, in the ultrasound group, AC > p75 was the sole indication for insulin. The ultrasound-based strategy, compared with the maternal glycemia-only strategy, resulted in a different treatment assignment in 34% of women. Rates of cesarean section (19.0% vs 18.2%), LGA (10.0% vs 12.1%), SGA (13.0% vs 12.1%), hypoglycemia (16.0% vs 17.0%), and admission (15.0% vs. 14.1%) did not differ significantly. The authors concluded that GDM management based on fetal growth combined with high glycemic criteria provides outcomes equivalent to management based on strict glycemic criteria alone. Inclusion of fetal growth might provide the opportunity to reduce glucose testing in low-risk pregnancies.

B, Women with gestational diabetes mellitus are rarely treated with a sulfonylurea drug, because of concern about teratogenicity and neonatal hypoglycemia. There is little information about the efficacy of these drugs in this group of women. Recently, however, there was a randomized trial [43] of 404 women with singleton pregnancies and gestational diabetes that required treatment. The women were randomly assigned between 11 and 33 weeks of gestation to receive glyburide or insulin according to an intensified treatment protocol. The primary end point was achievement of the desired level of glycemic control. Secondary end points included maternal and neonatal complications. As can be seen by in this figure, the mean pretreatment blood glucose concentration and glucose during treatment as measured at home was not significantly different in the glyburide group compared with the insulin group. Eight women in the glyburide group (4%) required insulin therapy. There were no significant differences between the glyburide and insulin groups in the percentage of infants who were large for gestational age, who had macrosomia, defined as a birth weight of 4000 g or more, who had lung complications, who had hypoglycemia, or who were admitted to a neonatal intensive care unit. The cord-serum insulin concentrations were similar in the two groups, and glyburide was not detected in the cord serum of any infant in the glyburide group. The authors concluded that in women with gestational diabetes, glyburide is a clinically effective alternative to insulin therapy. Further studies are necessary, however, before glyburide can be safely prescribed in clinical practice. BMI—body mass index; NICU—neonatal intensive care unit.

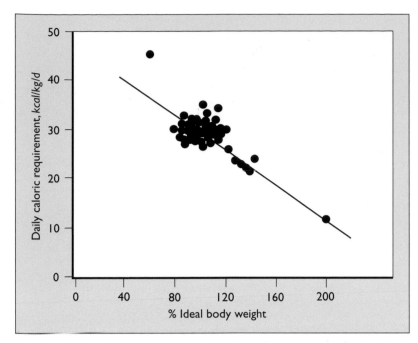

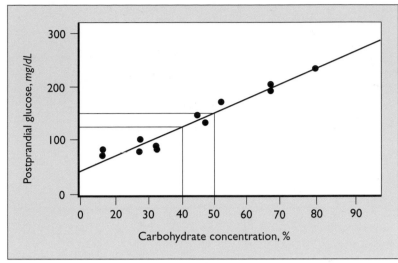

FIGURE 10-23. The caloric needs for pregnant women based on their ideal body weight. The main goal of treatment of women with gestational diabetes mellitus (GDM) is to prevent adverse effects to the mother and infant. Normalization of glucose levels is a proven factor to achieve this goal. In addition, postprandial glucose levels are more closely associated with macrosomia than are fasting levels. Women with GDM must follow an individually tailored diet prepared by a dietitian who also takes into account the amount, time, and type of insulin injection (if necessary). The diet must satisfy the minimum daily nutritional requirements for all pregnant women. The caloric intake must be compatible with the state of pregnancy and ensure the proper weight gain according to the patient's ideal weight before and during pregnancy. In this figure, the caloric needs of pregnancy are related to maternal body weight. The *closed circles* show that for a woman who is of normal body weight (80% to 120% ideal body weight), the caloric requirement is 30 kcal/kg/day (present pregnant weight). For overweight women, fewer calories are needed. Most overweight women are 130% above ideal body weight, and they require 24 kcal/kg/day. Morbidly obese women (> 150% above ideal body weight) may require as few as 12 kcal/kg/day (present pregnant weight) [44]. (*Adapted from* Jovanovic [45].)

FIGURE 10-24. The relationship between carbohydrate concentration, the meal plan, and the peak postprandial response. The calories are divided into frequent small feedings with the caveat that breakfast needs to be the smallest meal of the day, with less than 33% carbohydrate. This degree of carbohydrate restriction is necessary because the hypercortisolemia seen normally in early waking hours is potentiated in pregnancy. After the cortisol levels wane, then the other meals can be composed of 40% carbohydrate. This figure clearly shows that when the carbohydrate concentration in lunch and dinner is greater than 40%, then the peak postprandial glucose level is greater than 120 mg/dL or that level reported to be associated with a rapidly increasing risk of neonatal macrosomia [17]. (*Adapted from* Peterson and Jovanovic [16].)

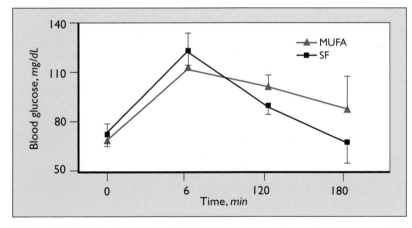

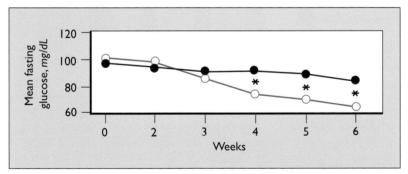

FIGURE 10-25. The postprandial glucose concentrations after a saturated fat (SF) meal compared with those concentrations after a monounsaturated fat (MUFA) meal. This figure demonstrates that the addition of SF or MUFA to the meal plan has different effects on the postprandial glucose concentrations. Despite the near-equal peak of the postprandial response at the 1-hour timepoint with SF compared with MUFA, by the 2- and 3-hour time points, the blood glucose levels are significantly lower with an SF meal. If macrosomia is caused by the total postprandial glucose load, then SF meal plans may actually be a means to minimize the need for insulin therapy in patients with gestational diabetes mellitus. (*Adapted from* Ilic *et al.* [47].)

FIGURE 10-26. Weekly fasting glucose concentrations during a cardiovascular training program compared with no exercise program in women with gestational diabetes mellitus (GDM). An arm exercise has been shown to be a safe and effective mode of therapy for treating these women. Our group documented that women with GDM can train using arm ergometry and that a program of this kind of cardiovascular conditioning exercise results in lower levels of glycemia than a program of diet alone. The effects of exercise on fasting glucose concentrations became apparent after 4 weeks of training, as shown by the *solid circles*. (*Adapted from* Jovanovic *et al.* [48].)

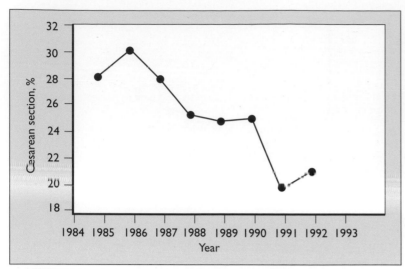

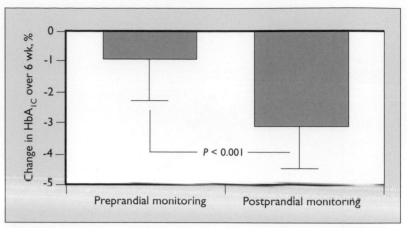

FIGURE 10-27. The decrease in the cesarean section rate in Santa Barbara County concomitant with the introduction of a program of universal screening and treatment of hyperglycemia in pregnancy. When the glucose level cannot be maintained within recommended limits (90 mg/dL before meals and no higher than 120 mg/dL at 1 hour after meals) by diet and exercise, then insulin treatment is needed. Rapid-acting insulin analogues can improve glycemic levels, and their use is increasing in most leading centers in the United States and Europe. Our experience in Santa Barbara County Health Care Service [39] with a program of universal screening and treatment of postprandial glucose by targeting the blood glucose level to be less than 120 mg/dL (with diet, exercise, and initiation of insulin when blood glucose levels are elevated) has shown that the birth weight is normalized. This degree of intensive care for all gestational diabetic women results in more than $2000 saved per pregnancy by avoiding cesarean sections necessitated to deliver macrosomic infants and neonatal intensive care admissions of sick infants. (*Adapted from* Jovanovic and Bevier [39].)

FIGURE 10-28. The glycosylated hemoglobin levels after 6 weeks of monitoring only preprandial glucose concentrations in women with gestational diabetes mellitus (GDM) needing insulin therapy compared with the glycosylated hemoglobin levels achieved in a matched population of women who were also monitoring postprandial glucose concentrations. de Veciana *et al.* [18] have also shown that when insulin-requiring women with GDM measure their preprandial glucose levels alone, the prevalence of macrosomia is 42%. When the postprandial glucose levels are measured and the treatment designed to maintain the levels at lower than 120 mg/dL, the prevalence of macrosomia was decreased to 12%. With only 6 weeks of treatment designed to blunt the postprandial glucose levels, the glycosylated hemoglobin level was significantly lower than in the group of gestational diabetes patients who were only monitoring glucose preprandially.

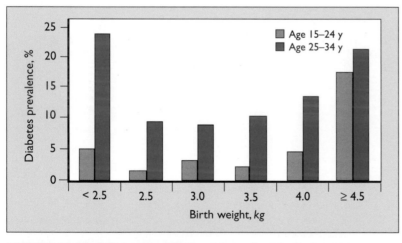

FIGURE 10-29. Relationship of birth weight to the risk of subsequent diabetes. Women who have had gestational diabetes mellitus previously should be advised to undergo repeated oral glucose tolerance tests once yearly and maintain a healthy lifestyle with regular exercise and normal body weight. They should seek consultation before their next pregnancy [22]. The follow-up of the offspring of diabetic mothers should include careful measurement of growth and development and concern for glucose intolerance during childhood. Children of diabetic mothers are at higher risk of obesity and glucose intolerance. Evidence is accumulating that good metabolic control in the mother during pregnancy can decrease this risk. There appears to be a U-shaped curve that relates birth weight to the risk of subsequent diabetes. Both at the low and high birth weights, it appears that the infants have a lack of pancreatic reserve of insulin; thus, as they grow and develop, they cannot increase their insulin secretion sufficiently to maintain glucose homeostasis. (*Adapted from* McCance *et al.* [49].)

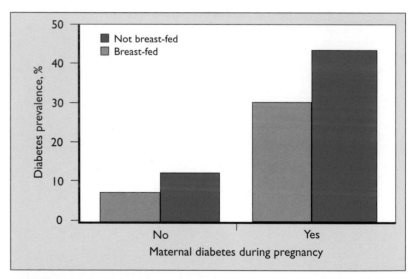

FIGURE 10-30. Predictors of subsequent diabetes in the offspring in Pima Indians. Pettitt and Knowler [9] reported that there is a long-term consequence of the intrauterine environment. When they adjusted for age, gender, birth weight, presence of diabetes in either parent, and whether or not the child was breastfed for at least 2 months after birth, the strongest predictors of subsequent diabetes in the child was the presence of maternal diabetes and not being breastfed. The *dark bars* represent the children who were not breastfed; the *light bars* represent the children who were breastfed. Thus, it is clear that the intrauterine environment must be normalized and sufficient nutrition must be provided (but not overnutrition). Maintaining the nutritional status of the child after birth is paramount in decreasing the rapidly increasing rate of diabetes. (*Adapted from* Pettitt and Knowler [9].)

References

1. American Diabetes Association: Clinical practice recommendations 2001: gestational diabetes. *Diabetes Care* 2001, 24(suppl):S77–S79.

2. Hod M, Diamant YZ: Diabetes in pregnancy. Norbert Freinkel Memorial Issue. *Isr J Med Sci* 1991, 27:421.

3. Mills JL, Simpson JL, Driscoll SG, et al.: Incidence of spontaneous abortion among normal women and insulin dependent diabetic women whose pregnancies were identified within 21 days of conception. *N Engl J Med* 1988, 319:1617.

4. Mills JL, Knopp RH, Simpson JL, et al.: Lack of relation of increased malformation roles in infants of diabetic mothers to glycemic control during organogenesis. *N Engl J Med* 1988, 318:671.

5. Petersen M, Pedersen SA, Greisen G, et al.: Early growth delay in diabetic pregnancy: relation to psychomotor development at age 4. *Br Med J* 1988, 296:598.

6. van Dijk DJ, Axer-Siegel R, Erman A, Hod M: Diabetic vascular complications and pregnancy. *Diabetes Rev* 1995, 3:632.

7. Catalano PM, Drago NM, Amini S: Maternal carbohydrate metabolism and its relationship to fetal growth and body composition. *Am J Obstet Gynecol* 1995, 172:14640.

8. Hod M, Diamant YZ: The offspring of a diabetic mother—short- and long-range implications. *Isr J Med Sci* 1992, 28:81

9. Pettitt DJ, Knowler WC: Long-term effects of the intrauterine environment, birth weight, and breast-feeding in Pima Indians. *Diabetes Care* 1998, 21:B138–B141.

10. Pedersen J: Fetal mortality in diabetes in relation to management during the latter part of pregnancy. *Acta Endocrinol* 1954, 15:282.

11. Freinkel N: Banting Lecture 1980: of pregnancy and progeny. *Diabetes* 1980, 29:10235.

12. Jovanovic L, Peterson CM: Moment in history: turning point in blood glucose monitoring of diet and insulin dosing. *Trans Am Soc Artif Intern Organs* 1990, 36:799.

13. Buchanan TA, Unterman T, Metzger BE: The medical management of diabetes in pregnancy. *Clin Perinatol* 1985, 12:625.

14. Pedersen J, Pedersen LM: Diabetes mellitus and pregnancy: the hyperglycemia, hyperinsulinemia theory and the weight of the newborn baby. In *Proceedings of the 7th Congress of the International Diabetes Federation*. Edited by Rodriguez RR, Vallance-Owen J. Amsterdam: Excerpta Medica; 1971:678.

15. Jovanovic L, Druzin M, Peterson CM: The effect of euglycemia on the outcome of pregnancy in insulin-dependent diabetics as compared to normal controls. *Am J Med* 1981, 71:921.

16. Jovanovic L, Peterson CM: Rationale for prevention and treatment of glucose-mediated macrosomia: A protocol for gestational diabetes. *Endocrinol Pract* 1996, 2:118.

17. Jovanovic L, Peterson CM, Reed GF, et al.: Maternal postprandial glucose levels and infant birth weight: the Diabetes in Early Pregnancy Study. The National Institute of Child Health and Human Development—Diabetes in Early Pregnancy Study. *Am J Obstet Gynecol* 1991, 164:103.

18. de Veciana M, Major CA, Morgan MA, et al.: Postprandial versus preprandial blood glucose monitoring in women with gestational diabetes mellitus requiring insulin therapy. *N Engl J Med* 1995, 333:12371.

19. Mills JL, Baker L, Goldman A: Malformations in infants of diabetic mothers occur before the seventh gestational week: implications for treatment. *Diabetes* 1979, 23:292.

20. Steel JM, Johnstone FD, Hepburn DA, Smith AF: Can prepregnancy care of diabetic women reduce the risk of abnormal babies? *Br Med J* 1990, 301:10703.

21. Kitzmiller JL, Gavin LA, Gin GD, et al.: Preconception care of diabetes: glycemic control prevents congenital anomalies. *JAMA* 1991, 265:731.

22. Metzger BE, Coustan DR: Proceedings of the Fourth International Workshop-Conference on Gestational Diabetes Mellitus. *Diabetes Care* 1998, 21(suppl):B1–B167.

23. Ylinen K, Aula P, Stenman UH, et al.: Risk of minor and major fetal malformations in diabetics with high hemoglobin A_{1c} values in early pregnancy. *Br Med J* 1984, 289:345.

24. Jovanovic L, Peterson CM: Management of the pregnant diabetic woman. *Diabetes Care* 1980, 3:63

25. Parretti E, Mecacci F, Papini M, et al.: Third trimester maternal glucose levels from diurnal profiles in non-diabetic pregnancies: correlation with sonographic parameters of fetal growth. *Diabetes Care* 2001, 24:13193.

26. Jovanovic L, Saxena BB, Dawood MY, et al.: Feasibility of maintaining euglycemia in insulin-dependent diabetic women. *Am J Med* 1980, 68:105.

27. Greene MF, Hare JW, Cloherty JP, et al.: First-trimester hemoglobin A1 and risk for major malformation and spontaneous abortion in diabetic pregnancy. *Teratology* 1989, 39:225.

28. Jovanovic L: *Medical Management of Pregnancy Complicated by Diabetes*. Alexandria: American Diabetes Association; 1993, revised 1995 and 2000.

29. Jovanovic L, Crues J, Durak E, Peterson CM: Magnetic resonance imaging in pregnancies complicated by gestational diabetes predicts infant birth weight ratio and neonatal morbidity. *Am J Perinatol* 1993, 10:432.

30. Holden KP, Jovanovic L, Druzin ML, Peterson CM: Increased fetal activity with low maternal blood glucose levels in pregnancies complicated by diabetes. *Am J Perinatol* 1984, 1:161.

31. Hanson U, Persson B, Thunell S: Relationship between haemoglobin A1c in early type 1 (insulin-dependent) diabetic pregnancy and the occurrence of spontaneous abortion and fetal malformation in Sweden. *Diabetologia* 1990, 33:100.

31. Jovanovic L, Knopp RH, Brown A, et al.: Declining insulin requirements in the late first trimester of diabetic pregnancy. *Diabetes Care* 2001, 24:11306.

32. Menon RK, Cohen RM, Sperling MA, et al.: Transplacental passage of insulin in pregnant women with insulin-dependent diabetes mellitus. Its role in fetal macrosomia. *N Engl J Med* 1990, 323:309.

33. Jovanovic L, Kitzmiller JL, Peterson CM: Randomized trial of human versus animal species insulin in diabetic pregnant women: improved glycemic control, not fewer antibodies to insulin, influences birth weight. *Am J Obstet Gynecol* 1992, 167:13250.

34. Jovanovic L, Mills JL, Peterson CM: Anti-insulin titers do not influence control or insulin requirements in early pregnancy. *Diabetes Care* 1984, 7:68

35. Jovanovic L, Ilic S, Pettitt DJ, et al.: The metabolic and immunologic effects of insulin lispro in gestational diabetes. *Diabetes Care* 1999, 22:14226.

36. Pettitt DJ, Ospina P, Kolaczynski JW, Jovanovic L: Comparison of an insulin analog, insulin aspart, and regular human insulin with no insulin in gestational diabetes mellitus. *Diabetes Care* 2003, 26:183–186.

37. Jovanovic L, Peterson CM: The art and science of maintenance of normoglycemia in pregnancies complicated by type 1 diabetes mellitus. *Endocrinol Pract* 1996, 2:130.

38. White P: Pregnancy and diabetes. In *Joslin's Diabetes Mellitus*, edn 11. Edited by Marble A, White P, Bradley RF, Krall LP. Philadelphia: Lea & Febiger; 1971:50.

39. Jovanovic L, Bevier W: The Santa Barbara County Health Care Services Program: birth weight change concomitant with screening for and treatment of glucose-intolerance of pregnancy: a potential cost-effective intervention. *Am J Perinatol* 1997, 14:221.

40. Buchanan TA, Kjos SL, Montoro MN, et al.: Use of fetal ultrasound to select metabolic therapy for pregnancies complicated by mild gestational diabetes. *Diabetes Care* 1994, 17:275–283.

41. Kjos SL, Schaefer-Graf U, Sardesi S, et al.: A randomized controlled trial using glycemic plus fetal ultrasound parameters versus glycemic parameters to determine insulin therapy in gestational diabetes with fasting hyperglycemia. *Diabetes Care* 2001, 24:1904–1910.

42. Schaefer-Graf UM, Kjos SL, Fauzan OH, et al.: A randomized trial evaluating a predominantly fetal growth-based strategy to guide management of gestational diabetes in Caucasian women. *Diabetes Care* 2004, 27:297–302.

43. Langer O, Conway DL, Berkus MD, et al.: A comparison of glyburide and insulin in women with gestational diabetes mellitus. *N Engl J Med* 2000, 343:1134–1138.

44. Jovanovic L: Nutritional management of the obese gestational diabetic woman [guest editorial]. *J Am Coll Nutr* 1992, 11:246.

45. Jovanovic L: Time to reassess the optimal dietary prescription for women with gestational diabetes [editorial]. *Am J Clin Nutr* 1999, 70:3.

46. Peterson CM, Jovanovic L: Percentage of carbohydrate and glycemia response to breakfast, lunch, and dinner in women with gestational diabetes. *Diabetes* 1991, 40(suppl):172.

47. Ilic S, Jovanovic L, Pettitt DJ: Comparison of the effect of saturated and monounsaturated fat on postprandial plasma glucose and insulin concentration in women with gestational diabetes mellitus. *Am J Perinatol* 2000, 16:489.

48. Jovanovic L, Durak EP, Peterson CM: Randomized trial of diet versus diet plus cardiovascular conditioning on glucose levels in gestational diabetes. *Am J Obstet Gynecol* 1989, 161:415.

49. McCance DR, Pettitt DJ, Hanson RL, et al.: Birth weight and non-insulin dependent diabetes: thrifty genotype, thrifty phenotype, or surviving small baby genotype? *Br Med J* 1994, 308:942.

11

MECHANISMS OF HYPERGLYCEMIC DAMAGE IN DIABETES

Susanna Hofmann and Michael Brownlee

In the 21st century, the central therapeutic problem in diabetes mellitus is not management of its acute metabolic derangements but, rather, prevention and treatment of its chronic micro- and macrovascular complications. In the United States, diabetic microvascular complications are the leading cause of new blindness in people ages 20 to 74 years and are the leading cause of endstage renal disease. Diabetic patients are the fastest growing group of renal dialysis and transplant recipients. The life expectancy for patients with diabetic endstage renal failure is only 3 or 4 years. More than 60% of diabetic patients are affected by neuropathy, which includes distal symmetrical polyneuropathy; mononeuropathies; and a variety of autonomic neuropathies that cause erectile dysfunction, urinary incontinence, gastroparesis, and nocturnal diarrhea. Approximately 60% of type 2 diabetic patients have hypertension. Accelerated lower extremity arterial disease caused by diabetes, in conjunction with neuropathy, makes diabetes account for 50% of all nontraumatic amputations in the United States. Diabetic patients have a death rate from coronary heart disease that is two to four times that of nondiabetic

patients. A similar increased risk occurs with stroke. Heart disease in diabetic patients appears earlier in life and is more often fatal. Life expectancy is about 7 to 10 years shorter for diabetic patients than for people without diabetes [1].

Epidemiologic studies show a strong relationship between glycemia and diabetic microvascular complications in type 1 and type 2 diabetes. There is a continuous relationship between the level of glycemia and the risk of development and progression of complications. In contrast, hyperglycemia is not the primary initiating factor, although it does play a contributing role. Rather, insulin resistance and its consequences are primarily responsible for the progression of complications. This chapter reviews the mechanisms of hyperglycemic damage in diabetes. The discussion includes the specificity of target organ damage, major mechanisms of hyperglycemic tissue damage, relationship of various mechanisms to each other, potential role of insulin resistance, genetics of complication susceptibility, and development of complications during posthyperglycemic euglycemia.

Target-organ Specificity of Hyperglycemic Damage

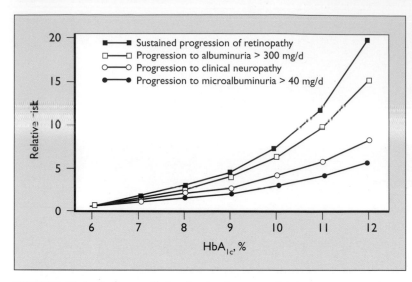

FIGURE 11-1. Relative risks for the development of diabetic microvascular complications at different levels of mean hemoglobin A_{1c} (HbA$_{1c}$, glycated hemoglobin), obtained from the Diabetes Control and Complications Trial. Patients with insulin-dependent diabetes whose intensive insulin therapy resulted in HbA$_{1c}$ values 2% lower than those receiving conventional insulin therapy had a 76% lower incidence of retinopathy, a 54% lower incidence of nephropathy, and a 60% reduction in neuropathy. (*Adapted from* Skyler [1].)

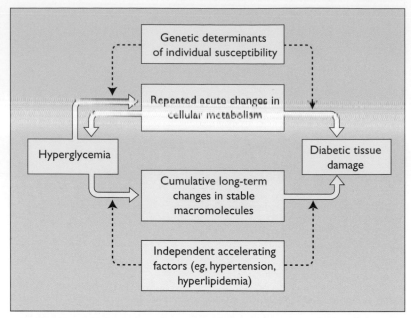

FIGURE 11-2. The mechanisms by which hyperglycemia and independent risk factors interact to cause chronic diabetic complications. One group of mechanisms involves repeated acute changes in cellular metabolism that are reversible when euglycemia is restored. Another group of mechanisms involves cumulative changes in long-lived macromolecules that persist despite restoration of euglycemia. These mechanisms are influenced by genetic determinants of susceptibility or resistance to hyperglycemic damage and by independent risk factors such as hypertension. (*Adapted from* Giardino and Brownlee [2].)

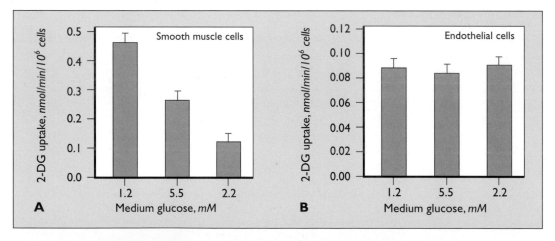

FIGURE 11-3. Lack of downregulation of glucose transport in cells affected by diabetic complications. Vascular smooth muscle cells, which are not damaged by hyperglycemia, show an inverse relationship between glucose concentration and glucose transport, measured as 2-deoxyglucose (2-DG) uptake (**A**). In contrast, vascular endothelial cells, a major target of hyperglycemic damage, show no significant change in glucose transport when the glucose level is elevated (**B**). Thus, intracellular hyperglycemia appears to be the major determinant of diabetic tissue damage. (*Adapted from* Kaiser et al. [3].)

Major Mechanisms of Hyperglycemic Damage

MECHANISMS OF HYPERGLYCEMIA-INDUCED TISSUE DAMAGE

Increased polyol pathway flux

Increased advanced glycation endproduct formation

Activation of protein kinase C isoforms

Increased hexosamine pathway flux

FIGURE 11-4. Mechanisms of hyperglycemia-induced tissue damage. Four major hypotheses about how hyperglycemia causes diabetic complications have generated extensive data, as well as several clinical trials based on specific inhibitors of these mechanisms. More than 1000 papers seemed to show that all were important, yet two things suggested that the something major was missing: there was no apparent common element linking these mechanisms to each other, and clinical trials of inhibitors of these pathways have all been disappointing.

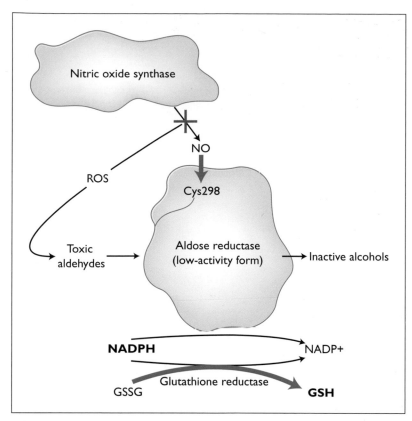

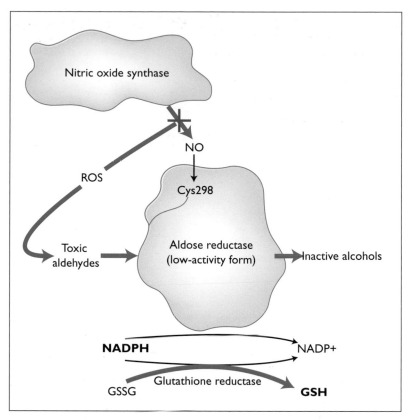

FIGURE 11-5. Potential function of aldose reductase in nondiabetic cells. The enzyme aldose reductase converts a variety of toxic aldehydes (such as 2-oxo-aldehydes and those derived from lipid peroxidation) to inactive alcohols. The reduced form of nicotinamide adenine dinucleotide phosphate (NADPH) is the cofactor in this reaction and in the regeneration of glutathione by glutathione reductase. Reactive oxygen species (ROS) appear to reduce nitric oxide (NO) levels. The activity of aldose reductase is reversibly downregulated by nitric oxide modification of a cysteine residue in the enzyme's active site. GSH—reduced glutathione; GSSG—oxidized glutathione; NADP—nicotinamide adenine dinucleotide phosphate, oxidized form. (*Adapted from* Chandra *et al.* [4], Pieper *et al.* [5], and King and Brownlee [6].)

FIGURE 11-6. Potential function of aldose reductase in nondiabetic cells under oxidative stress. In a euglycemic environment, reactive oxygen species (ROS) increase the concentration of toxic aldehydes. At the same time, nitric oxide (NO) levels are reduced, thereby converting aldose reductase to a high-activity form. Glutathione levels are unaffected. GSH—reduced glutathione; GSSG—oxidized glutathione; NADP—nicotinamide adenine dinucleotide phosphate, oxidized form; NADPH—nicotinamide adenine dinucleotide phosphate, reduced form. (*Adapted from* Chandra *et al.* [4], Pieper *et al.* [5], and King and Brownlee [6].)

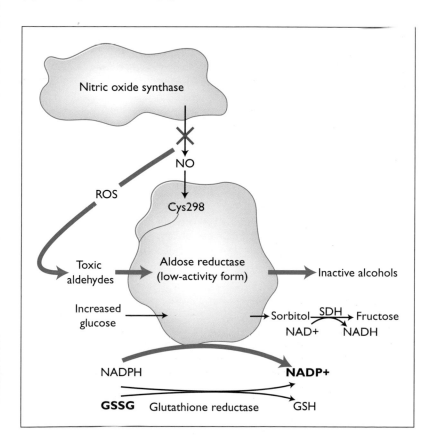

FIGURE 11-7. Potential function of aldose reductase in diabetic cells. In a hyperglycemic environment, reactive oxygen species (ROS) are increased, with the same consequences described in Figure 11-6. In addition, increased intracellular glucose levels result in increased enzymatic conversion to polyalcohol sorbitol and in concomitant decreases in levels of the reduced form of nicotinamide adenine dinucleotide phosphate (NADPH) and glutathione. In cells in which aldose reductase activity is sufficient to deplete glutathione, hyperglycemia-induced oxidative stress is augmented. Sorbitol is oxidized to fructose by the enzyme sorbitol dehydrogenase (SDH). GSH—reduced glutathione; GSSG—oxidized glutathione; NAD—nicotinamide adenine dinucleotide; NADH—nicotinamide adenine dinucleotide, reduced form; NO—nitric oxide. (*Adapted from* Chandra *et al.* [4], Pieper *et al.* [5], and King and Brownlee [6].)

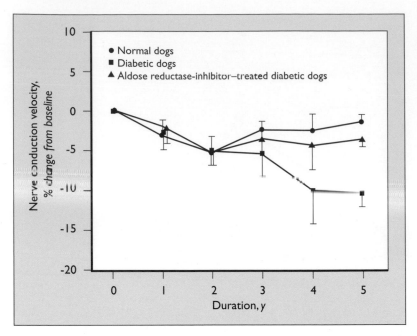

FIGURE 11-8. Effect of aldose reductase inhibition on diabetes-induced dogs decreases in nerve conduction velocity. In diabetic dogs, conduction became significantly less than normal within 42 months. Conduction velocity in dogs treated with aldose reductase inhibitors remained statistically equal to normal throughout the 5-year study. In contrast, aldose reductase inhibition had no effect on the development of diabetic retinopathy and of capillary basement thickening in the retina, kidney, or muscle. (*Adapted from* Engerman *et al.* [7].)

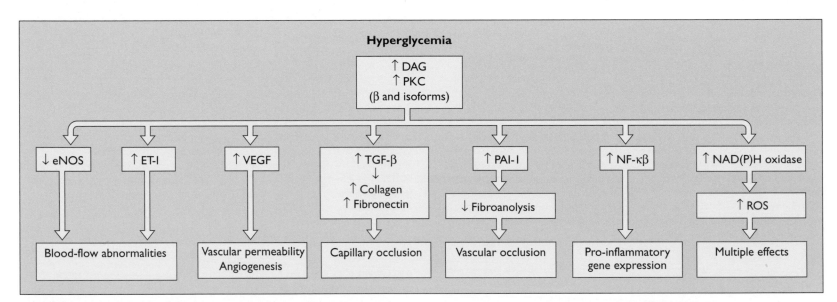

FIGURE 11-9. Potential consequences of hyperglycemia-induced diacylglycerol-protein kinase C activation. Hyperglycemia increases diacylglycerol (DAG) content, in part by de novo synthesis and possibly also by phosphatidylcholine hydrolysis. Increased DAG, its mimetics, and reactive oxygen all activate protein kinase C (PKC), primarily the beta and delta isoforms. Activated PKC increases the production of cytokines and extracellular matrix, the fibrinolytic inhibitor plasminogen activator inhibitor-1 (PAI-1), and the vasoconstrictor endothelin-1 (ET-1). PKC is also a mediator of vascular endothelial growth factor (VEGF) activity. These changes contribute to basement membrane thickening, vascular occlusion, increased permeability, and activation of angiogenesis. ANP—atrial natriuretic peptide; eNOS—endothelial nitric oxide synthase; NADH—nicotinamide adenine dinucleotide; NF-κB—nuclear factor κB; ROS—reactive oxygen species; TGF—transforming growth factor. (*Adapted from* Koya and King [8].)

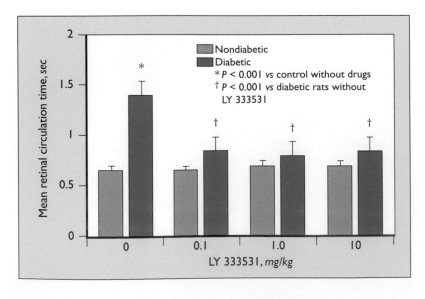

FIGURE 11-10. Amelioration of diabetes-induced retinal vascular dysfunction by an inhibitor of protein kinase C (PKC)-β. In rats, diabetes increased mean retinal circulation time from 0.67 to 1.40 seconds. In diabetic patients, treatment with the highest dose of the PKC beta inhibitor LY 333531 reduced the time to 0.87 seconds. (*Adapted from* Ishii *et al.* [9].)

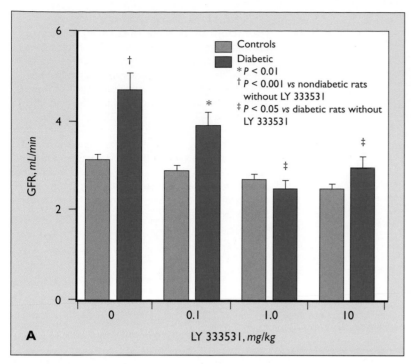

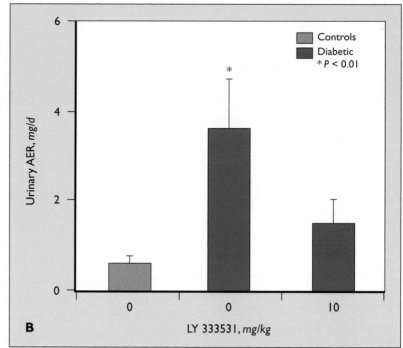

FIGURE 11-11. Amelioration of diabetes-induced renal dysfunction by an inhibitor of protein kinase C (PKC)-β. In rats, diabetes increased the glomerular filtration rate (GFR) from a mean of 3.0 to 4.6 mL/min. In diabetic patients, treatment with the highest dose of the PKC-β inhibitor LY 333531 normalized the mean GFR (**A**). Similarly, diabetes increased the albumin excretion rate in rats from a mean of 1.6 to 11.7 mg/d. Treatment of diabetic patients with the highest dose of LY 333531 reduced the mean albumin excretion rate to 4.9 mg/d (**B**). AER—albumin excretion rate. (*Adapted from* Ishii *et al.* [9].)

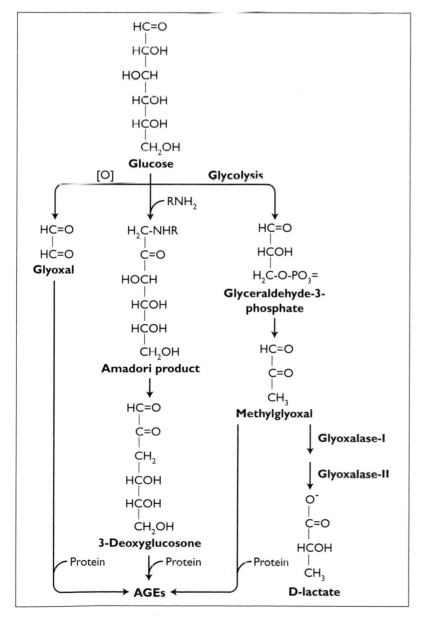

FIGURE 11-12. Potential pathways leading to the formation of advanced glycation endproducts (AGEs). The latter can arise from autoxidation of glucose to glyoxal, decomposition of the Amadori product to 3-deoxyglucosone, and fragmentation of glyceraldehyde-3-phosphate to methylglyoxal. These reactive dicarbonyls react with amino groups of proteins to form AGEs. Methylglyoxal and glyoxal are detoxified by the glyoxalase system. All three AGE precursors are also substrates for other reductases. (*Adapted from* Shinohara *et al.* [10] and Vander Jagt *et al.* [11].)

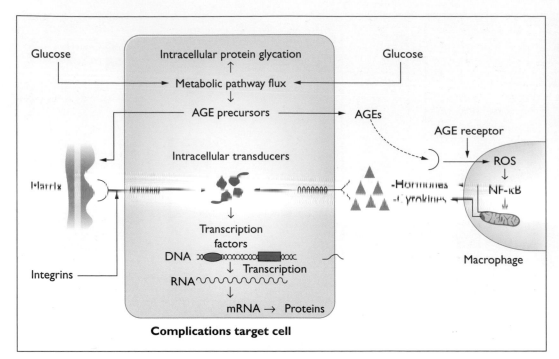

Complications target cell

FIGURE 11-13. Intracellular production of advanced glycation endproduct (AGE) precursors damages target cells by three general mechanisms. First, intracellular protein glycation alters protein function. Second, extracellular matrix modified by AGE precursors has abnormal functional properties. Third, plasma proteins modified by AGE precursors bind to the AGE receptors RAGE (receptor for AGE) on adjacent cells, such as macrophages, thereby inducing receptor-mediated production of reactive oxygen species (ROS). The latter, in turn, activates nuclear factor κB (NF-κB) and expression of pathogenic gene products, including cytokines and hormones. mRNA—messenger RNA. (*Adapted from* Brownlee [12].)

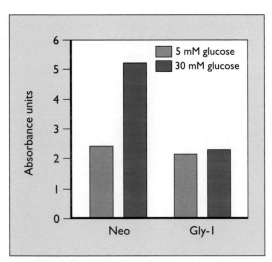

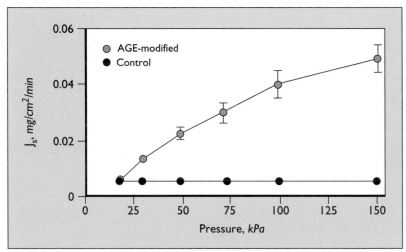

FIGURE 11-14. Intracellular protein glycation by the advanced glycation endproduct precursor methylglyoxal increases macromolecular endocytosis in endothelial cells. After exposure to 30 mmol of glucose/L, macromolecular endocytosis by GM7373 endothelial cells that were stably transfected with neomycin-resistance gene (Neo) were increased 2.2-fold. In contrast, when increased methylglyoxal accumulation was prevented by overexpressing the enzyme glyoxalase I (Gly-1) in these cells, 30 mmol/L of glucose did not increase macromolecular endocytosis. (*Adapted from* Shinohara *et al.* [10].)

FIGURE 11-15. Glomerular basement membrane modified by advanced glycation endproducts (AGEs) has increased permeability to albumin. Ultrafiltration of albumin (Js) by AGE-modified glomerular basement membrane is significantly increased compared with ultrafiltration of albumin by unmodified glomerular basement membrane over a range of different filtration pressures. (*Adapted from* Cochrane and Robinson [13].)

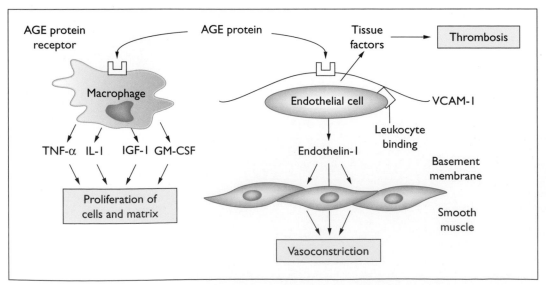

FIGURE 11-16. The mechanisms by which advanced glycation endproduct (AGE)–modified protein binding to specific receptors on macrophages and endothelial cells may cause pathologic changes in diabetic blood vessels. On macrophages and mesangial cells, binding stimulates production of tumor necrosis factor (TNF)-α, interleukin-1 (IL-1), insulin-like growth factor-1 (IGF-1), and granulocyte-macrophage colony-stimulating factor (GM-CSF) at levels that increase proliferation of smooth muscle cells and increase matrix production. On endothelial cells, binding induces procoagulatory changes in gene expression and increased expression of leukocyte-binding vascular adhesion molecule-1 (VCAM-1). (*Adapted from* Brownlee [14].)

EFFECT OF AMINOGUANIDINE TREATMENT ON DIABETIC TARGET TISSUE

Variable	Nondiabetic Animals	Diabetic Animals	Diabetic Animals Receiving Aminoguanidine Treatment
Retinal acellular capillaries, mm^2	9 ± 2	167 ± 27	33 ± 11
Retinal microaneurysms, % positive	0	37.5	0
Urinary albumin excretion, mg/24 h	2.4 ± 1.3	38.9 ± 1.4	5.1 ± 1.5
Mesangial volume fraction, %	12.5 ± 2.5	18.8 ± 2.5	13.7 ± 0.6
Motor nerve conduction velocity, m/sec	65.5 ± 2	52.4 ± 3	64 ± 2
Nerve action potential amplitude, %	100	63	97
Arterial elasticity, nL/mm Hg/mm	—	7.5 ± 1.5	10.8 ± 3
Arterial fluid filtration, nL/mm	—	0.9	0.45

FIGURE 11-17. Amelioration of abnormalities in diabetic target tissues by an advanced glycation endproduct inhibitor. The effects of this inhibitor (aminoguanidine) on diabetic abnormalities have been investigated in the retinas, kidneys, nerves, and arteries. In experimental animals, the development of all pathognomonic abnormalities examined was inhibited by 85% to 90%. In a large randomized, double-blind, placebo-controlled, multicenter study of type 1 diabetic patients with overt nephropathy, aminoguanidine treatment lowered total urinary protein and slowed progression of nephropathy. In addition, aminoguanidine reduced the progression of diabetic retinopathy (Bolton et al., Unpublished data). (Adapted from Brownlee [12].)

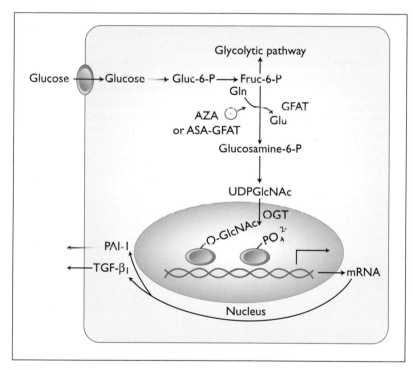

FIGURE 11-18. Hyperglycemia increases flux through the hexosamine pathway. Under hyperglycemic conditions, glucose is metabolized through glycolysis, first to glucose-6 phosphate, then fructose-6 phosphate, and then through the rest of the glycolytic pathway. Some of that fructose-6-phosphate is diverted into a signaling pathway in which the enzyme called glutamine: fructose-6-phosphate amidotransferase (GFAT) converts fructose-6 phosphate to glucosamine-6 phosphate and finally to uridine diphosphate (UDP) N-acetyl glucosamine. Subsequently, the N-acetyl glucosamine is transferred onto transcription factors. Modification by this glucosamine results in increased expression of transforming growth factor (TGF)-β1 and plasminogen activator inhibitor-1 (PAI-1). mRNA—messenger RNA; PAI-1— plasminogen activator inhibitor-1. (Adapted from Brownlee [15].)

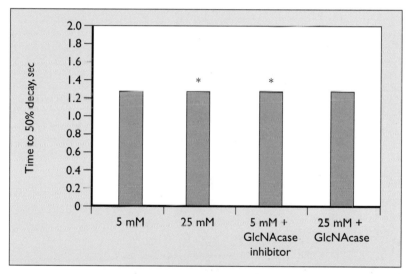

FIGURE 11-19. Hexosamine pathway inhibition prevents impaired cardiomyocyte diastolic dysfunction. Concentrations of 25-mM glucose increase diastolic dysfunction in the cardiomyocytes. Inhibition of the enzyme GlcNAcase that normally removes the N-acetylglucosamine from transcription factors causes the same degree of dysfunction in physiologic glucose (5 mM). Of note, increased removal of the latter by overexpression of the removal enzyme prevents the hyperglycemia-induced defect.

Interrelationship of Mechanisms of Hyperglycemic Damage

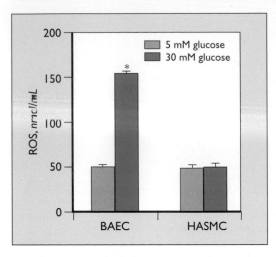

FIGURE 11-20. Hyperglycemia increases intracellular reactive oxygen species (ROS) in cells whose glucose transport rate is not downregulated by hyperglycemia. Hyperglycemia increases intracellular ROS formation in aortic endothelial cells, unable to downregulate glucose transport under hyperglycemic conditions (measured as dichlorofluorescein [DCF]). In contrast, vascular smooth muscle cells, capable of reducing glucose transport (as shown in Fig. 11-3B), do not increase ROS production with hyperglycemia. Thus, hyperglycemia rapidly increases intracellular ROS production in all cell types affected by diabetic complications, which share the ability to protect themselves from intracellular hyprglycemia by downregulating glucose transport (Brownlee, Unpublished data). BAEC— bovine aortic endothelial cell; HASMC—human aortic smooth muscle cell.

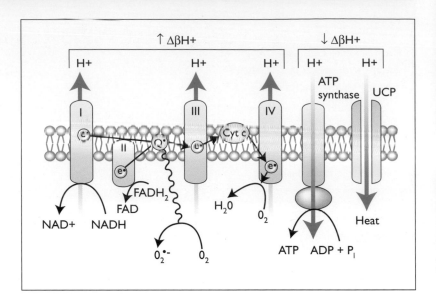

FIGURE 11-21. Production of superoxide by the mitochondrial electron transport chain. Increased hyperglycemia-derived electron donors from the tricarboxylic acid cycle (nicotinamide adenine dinucleotide, reduced form and flavin adenine dinucleotide reduced form [$FADH_2$]) generate a high mitochondrial membrane potential (H^+) by pumping protons across the mitochondrial inner membrane. This inhibits electron transport at complex III, increasing the half-life of free radical intermediates of coenzyme Q (ubiquinone), which reduce O_2 to superoxide. FAD—flavin adenine dinucleotide; NAD—nicotinamide adenine dinucleotide; NADH—nicotinamide adenine dinucleotide, reduced form; UCP—uncoupling protein. (*Adapted from* Brownlee [15].)

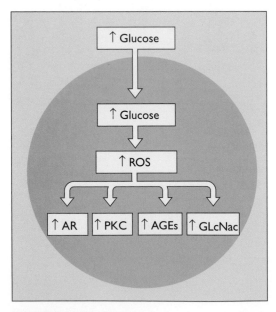

FIGURE 11-22. Overproduction of superoxide by the mitochondrial electron transport chain. Until recently, there has been no apparent common element linking the different biochemical mechanisms underlying diabetic complications. This issue has now been resolved by the recent discovery that each of the different pathogenic mechanisms reflects a single hyperglycemia-induced process: overproduction of superoxide by the mitochondrial electron transport chain. In cells in which intracellular glycemia reflects blood glucose (*eg*, endothelial cells), increased generation of nicotinamide adenine dinucleotide in the tricarboxylic acid cycle results in excess mitochondrial superoxide generation. This superoxide increases flux through aldose reductase (AR), activates protein kinase C (PKC), increases intracellular formation of advanced glycation endproduct (AGE) precursors, and increases flux through the hexosamine pathway (GlcNAc) [15]. ROS—reactive oxygen species.

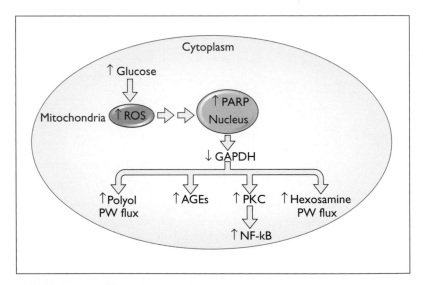

FIGURE 11-23. Hyperglycemia-induced mitochondrial overproduction of reactive oxygen species (ROS) activates all major pathways (PWs) of diabetic cellular damage. This scheme summarizes the unifying mechanism. In cells that are unable to downregulate glucose transport, hyperglycemia-induced mitochondrial overproduction of reactive oxygen activates all major PWs of diabetic cellular damage. This excess of ROS causes strand breaks in nuclear DNA and subsequently activates Poly (ADP-ribose) polymerase (PARP), a DNA repair enzyme, which then modifies glyceraldehyde-phosphate dehydrogenase (GAPDH), reducing its activity. Low GAPDH activity activates the polyol PW, increases intercellular advanced glycation endproduct (AGE) formation, activates protein kinase C (PKC) and subsequently nuclear factor κB (NF-κB), and furthermore increases hexosamine PW flux.

Potential Role of Insulin Resistance

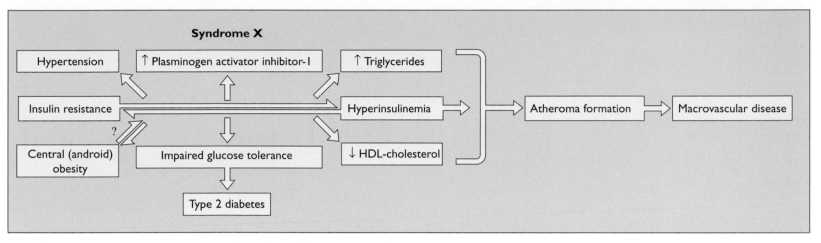

FIGURE 11-24. Insulin resistance may exacerbate known risk factors for vascular damage. Insulin resistance is associated with atherogenic changes in plasma lipoproteins, increased plasminogen activator inhibitor-1 levels, and hypertension. This association has been termed "syndrome X." HDL—high-density lipoprotein. (*Adapted from* Gray and Yudkin [16].)

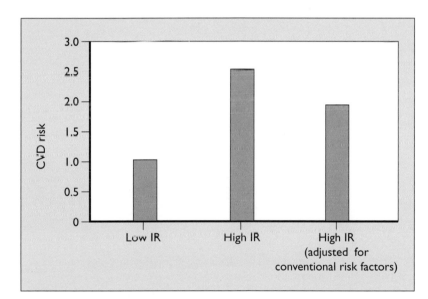

FIGURE 11-25 Conventional metabolic syndrome risk factors are not the major determinants of diabetic macrovascular disease. Data from the San Antonio Heart Study show that in men without diabetes or impaired glucose tolerance, high insulin resistance (IR) increases cardiovascular risk by 2.5-fold. Surprisingly, after adjustment for 11 known cardiovascular disease (CVD) risk factors, including high-density lipoprotein, triglycerides, systolic blood pressure, and smoking, CVD risk remained twofold in insulin-resistant subjects. Thus, a large part of the increased CVD risk conferred by IR reflects a previously unidentified consequence of IR (*Adapted from* Hanley *et al.* [17].).

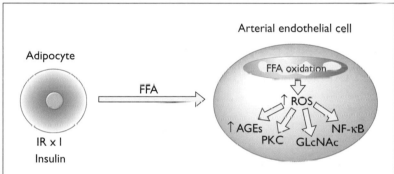

FIGURE 11-26. Increased free fatty acids (FFAs) attributable to insulin resistance cause mitochondrial overproduction of reactive oxygen species (ROS) in macrovascular (but not in microvascular) endothelial cells. Using both cell culture and animal models, Hofmann *et al.* [18] found that the unidentified consequence of insulin resistance is increased FFA flux from adipocytes into arterial endothelial cells. In macrovascular (but not in microvascular) endothelial cells, increased FFA oxidation in the mitochondria causes overproduction of ROS by exactly the same mechanism as previously described for hyperglycemia. The increased ROS generated by FFAs in the arterial endothelial cells activates the same damaging mechanisms as glucose, resulting in a variety of well-described proatherogenic changes. Although more investigations are needed to confirm this hypothesis, at present, it seems that the unified mechanism may explain diabetic macrovascular, as well as microvascular complications. AGE—advanced glycation endproduct; IR—insulin resistance; NF-κB—nuclear factor κB; PKC—protein kinase C. (*Adapted from* Hofmann *et al.* [18].).

Genetics of Susceptibility to Complications

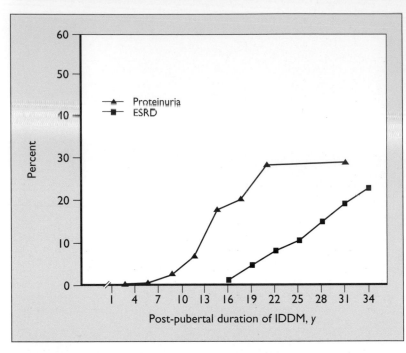

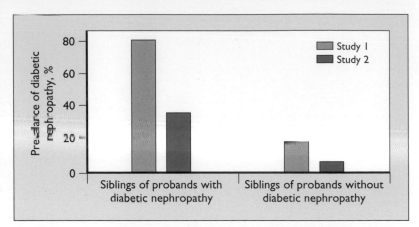

FIGURE 11-28. Familial clustering of diabetic nephropathy suggests a major genetic effect. In one study [20], the risk for nephropathy was 83% in diabetic siblings of an affected patient compared with 16% in diabetic siblings of an unaffected patient. In another study, the risks were 33% and 10%, respectively. Familiar clustering has also been reported for diabetic retinopathy and for coronary artery calcification. (*Adapted from* Trevisan *et al.* [20].)

FIGURE 11-27. Prevalence of clinically significant diabetic nephropathy in patients with insulin-dependent diabetes mellitus (IDDM) according to diabetes duration. The cumulative incidence of overt proteinuria levels off at 27%. After 34 years of diabetes, the cumulative incidence of endstage renal disease (ESRD) is 21.4%. These data suggest that only a subset of patients are susceptible to the development of clinical nephropathy. (*Adapted from* Krolewski *et al.* [19].)

Development of Complications During Posthyperglycemic Euglycemia

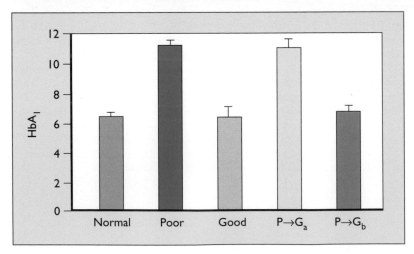

FIGURE 11-29. Development of retinopathy during posthyperglycemic normoglycemia ("hyperglycemic memory"). Shown are mean hemoglobin A (HbA_1) values for dogs in one study [21]. Normal dogs were compared with diabetic dogs who had had poor control for 5 years, good control for 5 years, or poor control for 2.5 years (P-G_a) followed by good control for the next 2.5 years (P-G_b). Values for both the good control group and the P-G_b group were identical to those in the normal group. (*Adapted from* Engerman and Kern [21].)

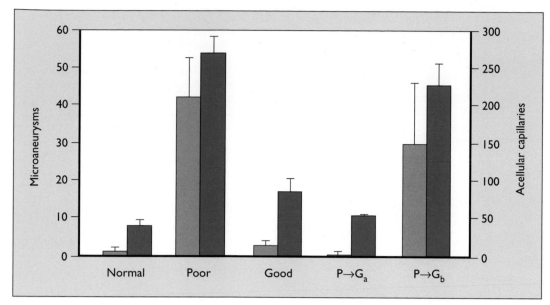

FIGURE 11-30. Development of retinopathy during posthyperglycemic normoglycemia ("hyperglycemic memory"). Shown is quantitation of retinal microaneurysms and acellular capillaries in one study [21]. Lesions of diabetic retinopathy developed during 5 years of poor control. Good control almost always prevented this abnormality. After 2.5 years of poor control (P-Ga), retinopathy was absent. However, despite the institution of good control (P-Gb) in this group after 2.5 years (P-Ga), retinopathy developed over the next 2.5 years to an extent almost equal to that seen in the 5-year poor control group.

This phenomenon has now been confirmed in human diabetes. In the Diabetes Control and Complications Trial (DCCT) follow-up study (EDIC), the mean hemoglobin A_{1c} (HbA$_{1C}$) of the standard therapy group came down, and the mean HbA$_{1c}$ of the intensive therapy group went up to values that were identical for the two groups. These HBA$_{1c}$ values of the two groups have remained identical for nearly 10 years. However, in contrast to expectations, the effects of previous high HbA$_{1c}$ on poststudy retinopathy and nephropathy have persisted, as if there had been no improvement in HbA$_{1c}$ at all. This phenomenon of "metabolic memory" has major implications for the majority of people with diabetes (type 2 diabetics) because the average duration of hyperglycemia before diagnosis is 8 to 10 years, close to the time frame for establishment of "metabolic memory" in the DCCT [22]. (*Adapted from* Engerman and Kern [21].)

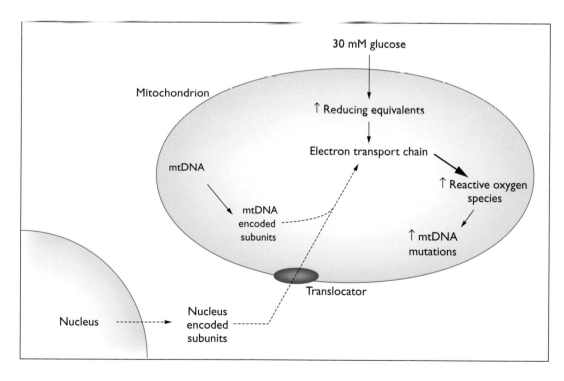

FIGURE 11-31. Potential mechanism for hyperglycemic memory. Hyperglycemia-induced increases in reactive oxygen species (ROS) are a consequence of increased reducing equivalents generated from increased glucose metabolism flowing through the mitochondrial electron transport chain. The increased production of ROS would not only increase aldose reductase activity, protein kinase C activity, and formation of advanced glycation endproducts but would also induce mutations in mitochondrial DNA (mtDNA). (*Adapted from* Wei [23] and Nishikawa *et al.* [24].)

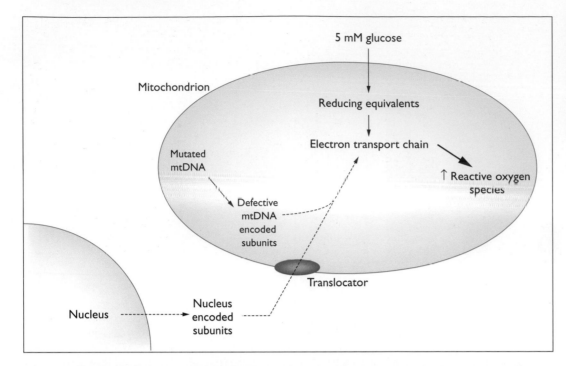

FIGURE 11-32. Potential mechanism for hyperglycemic memory. Mitochondrial DNA (mtDNA) mutated by hyperglycemia-induced reactive oxygen species (ROS) would encode defective electron transport chain subunits. These defective subunits would cause increased production of ROS by the electron transport chain at physiologic concentrations of glucose and glucose-derived reducing equivalents. (*Adapted from* Wei [23] and Nishikawa *et al.* [24].)

References

1. Skyler J: Diabetic complications: the importance of glucose control. *Endocrinol Metab Clin North Am* 1996, 25:243–245.

2. Giardino J, Brownlee M: Mechanisms of chronic diabetic complications. In *Textbook of Diabetes*, vol 1. Edited by Pickup JC, Williams G. London: Blackwell Scientific; 1997.

3. Kaiser N, Sasson S, Feener EP: Differential regulation of glucose transport and transporters by glucose in vascular endothelial and smooth muscle cells. *Diabetes* 1993, 42:80–89.

4. Chandra A, Srivastava S, Petrash JM: Active site modification of aldose reductase by nitric oxide donors. *Biochim Biophys Acta* 1997, 131:217–222.

5. Pieper GM, Langenstroer P, Siebeneich W: Diabetic-induced endothelial dysfunction in rat aorta: role of hydroxyl radicals. *Cardiovasc Res* 1997, 34:145–156.

6. King GL, Brownlee MB: The cellular and molecular mechanisms of diabetic complications. *Endocrinol Metab Clin North Am* 1996, 25:255–270.

7. Engerman RL, Kern TS, Larson ME: Nerve conduction and aldose reductase inhibition during 5 years of diabetes or galactosaemia in dogs. *Diabetologia* 1994, 37:141–144.

8. Koya D, King GL: Protein kinase C activation and the development of diabetic complications. *Diabetes* 1998, 47:859–867.

9. Ishii H, Jirousek MR, Koya D, *et al.*: Amelioration of vascular dysfunctions in diabetic rats by an oral PKC beta inhibitor. *Science* 1996, 272:728–731.

10. Shinohara M, Thornalley PJ, Giardino I, *et al.*: Overexpression of glyoxalase-I in bovine endothelial cells inhibits intracellular advanced glycation endproduct formation and prevents hyperglycemia-induced increases in macromolecular endocytosis. *J Clin Invest* 1998, 101:1142–1147.

11. Vander Jagt DL, Torres JE, Hunsaker LA, *et al.*: Physiological substrates of human aldose and aldehyde reductases. *Adv Exp Med Biol* 1997, 414:491–497.

12. Brownlee M: Glycation and diabetic complications. *Diabetes* 1994, 43:836–841.

13. Cochrane SM, Robinson GB: In vitro glycation of glomerular basement membrane alters its permeability: a possible mechanism in diabetic complications. *FEBS Lett* 1995, 375:41–44.

14. Brownlee M: Advanced glycation end products in diabetic complications. *Curr Opin Endocrinol Diabetes* 1998, 3:291–297.

15. Brownlee M: Biochemistry and molecular cell biology of diabetic complications. *Nature* 2001, 414:813–820.

16. Gray RP, Yudkin JS: Cardiovascular disease in diabetic mellitus. In *Textbook of Diabetes*, vol. 1. Edited by Pickup JC, Williams G. London: Blackwell Scientific; 1997.

17. Hanley AJ, Williams K, Stern MP, Haffner SM: Homeostasis model assessment of insulin resistance in relation to the incidence of cardiovascular disease: the San Antonio Heart Study. *Diabetes Care* 2002, 25:1177–1184.

18. Hofmann S, Brownlee M: *Diabetes Mellitus: A Fundamental and Clinical Text*, edn 3. Edited by LeRotih D, Olefsky JM, Taylor SI. Philadelphia: Lippincott Williams & Wilkins; 2003.

19. Krolewski SA, Warram JH, Freire MB, *et al.*: Epidemiology of late diabetic complications: a basis for the development and evaluation of prevention programs. *Endocrinol Metab Clin North Am* 1996, 25:217–242.

20. Trevisan R, Barnes DJ, *et al.*: Pathogenesis of diabetic nephropathy. In *Textbook of Diabetes*, vol 2. Edited by Pickup JC, Williams G. London: Blackwell Scientific; 1997.

21. Engerman RL, Kern TS: Progression of incipient diabetic retinopathy during good glycemic control. *Diabetes* 1987, 36:808–812.

22. Writing Team for the Diabetes Control and Complications Trial: Effect of intensive therapy on the microvascular complications of type 1 diabetes mellitus. *JAMA* 2002, 287:2563–2569.

23. Wei Y: Oxidative stress and mitochondrial DNA mutations in human aging. *Soc Exp Biol Med* 1998, 217:53–63.

24. Nishikawa T, Edelstein D, Brownlee MB, *et al.*: Reversal of hyperglycemia-induced PKC activation, intracellular AGE formation, and sorbitol accumulation by inhibition of electron transport complex II. *Diabetes* 1999, 48(suppl):A73.

MANAGEMENT AND PREVENTION OF DIABETIC COMPLICATIONS

Sunder Mudaliar and Robert R. Henry

12

Type 2 diabetes is a chronic disease characterized by insulin resistance, impaired insulin secretion, and hyperglycemia. The long-term complications of diabetic retinopathy, nephropathy, neuropathy, and accelerated atherosclerosis lead to significant morbidity in the form of preventable blindness, endstage renal disease, limb amputations, and premature cardiovascular disease [1]. Diabetics suffer from the morbidity of their microvascular complications, and most of them ultimately die from the complications of macrovascular coronary artery disease.

A pathophysiologic hallmark of type 2 diabetes is insulin resistance, which has genetic and acquired components [2]. Glucose intolerance and hyperglycemia supervene only when the pancreatic β cell is unable to maintain compensatory hyperinsulinemia to overcome tissue resistance to insulin action [3]. In addition to having hyperglycemia and insulin resistance, nearly 80% of diabetics are obese and have a host of other metabolic abnormalities, including dyslipidemia (increased small dense low-density lipoprotein cholesterol, decreased high-density lipoprotein cholesterol, and raised triglyceride levels), hypertension, and abnormalities of coagulation and the fibrinolytic system. This cluster of metabolic abnormalities, which has been termed the *metabolic syndrome* [4] or the *cardiovascular dysmetabolic syndrome* [5], is associated with a higher incidence of cardiovascular morbidity and mortality [6].

The major cause of tissue damage in diabetes is vascular disease in the micro- and macrovasculature [7,8]. Four major molecular mechanisms have been implicated in glucose-mediated vascular damage. These include increased polyol pathway flux, increased flux through the hexosamine pathway, increased formation of diacylglycerol with subsequent activation of specific protein kinase C isoforms, and accelerated nonenzymatic formation of advanced glycation endproducts. Recent evidence seems to suggest that each of these mechanisms is triggered by a single hyperglycemia-induced process of overproduction of superoxide by the mitochondrial electron transport chain [8]. The net result of these changes induced by hyperglycemia in diabetes is overproduction of potentially damaging reactive oxygen species and upregulation of cytokines and tissue growth factors. In insulin-resistant patients with type 2 diabetes, in addition to hyperglycemia, insulin resistance also plays a major role in the induction of macrovascular abnormalities and atherosclerotic cardiovascular disease [4,5].

The development of diabetic complications is no longer inevitable. Results from the United Kingdom Prospective Diabetes Study clearly demonstrate that tight glucose and blood pressure control in patients with type 2 diabetes prevents the development of and delays the progression of microvascular complications and possibly macrovascular disease [9–11]. In addition, results from the United Kingdom Prospective Diabetes Study and other studies have shown that treatment of concomitant risk factors such as lipids and blood pressure and the use of aspirin have favorable effects on cardiovascular complications in patients with type 2 diabetes [12]. However, the ultimate goal in the management of diabetes is the prevention of diabetes. Recent results from the Diabetes Prevention Program have shown that with intensive lifestyle modification, it is possible to delay or prevent the onset of type 2 diabetes in high-risk individuals [13].

Complications of Diabetes

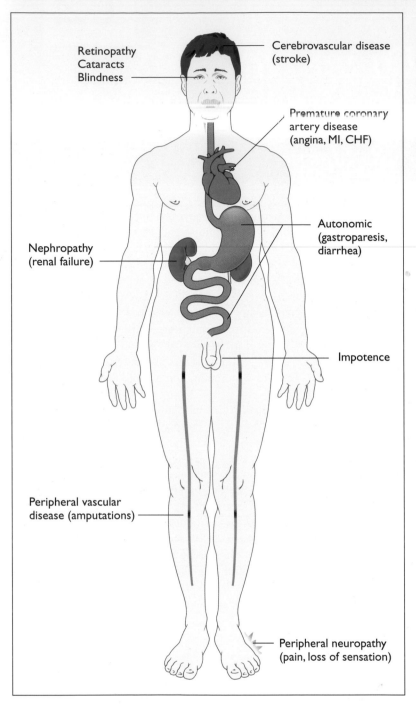

FIGURE 12-1. Clinical manifestations of diabetes. The complications of diabetes are protean and encompass nearly all organ systems. Diabetes is currently the leading cause of adult-onset blindness in the United States, and it accounts for more than one third of new cases of endstage renal disease. Accelerated lower extremity arterial disease in diabetics with neuropathy is responsible for 50% of all nontraumatic amputations, and the death rate for cardiovascular disease in diabetes patients is at least 2.5 times that in nondiabetic patients [1]. Heart disease appears earlier in type 2 diabetes and is more often fatal. Throughout their lives, diabetic individuals suffer from the microvascular complications of blindness, endstage renal disease, and neuropathy, and, sooner rather than later, most diabetics ultimately die from the complications of macrovascular cardiovascular disease. CHF—congestive heart failure; MI—myocardial infarction.

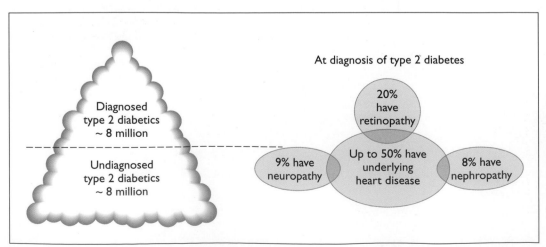

FIGURE 12-2. The epidemiology of diabetes and its complications. Diabetes mellitus is an important clinical and public health problem in the United States. Nearly 8 million adults have been diagnosed with diabetes—90% to 95% of whom have type 2 diabetes. In addition, it is estimated that an additional 8 million individuals who meet the diagnostic criteria for diabetes remain undiagnosed. It has been estimated that among patients in the United States, type 2 diabetes may have been present for up to 12 years before clinical diagnosis. During this period of undiagnosed and untreated diabetes, micro- and macrovascular disease progress. By the time of diagnosis, 20% of patients have retinopathy, 8% have nephropathy, 9% have neuropathy, and up to 50% have cardiovascular disease [1,14].

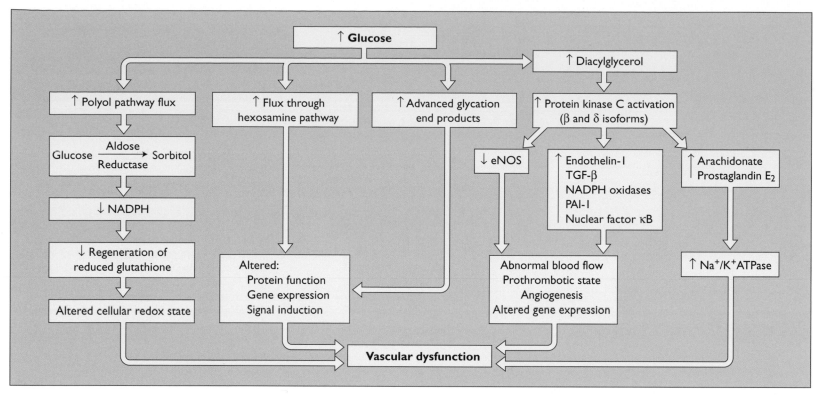

FIGURE 12-3. Possible cellular and molecular mechanisms of vascular disease in diabetes. Hyperglycemia in diabetes causes damage to many tissues, including the retina, kidneys, nerves, heart, brain, and skin. A major cause of tissue damage is vascular disease, which affects the microvasculature and the macrovasculature. Hyperglycemia-induced mechanisms that induce vascular damage include increased polyol pathway flux, increased flux through the hexosamine pathway, increased formation of diacylglycerol and the subsequent activation of specific protein kinase C isoforms, and accelerated nonenzymatic formation of advanced glycation endproducts (AGEs). Each of these mechanisms contributes to vascular dysfunction through a number of mechanisms, including the production of vasodilatory prostaglandins, overproduction of potentially damaging reactive oxygen species, and upregulation of cytokines and growth factors. eNOS— endothelial nitric oxide synthase; NADPH—nicotinamide adenine dinucleotide phosphate; PAI-1—plasminogen activator inhibitor-1; TGF-β—transforming growth factor–β. (*Adapted from* King [7] and Brownlee [8].)

Diabetic Retinopathy

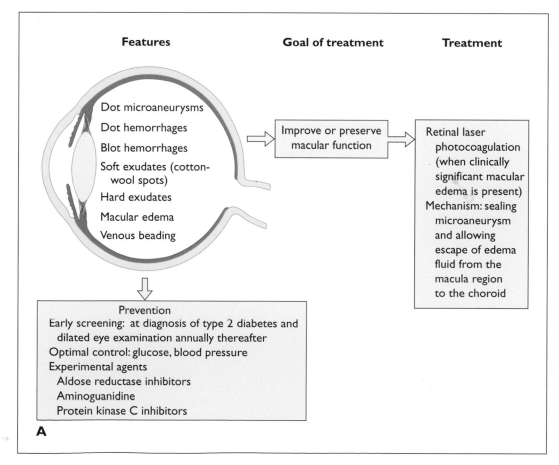

Features	Goal of treatment	Treatment

Dot microaneurysms
Dot hemorrhages
Blot hemorrhages
Soft exudates (cotton-wool spots)
Hard exudates
Macular edema
Venous beading

Improve or preserve macular function

Retinal laser photocoagulation (when clinically significant macular edema is present)
Mechanism: sealing microaneurysm and allowing escape of edema fluid from the macula region to the choroid

Prevention
Early screening: at diagnosis of type 2 diabetes and dilated eye examination annually thereafter
Optimal control: glucose, blood pressure
Experimental agents
  Aldose reductase inhibitors
  Aminoguanidine
  Protein kinase C inhibitors

A

FIGURE 12-4. Clinical features and management of diabetes. Diabetes is the leading cause of new blindness in adults. Retinopathy is present in a considerable proportion of type 2 diabetics at the time of diagnosis. After 15 or more years of disease, the risk of any retinopathy is approximately 78%, with approximately one third of patients having macular edema and approximately one sixth of patients having proliferative retinopathy [15]. Diabetic retinopathy may be classified as nonproliferative diabetic retinopathy (NPDR) or proliferative diabetic retinopathy (PDR). **A**, NPDR. NPDR is characterized by structural abnormalities of the retinal vessels (primarily, the capillaries but also the venules and arterioles), varying degrees of retinal nonperfusion, retinal edema, lipid exudates, and intraretinal hemorrhage. NPDR may be mild, moderate, or severe.

(Continued on next page)

Features

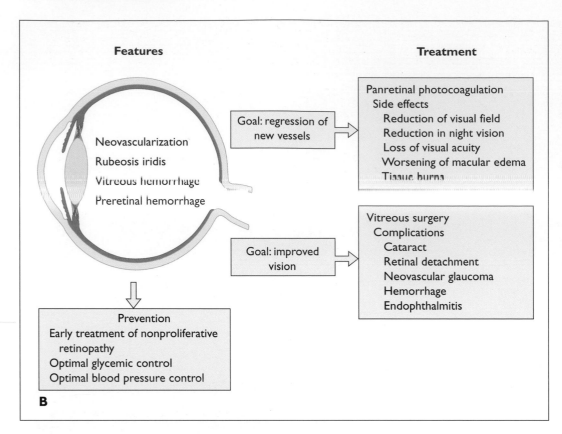

Neovascularization
Rubeosis iridis
Vitreous hemorrhage
Preretinal hemorrhage

Goal: regression of new vessels →

Treatment

Panretinal photocoagulation
Side effects
Reduction of visual field
Reduction in night vision
Loss of visual acuity
Worsening of macular edema
Tissue burns

Goal: improved vision →

Vitreous surgery
Complications
Cataract
Retinal detachment
Neovascular glaucoma
Hemorrhage
Endophthalmitis

Prevention
Early treatment of nonproliferative
retinopathy
Optimal glycemic control
Optimal blood pressure control

B

FIGURE 12-4. *(Continued)* **B,** PDR. The presence of extensive areas of hemorrhages, microaneurysms, venous beading, or intraretinal microvascular abnormalities (tortuous dilated vessels adjacent to nonperfused areas of the retina) predicts the progression to PDR. For patients with mild, moderate, or severe NPDR, the risk of developing PDR is 5%, 12% to 24%, and 50%, respectively [15].

All patients with type 2 diabetes should have a dilated eye examination at the time of diagnosis and annually or more often thereafter [16]. Prevention of retinopathy is best accomplished by maintaining near normal glycemia. After NPDR develops, intensive attempts should be made to optimize glucose and blood pressure (BP) control, and clinically significant macular edema (*ie*, retinal edema that threatens the fovea) should be treated with focal or grid photocoagulation, which reduces the risk of moderate visual loss by approximately 50%. Panretinal photocoagulation may be beneficial in PDR, along with measures to optimize glucose and BP control [15]. The United Kingdom Prospective Diabetes Study has confirmed that intensive blood glucose and BP control reduces the risk of retinopathy progression [9–11].

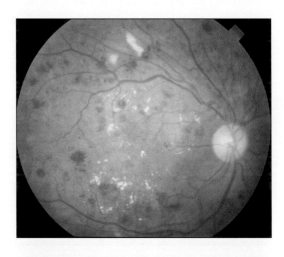

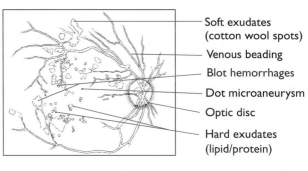

Soft exudates
(cotton wool spots)
Venous beading
Blot hemorrhages
Dot microaneurysm
Optic disc
Hard exudates
(lipid/protein)

FIGURE 12-5. Nonproliferative diabetic retinopathy (NPDR). The characteristic features of NPDR include dot aneurysms (hypercellular, saccular outpouchings of the capillary wall), blot hemorrhages resulting from vascular occlusion, cotton-wool spots (retinal nerve fiber infarcts caused by ischemia), hard exudates (lipid and protein exudates caused bexcessive vascular permeability), and venous beading (abnormal appearance of retinal veins with localized swellings and constrictions resembling sausage links). (*Courtesy of* Dr. M. Goldbaum, UCSD/VA San Diego Health Care System, San Diego, CA.)

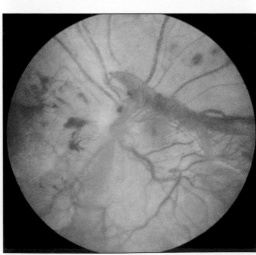

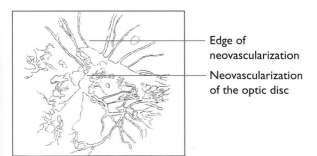

Edge of
neovascularization
Neovascularization
of the optic disc

FIGURE 12-6. Classical features of proliferative diabetic retinopathy (PDR). The development of neovascularization is pathognomonic of this stage. The presence of new vessels on the optic nerve head or on more than one fourth of the disc area, together with preretinal or vitreous hemorrhages, is indicative of high-risk PDR and is an absolute indication for panretinal photocoagulation, if technically possible. (*Courtesy of* Dr. M. Goldbaum, UCSD/VA San Diego Health Care System, San Diego, CA.)

Nephropathy

URINARY ALBUMIN EXCRETION RATE

	Urinary AER, 24-h Collection, mg	Timed Collection, µg/min	Spot Collection, µg/mg Creatinine
Normal	< 30	< 20	< 30
Microalbuminuria	30–299	20–199	30–299
Macroalbuminuria (overt neuropathy)	300 or greater	200 or greater	300 or greater

FIGURE 12-7. Urinary albumin excretion rate (AER). The incidence of endstage renal disease (ESRD) in type 2 diabetes ranges from 4% to 20%. Because type 2 diabetes is 10 times or more prevalent than type 1 diabetes, the incidence of ESRD is approximately the same in both types of diabetes [1]. The cost of treatment for ESRD in diabetes in the United States exceeds $2 billion annually [17].

A nondiabetic patient with normal kidneys excretes less than 30 mg of albumin every 24 hours (20 µm/min) into the urine, and in a spot urine collection has an albumin:creatinine ratio of less than 30 (mg of albumin/mg of creatinine). Microalbuminuria is present at diagnosis in 3% to 30% of patients with type 2 diabetes. Without specific interventions, 20% to 40% of type 2 diabetes patients with microalbuminuria progress to overt nephropathy. However, 20 years after the onset of overt nephropathy, only approximately 20% have

progressed to ESRD [18]. There is substantial evidence that the onset of microalbuminuria and progression of nephropathy correlate closely with poor glycemic control and, more importantly, that improved glycemic and blood pressure control reduces the onset and progression of microalbuminuria and nephropathy [9–11,19]. Screening for microalbuminuria should be performed at the time of diagnosis and annually thereafter by a random/spot urine albumin and creatinine measurement. (This test has good correlation with 24-hour albumin measurements.) Because the urine albumin excretion rate is variable, two of three specimens collected within a 3- to 6-month period should be abnormal before a patient is considered to have crossed a diagnostic threshold. Exercise within the preceding 24 hours, fever, heart failure, marked hyperglycemia, and marked hypertension may elevate urine albumin excretion rate over borderline values [18].

STAGES OF DIABETIC NEUROPATHY IN TYPE 2 DIABETES

Asymptomatic	Renal Insufficiency	Endstage Renal Disease
Normal GFR/creatinine	Decreasing GFR	Uremia
Hypertension	Increasing creatinine	Greatly increased creatinine
Microalbuminuria (30–300 mg/d)	Proteinuria > 500 mg/d	Greatly decreased GFR (< 15 mL/min)

FIGURE 12-8. Stages of diabetic nephropathy in type 2 diabetes. The natural history of nephropathy In type 2 diabetes is not as clear as it is in type 1 diabetes, for which five stages of nephropathy have been described: 1) an early stage of increased glomerular filtration, progressing through 2) a stage of early glomerular lesions with glomerular basement thickening and mesangial matrix expansion, and on to 3) incipient diabetic nephropathy with microalbuminuria (urinary albumin 30 to 300 mg/day). Ultimately, 4) clinical nephropathy with overt proteinuria over 500 mg/day and declining glomerular filtration rate (GFR) develops and culminates in 5) endstage renal disease. The early stages of nephropathy have not yet been well documented in type 2 diabetes. (*Data from* Friedman [20].)

MEASURES TO PREVENT OR RETARD DIABETIC NEUROPATHY

Optimal glycemic control: HbA$_{1C}$ < 7% (caution in the elderly)

Adequate BP control: < 130/80 mm Hg (caution in those with autonomic neuropathy)

ACE inhibitors (when microalbuminuria is present with urinary albumin 30–300 mg/d)

Dietary protein restriction (when overt neuropathy is present with urinary protein > 500 mg/d or when there is a strong family history of neuropathy)

Experimental

Aminoguanidine (inhibits AGE formation)

Protein kinase C inhibitors

FIGURE 12-9. Measures to prevent or retard diabetic nephropathy. In the United Kingdom Prospective Diabetes Study (UKPDS), tight glycemic control (with a median hemoglobin A$_{1C}$ [HbA$_{1C}$] of < 7%) and blood pressure (BP) control (with a mean BP of 144/82 mm Hg) were associated with reductions in the progression of microalbuminuria [9–11]. More recently, in the MICRO-HOPE (Microalbuminuria, Cardiovascular, and Renal Outcomes Heart Outcomes Prevention Evaluation Study) study [21], 3577 subjects with type 2 diabetes were randomized to placebo or 10 mg/d of ramipril, an angiotensin-converting enzyme inhibitor. The study was stopped 6 months early (after 4.5 years) because ramipril had consistent benefits in not only reducing the risk of overt nephropathy by 16% but also was associated with significant reductions in the risk of myocardial infarction, stroke, cardiovascular mortality, and all-cause mortality by approximately 30%. ACE—angiotensin-converting enzyme; AGE—advanced glycation endproduct.

Diabetic Neuropathy

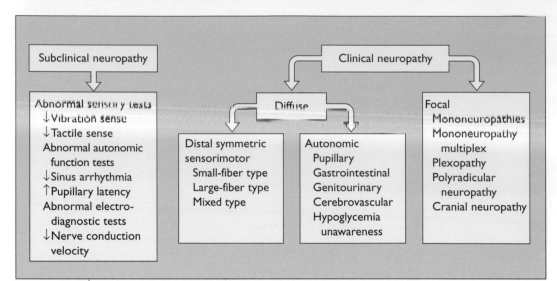

FIGURE 12-10. Clinical features of diabetic neuropathy. Diabetic neuropathy is one of the most common complications of diabetes. Its clinical manifestations cause much suffering among diabetic patients. Acute hyperglycemia decreases nerve function, and chronic hyperglycemia is characterized by progressive loss of nerve fibers, a loss that can be assessed noninvasively by several tests of nerve function, including quantitative sensory tests, autonomic function tests, and electrophysiologic testing [22].

CLINICAL FEATURES OF DISTAL SENSORIMOTOR DIABETIC NEUROPATHY

Large Fiber Type	Small Fiber Type
Unsteady gait	Pain predominates
Absent reflexes	Variable reflexes
Decreased vibration/position sense	Variable position/vibration sense
Charcot's joints possible	Variable presence of Charcot's joints
Mimics posterior column lesions	Ultimately leads to sensory loss

FIGURE 12-11. Distal sensorimotor diabetic neuropathy.

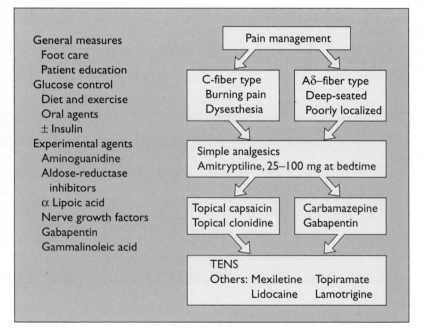

FIGURE 12-12. Management of peripheral diabetic neuropathy. The pathophysiologic mechanisms underlying decreased nerve function and nerve fiber loss in diabetics still are not fully understood but may include the formation of sorbitol by aldose reductase and the formation of advanced glycation endproducts [22]. Similar to other diabetic complications, the progression of neuropathy is related to glycemic control. Chronic sensory neuropathy with moderate or severe sensory loss involving large-fiber sensation (touch, vibration, and joint position sense) or small-fiber sensation (pain and temperature sense) is associated with a high risk of ulceration.

Current approaches to the prevention and treatment of diabetic neuropathy include measures to optimize glucose coes for pain control; and use of aldose reductase inhibitors, which appear to slow the progression of neuropathy rather than provide symptomatic relief [23]. TENS—transcutaneous electrical nerve stimulation.

Diabetic Foot Disease

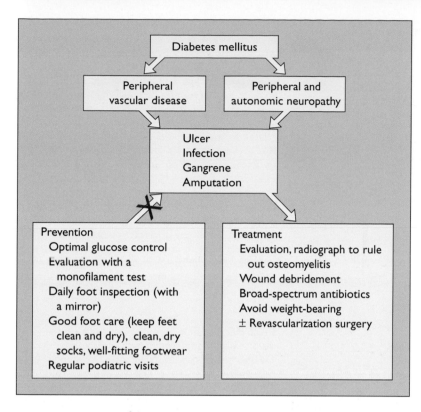

FIGURE 12-13. Clinical features and management of diabetic foot disease. Diabetic foot lesions are a major cause of hospitalization, with approximately 20% of all diabetics entering the hospital because of foot problems. Nearly 55,000 lower extremity amputations are performed each year in the United States on diabetic individuals, accounting for 50% of all nontraumatic amputations [24]. Diabetic foot lesions are the result of a combination of peripheral and autonomic neuropathy and peripheral vascular disease (ischemia). The cascade of events begins with foot ulcers, infection, and gangrene, and ultimately results in amputation. Management of diabetic foot ulcers should be aggressive and should include detailed evaluation of the ulcer and the foot, radiography to exclude osteomyelitis, broad-spectrum antibiotics, wound debridement (if indicated), and avoidance of weight-bearing. Topical application of antibacterial agents and platelet-derived growth factors may be useful adjunctive measures. Preventive measures include optimal glycemic control; daily foot inspections (with the aid of a mirror); good foot care (keeping the feet clean and dry); wearing clean socks and appropriate, well-fitting shoes; and regular podiatric visits. Good patient education and a team approach are the keys to the prevention and treatment of diabetic foot disease.

Diabetic individuals are particularly prone to foot deformities and the development of cocked-up toes, which results in pressure at the tips of the toes and under the first metatarsal head, leading to ulceration and infection. The ideal treatment is prophylactic surgery to straighten the toes. If this is not feasible, special shoes with a cushioned insole to protect the toes and metatarsal head should be worn. All diabetics should have the protective sensory function in their feet evaluated with a 10-g Semmestel-Weinstein monofilament. If a patient cannot consistently feel a 10-g monofilament, protective sensory function has been lost, and the patient is at high risk of developing foot ulcers [25].

Diabetic Male Sexual Dysfunction

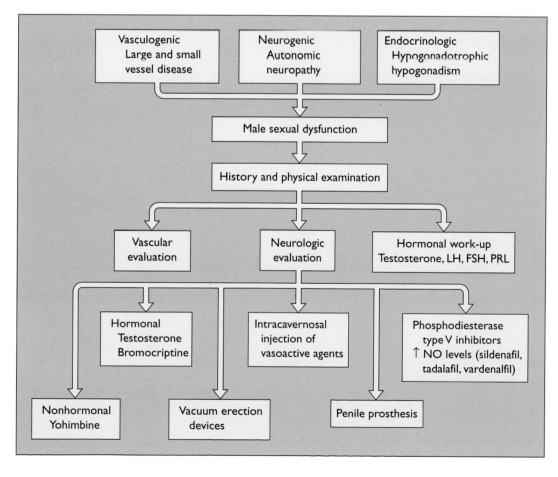

FIGURE 12-14. Evaluation and management of diabetic male sexual dysfunction. The prevalence of erectile dysfunction in diabetic men ranges from 35% to 75%, significantly higher than that in the general population [26]. Its onset is insidious, and it may occur early in the disease. The major underlying abnormalities are vascular (cavernosal artery insufficiency, corporal veno-occlusive dysfunction) and neurologic (autonomic neuropathy). The role of hormonal abnormalities is controversial. All diabetic men with erectile dysfunction require a detailed endocrinologic workup (luteinizing hormone [LH], follicle-stimulating hormone [FSH], prolactin [PRL], and testosterone levels) and, in select cases, vascular evaluation (intracavernosal injection test, visual sexual stimulation, and penile duplex ultrasonography) and neurologic evaluation (nocturnal penile tumescence test, cavernosal electrical activity potential, somatosensory evoked potentials, and sacral latency test). Treatment options include nonhormonal α-2-adrenergic blocking agents (yohimbine); hormonal therapy, if indicated (testosterone replacement in hypogonadism, bromocriptine or surgery for prolactinomas, discontinuation of medications causing hyperprolactinemia); vacuum erection devices; intracavernosal injection of vasoactive agents; penile prostheses (in selected cases); and the recently introduced phosphodiesterase V inhibitors sildenafil, vardenafil, and tadalafil, which act by increasing nitric oxide (NO) levels.

Cardiovascular Disease in Diabetes

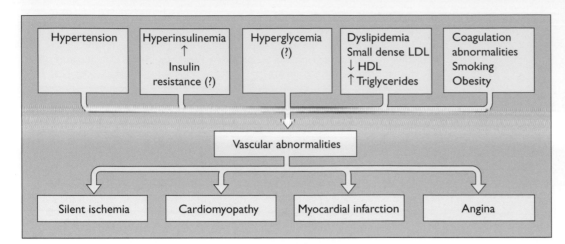

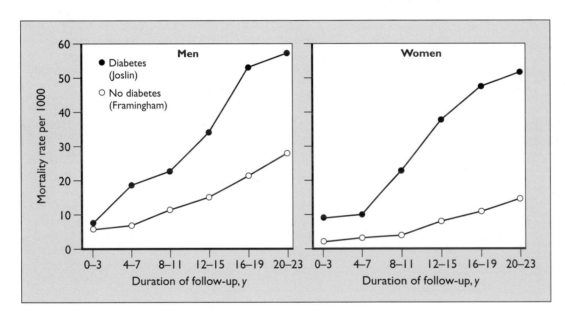

FIGURE 12-15. Pathogenesis and clinical features of heart disease in diabetes. The risk for cardiovascular disease in patients with diabetes is two to five times that in nondiabetic persons [27]. At the time of diagnosis of type 2 diabetes, more than 50% of patients have preexisting coronary artery disease [14]. Numerous risk factors contribute to macrovascular dysfunction in type 2 diabetes. Some appear related to the insulin resistance and hyperinsulinemia that is characteristic of the early stages of type 2 diabetes before the onset of pancreatic β-cell exhaustion and overt hyperglycemia. These include the various components of the cardiovascular dysmetabolic syndrome (ie, hypertension, central obesity, dyslipidemia, glucose intolerance, and coagulation abnormalities) [5]. Heart disease in diabetics may result in silent myocardial ischemia or manifest as angina, myocardial infarction, or congestive heart failure (diabetic cardiomyopathy). HDL—high-density lipoprotein; LDL—low-density lipoprotein.

FIGURE 12-16. Cardiovascular disease is the major cause of mortality in type 2 diabetics. Comparison of data from the Joslin Study and the Framingham Study show that the mortality rate attributable to coronary artery disease (CAD) is doubled in men with diabetes and nearly quadrupled in women with diabetes as compared with the nondiabetic population [28]. Moreover, within the diabetic population, glucose control is an important predictor of CAD mortality and all CAD events [29].

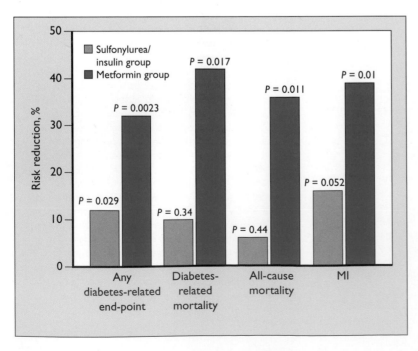

FIGURE 12-17. The United Kingdom Prospective Diabetes Study (UKPDS) was a large study in which 5102 subjects with newly diagnosed type 2 diabetes were followed for an average of 10 years to determine whether intensive glucose lowering reduces cardiovascular and microvascular complications and to determine the benefits and disadvantages of sulfonylureas, metformin, and insulin [9,10]. The UKPDS results demonstrated that although microvascular complications are decreased by nearly 25% by lowering hemoglobin A_{1C} (HbA_{1C}) to a median of 7% (compared with 7.9% in the conventional group), there was no significant effect on cardiovascular complications, with only a nonsignificant 16% reduction in the risk of combined fatal or nonfatal myocardial infarction (MI). However, an epidemiologic analysis showed a continuous association between the risk of cardiovascular complications and glycemia, such that for every percentage point decrease in HbA_{1C} (eg, 9% to 8%), there was a 25% reduction in diabetes related deaths, a 7% reduction in all-cause mortality, and an 18% reduction in fatal or nonfatal MI.

In the subgroup of obese diabetic subjects treated with metformin, intensive glucose lowering with a median HbA_{1C} of 7.4% (compared with 8.0% in the conventional group) was associated with significantly decreased risks of diabetes-related deaths, all-cause mortality, and MI [10]. However, in a surprise outcome, in obese diabetic subjects in this substudy who had metformin added to existing sulfonylurea treatment, there was a significant increase in all-cause and diabetes-related mortality and no beneficial effects on cardiovascular or microvascular outcomes. In the UKPDS, reassuringly, tight blood pressure control (144/82 vs 154/87 mm Hg) was associated with significant reductions in virtually all cardiovascular and microvascular outcomes [11].

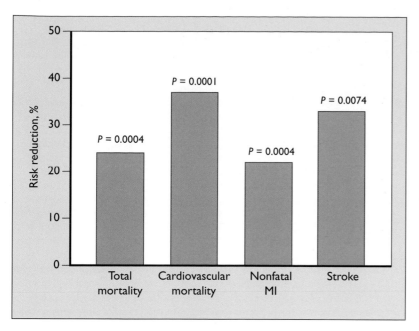

FIGURE 12-18. In contrast to the United Kingdom Prospective Diabetes Study, which studied patients with newly diagnosed diabetes, the recently concluded MICRO-HOPE (Microalbuminuria, Cardiovascular, and Renal Outcomes Heart Outcomes Prevention Evaluation Study) study randomized 3577 patients with long-standing type 2 diabetes (12 years' duration) to treatment with placebo or ramipril (an angiotensin-converting enzyme inhibitor) [21]. The study was stopped 6 months early (after 4.5 years) because 10 mg/day of ramipril significantly lowered the risk of all the measured cardiovascular outcomes, including fatal and nonfatal myocardial infarction (MI), stroke, nephropathy, and all-cause and cardiovascular mortality by 22% to 37%. The cardiovascular benefit in this study was greater than that attributable to the small decrease in blood pressure (BP) seen in this study and also additive to those of baseline therapeutic agents, which included aspirin, lipid-lowering agents, and other BP-lowering drugs.

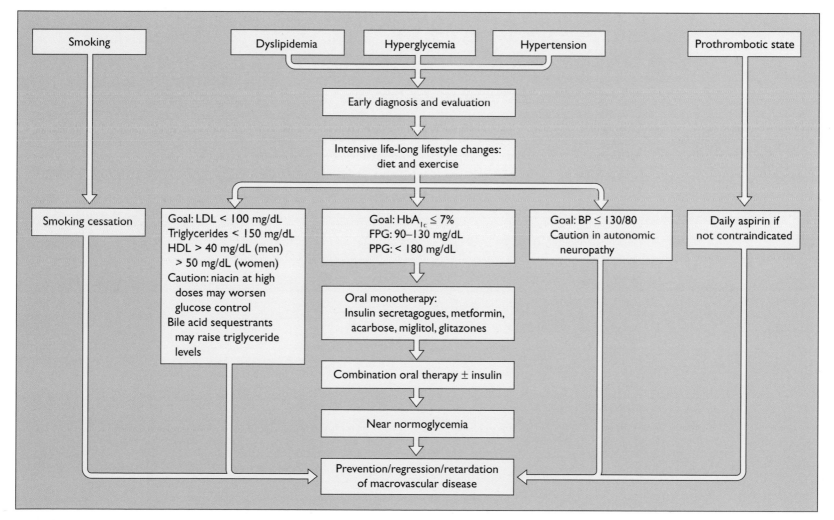

FIGURE 12-19. A multifactorial approach to management of cardiovascular disease in diabetes. Multiple risk factors contribute to accelerated atherosclerosis and premature coronary artery disease (CAD) in patients with diabetes. The cornerstone of prevention is aggressive intervention to identify and favorably modify established risk factors, including hyperglycemia, hyperlipidemia, and hypertension. Because of the extremely high risk of macrovascular disease in diabetes, the National Cholesterol Education Program has recently designated diabetes as a "CAD risk equivalent" [4] and, hence, in patients with diabetes, the target low-density lipoprotein (LDL) cholesterol level should be less than 100 mg/dL; the target high-density lipoprotein (HDL) cholesterol goal should be above 40 mg/dL in men and 50 mg/dL in women; and the triglyceride goal should be less than 150 mg/dL [30]. Unless contraindicated, all eligible diabetics should take aspirin daily [31]. The importance of lifestyle changes and strict adherence to dietary and exercise recommendations should be emphasized at all times. The success of a focused, multifactorial intervention approach with continued patient education and motivation and strict targets was demonstrated in the recently concluded Steno-2 study. In this study, those in the group assigned to intensive multifactorial intervention not only achieved significantly better glycemic control, blood pressure (BP), and lipid parameters but also had a significantly lower risk of cardiovascular and microvascular events by approximately 50% [32]. FPG—fasting plasma glucose; HbA_{1C}—hemoglobin A_{1C}; PPG—postprandial glucose.

Economic Implications of Diabetic Complications

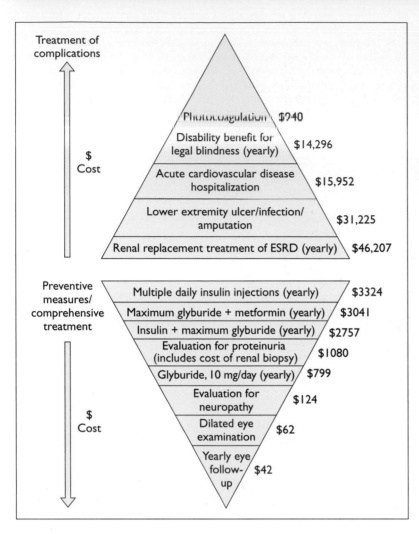

FIGURE 12-20. Dollar cost of diabetic complications: prevention versus treatment. The annual expense of treating diabetes and its complications in the United States (most of which is for treatment of type 2 diabetes) is estimated at about $100 billion [17]. Not only is type 2 diabetes costly, but it also causes excessive morbidity and mortality. Analysis of data has shown that prevention of this disease is not only preferable to treatment but is also more cost effective. This figure compares the cost of comprehensive treatment of diabetes with medications and preventive measures with the monumental costs of treating disease complications such as retinopathy, nephropathy, neuropathy, foot disease, and cardiovascular disease. It has been estimated that comprehensive treatment of type 2 diabetes with hemoglobin A_{1C} values maintained at 7.2% will reduce the cumulative incidence of blindness by 72%, endstage renal disease (ESRD) by 87%, and lower extremity amputation by 67%. Cardiovascular disease risk is increased by 3%, and life expectancy is increased by 1.39 years. The estimated incremental cost per quality-adjusted life-year gained is $16,002. This efficiency of treating type 2 diabetes is similar to that for screening and treating hypertension and is in the range of interventions considered cost effective. Treatment is more cost effective for those with earlier onset of diabetes, minorities, and those with higher hemoglobin A_{1C} under standard care. (*Data from* Eastman *et al.* [33].)

Future Directions: Prevention of Type 2 Diabetes

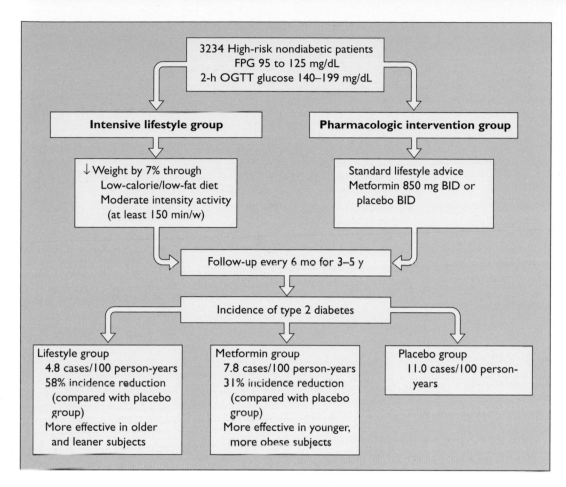

FIGURE 12-21. Prevention of type 2 diabetes. It is now clear that type 2 diabetes is not a milder form of diabetes. Its complications can be the same as or more severe than those of type 1 diabetes. Moreover, these complications occur early during the natural course of the disease, even before the disease's clinical onset. At the time of diagnosis of type 2 diabetes, 20% of patients have retinopathy, 8% have nephropathy, 9% have neuropathy [5], and up to 50% have underlying coronary artery disease (CAD) [27]. Results from several large randomized studies, including the United Kingdom Prospective Diabetes Study, have confirmed that treatment of hyperglycemia, hypertension, and hyperlipidemia may prevent or retard the progression of diabetic complications [9–12].

However, even with early intervention and intensive treatment, type 2 diabetes has significant morbidity and high costs. Ultimately, preventing or delaying the onset of diabetes may be more cost effective than treatment [13]. Impaired glucose tolerance ([IGT] with fasting plasma glucose: 110 to 125 mg/dL, or 2-hour post oral glucose tolerance test (OGTT) glucose 140 to 199 mg/dL) has been shown to be a strong risk factor for development of type 2 diabetes and a possible risk factor for CAD. Data suggest that at this stage of IGT, patients are at high risk for diabetes and CAD but have not yet developed end-organ disease.

The Diabetes Prevention Program (DPP), which was supported by the National Institutes of Health, was designed to determine if it is possible to prevent or delay the progression to type 2 diabetes through lifestyle changes or pharmacologic intervention in high-risk patients with IGT [13]. The DPP study randomized 3234 high-risk subjects with IGT to an intensive lifestyle intervention arm or pharmacologic or placebo treatment with standard lifestyle advice. The study was stopped 1 year early (average follow-up 2.8 years) because of a significant reduction in the incidence of diabetes in the lifestyle arm of the study. Subjects randomized to a low-calorie and low-fat diet combined with moderate-intensity physical activity lost an average of 5.6 kg and had a 58% reduction in the incidence of diabetes over 2.8 years. However, pharmacologic treatment with metformin 850 mg twice daily (BID) resulted in only a 31% reduction in the incidence of diabetes compared with placebo.

Currently, studies are in progress to determine if other pharmacologic agents such as angiotensin-converting enzyme inhibitors, angiotensin receptor blockers, and thiazolidinediones are also effective in reducing the onset of type 2 diabetes in high-risk individuals.

References

1. Harris MI: Summary. In *Diabetes in America*. NIH Publication No. 95-1468. Edited by Harris MI, Cowie CC, Stern MP, *et al.* Washington, DC: US Government Printing Office; 1995:1–14.

2. De Fronzo RA: Lilly Lecture 1987: The triumvirate: b cell, muscle, liver. A collusion responsible for NIDDM. *Diabetes* 1988, 37:667–687.

3. Pratley RE, Weyer C: The role of impaired early insulin secretion in the pathogenesis of Type II diabetes mellitus. *Diabetologia* 2001, 44:929–945.

4. Expert Panel on Detection, Evaluation, And Treatment of High Blood Cholesterol in Adults: Executive Summary of the Third Report of the National Cholesterol Education Program (NCEP) Expert Panel on Detection, Evaluation, and Treatment of High Blood Cholesterol in Adults (Adult Treatment Panel III). *JAMA* 2001, 285:2486–2497.

5. Fagan TC, Deedwania PC: The cardiovascular dysmetabolic syndrome. *Am J Med* 1998, 105(suppl 1A):77S–82S.

6. Laaksonen DE, Lakka HM, Niskanen LK, *et al.*: Metabolic syndrome and development of diabetes mellitus: application and validation of recently suggested definitions of the metabolic syndrome in a prospective cohort study. *Am J Epidemiol* 2002, 156:1070–1077.

7. King GL, Brownlee M: The cellular and molecular mechanisms of diabetic complications. *Endocrinol Metab Clin North Am* 1996, 25:255–270.

8. Brownlee M: Biochemistry and molecular cell biology of diabetic complications. *Nature* 2001, 414:813–820.

9. UK Prospective Diabetes Study Group: Intensive blood-glucose control with sulfonylurea or insulin compared with conventional treatment and risk of complications in patients with type 2 diabetes (UKPDS 33). *Lancet* 1998, 352:837–853.

10. UK Prospective Diabetes Study Group: Effect of intensive blood-glucose control with metformin on complications in overweight patients with type 2 diabetes (UKPDS 34). *Lancet* 1998, 352:854–865.

11. UK Prospective Diabetes Study Group: Tight blood pressure control and risk of macrovascular and microvascular complications in type 2 diabetes: UKPDS 38. *BMJ* 1998, 7160:703–713.

12. Reaven GM: Multiple CHD risk factors in type 2 diabetes: beyond hyperglycemia. *Diabetes Obes Metab* 2002, 4(suppl 1):S13–S18.

13. Diabetes Prevention Program Research Group: Reduction in the incidence of type 2 diabetes with lifestyle intervention or metformin. *N Engl J Med* 2002, 346:393–403.

14. Garber AJ: Vascular disease and lipids in diabetes. *Med Clin North Am* 1998, 82:931–948.

15. Aiello LP, Cavallerano J, Bursell S: Diabetic eye disease. *Endocrinol Metab Clin North Am* 1996, 25:271–291.

16. American Diabetes Association: Position statement: Diabetic retinopathy. *Diabetes Care* 2004, 27:S84–S87.

17. Hogan P, Dall T, Nikolov P: American Diabetes Association. Economic costs of diabetes in the US in 2002. *Diabetes Care* 2003, 26:917–932.

18. American Diabetes Association: Position statement: Diabetic nephropathy. *Diabetes Care* 2002, 25:S85–S89.

19. Marks JB, Raskin P: Nephropathy and hypertension in diabetes. *Med Clin North Am* 1998, 82:877–907.

20. Friedman E: Renal syndromes in diabetes. *Endocrinol Metab Clin North Am* 1996, 25:293–324.

21. Heart Outcomes Prevention Evaluation Study Investigators: Effects of ramipril on cardiovascular and microvascular outcomes in people with diabetes mellitus: results of the HOPE study and MICRO-HOPE substudy. *Lancet* 2000, 355:253–259.

22. Harati Y: Diabetes and the nervous system. *Endocrinol Metab Clin North Am* 1996, 25:325–359.

23. Boulton AJM, Malik RA: Diabetic neuropathy. *Med Clin North Am* 1998, 82:909–929.

24. Levin ME: Foot lesions in patients with diabetes mellitus. *Endocrinol Metab Clin North Am* 1996, 25:447–462.

25. American Diabetes Association: Position statement: foot care in diabetes. *Diabetes Care* 2002, 25(suppl):S69–S70.

26. Hakim LS, Goldstein I: Diabetic sexual function. *Endocrinol Metab Clin North Am* 1996, 25:379–400.

27. Zimmet PZ, Alberti KGMM: The changing face of macrovascular disease in NIDDM: an epidemic in progress. *Lancet* 1997, 350(suppl 1):1–4.

28. Krowelski AS, Warram JH, Valsania P, *et al.*: Evolving natural history of coronary artery disease in diabetes mellitus. *Am J Med* 1991, 90(suppl 2A):56S–61S.

29. Kuusisito J, Mykannen L, Pyorala K, *et al.*: NIDDM and its metabolic control predict coronary artery disease in elderly subjects. *Diabetes* 1994, 43:960–967.

30. American Diabetes Association: Position statement: Management of dyslipidemia in adults with diabetes mellitus. *Diabetes Care* 2004, 27:S68–S71.

31. American Diabetes Association: Position statement: aspirin therapy in diabetes. *Diabetes Care* 2004, 27:S72–S73.

32. Gaede P, Vedel P, Larsen N, *et al.*: Multifactorial intervention and cardiovascular disease in patients with type 2 diabetes. *N Engl J Med* 2003, 348:383–393.

33. Eastman RC, Javitt JC, Herman WH, *et al.*: Model of complications in NIDDM: analysis of the health benefits and cost-effectiveness of treating NIDDM with the goal of normoglycemia. *Diabetes Care* 1997, 20:735–744.

EYE COMPLICATIONS OF DIABETES

Lloyd Paul Aiello

13

Diabetic retinopathy is a well-characterized, sight-threatening, chronic, ocular disorder that eventually develops to some degree in nearly all patients with diabetes mellitus. With experienced ophthalmic evaluation, diabetic retinopathy can be detected in its early stages. Existing therapies are remarkably effective at preventing some types of visual loss when administered at the appropriate time in the disease process. In addition, improvement of systemic glycemic control is associated with a delay in onset and slowing of progression of diabetic retinopathy. Nevertheless, diabetic retinopathy is the leading cause of new cases of legal blindness, as well as severe and moderate of visual loss among Americans between the ages of 20 and 74 years. The pathologic changes associated with diabetic retinopathy are similar in types 1 and 2 diabetes mellitus, although there is a higher risk of more frequent and severe ocular complications in type 1 diabetes [1]. However, because more patients have type 2 than type 1 disease, patients with type 2 disease account for a higher proportion of those with visual loss.

Most visual loss associated with diabetes results from either new vessel growth on the retina (proliferative diabetic retinopathy [PDR]) or increased retinal vascular permeability (diabetic macular edema). The clinical stage associated with the greatest risk of severe visual loss is termed *high-risk PDR*, while the stage with the greatest risk of moderate visual loss is termed *clinically significant macular edema* (CSME). In the United States, an estimated 700,000 persons have PDR, 130,000 have high-risk PDR, 500,000 have macular edema, and 325,000 have CSME [2–5]. An estimated 63,000 cases of PDR, 29,000 of high-risk PDR, 80,000 of macular edema, 56,000 of CSME, and 5000 new cases of legal blindness occur yearly as a result of diabetic retinopathy [1,6]. Blindness has been estimated to be 25 times more common in persons with diabetes than in those without the disease [7,8].

Estimates of the medical and economic impact of retinopathy-associated morbidity have been performed using computer simulations. The models predict that if patients with type 1 disease receive treatment as recommended in the clinical trials in the absence of good glycemic control, a savings of $624 million and 173,540 person-years of sight would be realized [3,4]. The Diabetes Control and Complication Trial (DCCT) showed that the rate of development of any retinopathy and, once present, the rate of retinopathy progression were significantly reduced after 3 years of intensive insulin therapy [9,10]. Subsequent studies have confirmed a continuing benefit of intensive insulin therapy [11]. Applying DCCT intensive insulin therapy to all persons with insulin-dependent diabetes mellitus in the United States would result in a gain of 920,000 person-years of sight, although the costs of intensive therapy are three times that of conventional therapy [12,13].

An understanding of the pathogenesis, natural history, and available treatment options for patients with diabetic retinopathy is critical for all health care providers, because current therapeutic options can be remarkably effective at preventing severe visual loss when administered in an appropriate and timely manner. Indeed, with appropriate medical and ophthalmologic care, over 90% of severe visual loss resulting from proliferative diabetic retinopathy can be prevented [14,15].

Anatomy, Symptoms, and Pathology

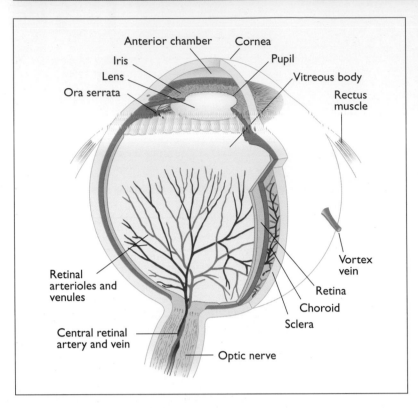

FIGURE 13-1. Normal ocular anatomy. This schematic cross-section shows the normal anatomy of the human eye. Diabetes can affect almost all ocular structures (*see* Fig. 13-2). However, the characteristic and most common changes occur in the retina and are termed diabetic retinopathy. Most of the severe sight-threatening complications involve either pathologic growth of vessels (neovascularization) in the retina or increased retinal vessel permeability [15]. These conditions are termed *proliferative diabetic retinopathy* and *diabetic macular edema*, respectively. Neovascularization also can arise at the iris, potentially leading to neovascular glaucoma.

OCULAR STRUCTURES AFFECTED BY DIABETES

Ocular Structure	Diabetes-associated with Pathology
Lids, nerves, and muscles	Palsy of cranial nerves III, IV, or VI
Cornea	Reduced sensitivity
	Increased susceptibility to corneal erosions
	Increased susceptibility to infection (corneal ulcers)
Anterior chamber	Hyphema (blood)
	Shallowing with longer disease duration
Iris	Neovascularization
	Depigmentation
Lens	Increased susceptibility to cataract
Vitreous	Vitreous hemorrhage
	Early posterior vitreous detachment
	Asteroid hyalosis
Retina	Retinal hemorrhage
	Microaneurysm
	Venous beading
	Intraretinal microvascular abnormalities
	Capillary loss
	Neovascularization
	Edema
	Lipid deposits
Optic disc	Neovascularization
	Diabetic papillopathy (swelling)
Sclera and other tissues	Delayed wound healing

FIGURE 13-2. Diabetes can affect most structures of the human eye [16]. Diabetes-induced ischemia of cranial nerves III, IV, and VI can result in drooping of the lids, ocular motility abnormalities, or both as a result of impaired innervation of the ocular muscles. Corneal erosions, corneal ulcers, cataracts, and delayed wound healing also reflect the general diabetic state. However, most visual loss associated with diabetes arises from complications involving neovascularization of the retina (or iris) or increased vasopermeability of the retinal vasculature.

CLINICAL PRESENTATIONS OF DIABETIC EYE COMPLICATIONS

Diabetes-associated Pathology	Clinical Symptoms
Palsy of cranial nerves III, IV, and VI	Diplopia (binocular)
	Ptosis
	Anisocoria
	"Blurred vision"
Reduced corneal sensitivity or corneal erosions or corneal infections	Ocular pain
	Ocular discharge
	Corneal opacification
	Decreased vision
Hyphema	Decreased vision
	Blood layering in anterior chamber
Angle closure glaucoma	Ocular pain
	"Halos" around light
	Decreased vision
Iris neovascularization	Ocular pain
	Decreased vision
	Blood layering in anterior chamber
Cataract	Decreased vision
	Glare with bright light
Vitreous hemorrhage	"Spots," "cobwebs," "lines" in vision (floaters)
	Decreased vision
Macular edema	Moderately decreased vision
	Image distortion
Proliferative diabetic retinopathy	Symptoms associated with vitreous hemorrhage and macular edema
Retina detachment	Photopsia
	Floaters
	Scotoma
	Decreased vision
	Image distortion
Diabetic papillopathy	Visual field change

FIGURE 13-3. Clinical presentations associated with diabetic eye complications. Each of the numerous diabetes-associated ocular pathologies can present with a diverse array of symptoms. Only a partial list is presented here. It is important to realize that serious diabetic eye disease may exist without any discernible symptoms. This fact underscores the essential need for regular, routine, lifelong follow-up regardless of the presence or absence of visual symptoms.

OCULAR PATHOLOGY ASSOCIATED WITH RETINOPATHY PROGRESSION

Disease Stage	Common Pathologic Changes
Preclinical stages	Alterations in cellular biochemistry
	Alterations in retinal blood flow
	Loss of retinal pericytes
	Thickening of basement membranes
Early stages Mild NPDR	Retinal vascular microaneurysms and blot hemorrhages
	Increased retinal vascular permeability
	Cotton wool spots
Middle stages	Venous caliber changes or beading
Moderate NPDR	IRMAs
Severe NPDR	Retinal capillary loss
Very severe NPDR	Retinal ischemia
	Extensive intraretinal hemorrhages and microaneurysms
Advanced stage PDR	Neovascularization of the disc
	Neovascularization elsewhere
	Neovascularization of the iris
	Neovascular glaucoma
	Pre-retinal and vitreous hemorrhage
	Fibrovascular proliferation
	Retinal traction, retinal tears, and retinal detachment

FIGURE 13-4. Ocular pathology associated with progression of diabetic retinopathy. Diabetic retinopathy generally progresses through well-characterized stages. Each stage is associated with typical pathologic changes. Some degree of clinically apparent retinopathy occurs in nearly all patients with diabetes of 20 or more years' duration, although preclinical alterations in blood flow, pericyte number, and basement membrane thickness can occur much earlier [17] The clinical stages before the development of neovascularization are termed *nonproliferative diabetic retinopathy* (NPDR). NPDR is subdivided into mild, moderate, severe, or very severe categories, depending on the type and extent of clinical pathology present. Increased vascular permeability can occur at this or any later stage. As the disease progresses, gradual loss of the retinal microvasculature results in retinal ischemia. Venous caliber abnormalities, intraretinal microvascular abnormalities (IRMAs), and more severe vascular leakage are common reflections of this increasing retinal nonperfusion (see Fig. 13-8). Once ischemia-induced neovascularization occurs, the disease is referred to as proliferative diabetic retinopathy (PDR) (see Fig. 13-10). Neovascularization can arise at the optic disc (neovascularization of the disc) or elsewhere in the retina (neovascularization elsewhere). The new vessels are fragile and prone to bleeding, resulting in vitreous hemorrhage. With time, the neovascularization tends to undergo fibrosis and contraction, resulting in retinal traction, retinal tears, vitreous hemorrhage, and retinal detachment (see Fig. 13-14). New vessels also can arise on the iris, resulting in neovascular glaucoma (see Fig. 13-15). (*Adapted from* Aiello et al. [15].)

INTERNATIONAL CLINICAL DIABETIC RETINOPATHY AND DIABETIC MACULAR EDEMA SCALE

Level of Diabetic Retinopathy	Findings
No apparent retinopathy	No abnormalities
Mild NPDR	Microaneurysms only
Moderate NPDR	More than microaneuysms, but less than severe NPDR
Severe NPDR	Any of the following:
	> 20 intraretinal hemorrhages in each four retinal quadrants; definite VB in two or more retinal quadrants; prominent IRMA in one or more retinal quadrants; and no PDR
PDR	

Level of DME	Findings
DME apparently absent	No apparent retinal thickening or hard exudates (HE) in posterior pole
DME apparently present	Mild DME: Some retinal thickening or HE in posterior pole, but distant from center of the macula
	Moderate DME: Retinal thickening or HE approaching the center, but not involving the center
	Severe DME: Retinal thickening or HE involving the center of the macula

FIGURE 13-5. To simplify classification and standardize communications between health care providers worldwide, in 2001 the American Academy of Ophthalmology initiated a project to establish a consensus International Classification of Diabetic Retinopathy and Diabetic Macular Edema [18,19]. The consensus panel relied on evidence-based studies including the Early Treatment Diabetic Retinopathy Study (ETDRS) and the Wisconsin Epidemiologic Study of Diabetic Patients.

Overall, the International Classification of Diabetic Retinopathy and Diabetic Macular Edema simplifies descriptions of the categories of diabetic retinopathy, but is not a replacement for ETDRS levels of diabetic retinopathy in large-scale clinical trials or studies in which precise retinopathy classification is required. DME—diabetic macular edema; IRMA—intraretinal microvascular abnormalities; NPDR—nonproliferative diabetic retinopathy; PDR—proliferative diabetic retinopathy; VB—venous beading.

Nonproliferative Diabetic Retinopathy

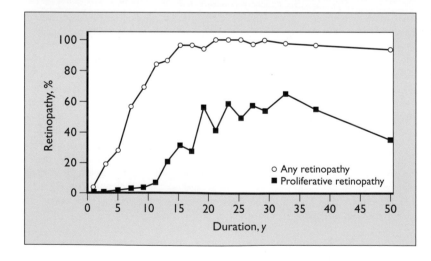

FIGURE 13-6. Incidence Prevalence of diabetic retinopathy by duration of diabetes. The percentage of patients developing with either any diabetic retinopathy or proliferative diabetic retinopathy is presented as a function of duration of type 1 diabetes in years. Note that almost all patients have some evidence of diabetic retinopathy once the duration of diabetes exceeds 15 years. In addition, the incidence prevalence of proliferative diabetic retinopathy (PDR) is negligible within 5 years of the onset of diabetes, although nearly 60% of patients eventually will develop PDR. These observations serve as the foundation for clinical care recommendations concerning the appropriate timing of initial ophthalmologic evaluation, as detailed in Figure 13-7. (*Adapted from* Krolewski *et al.* [20].)

INITIAL OPHTHALMOLOGIC EXAMINATION SCHEDULE

Age at Onset of Diabetes Mellitus	Recommended First Examination	Minimum Routine Follow-up*
29 years or younger	Within 3–5 years after diagnosis of diabetes Once patient is age 10 years or older	Yearly
30 years or older	At time of diagnosis of diabetes	Yearly
Patient becomes pregnant	Before conception and during the first trimester	Physician discretion pending results of first trimester examination

Abnormal findings necessitate more frequent follow-up.

FIGURE 13-7. Only approximately 25% of patients with type 1 diabetes will have any retinopathy after 5 years, although most eventually will develop the disease (see Fig. 13-6) [21]. The prevalence of PDR is less than 2% at 5 years. For patients with type 2 disease, however, the onset date of diabetes frequently is not known precisely, and thus, more severe disease can be observed soon after diagnosis. Up to 3% of patients first diagnosed after age 30 may have clinically significant macular edema or high-risk PDR at the time of initial diagnosis of diabetes [22]. Thus, in patients over age 10, the initial ophthalmic examination is recommended beginning 5 years after the diagnosis of type 1 diabetes mellitus and on diagnosis of type 2 diabetes mellitus [15]. The onset of vision-threatening retinopathy is rare in children before puberty, regardless of the duration of diabetes; however, if diabetes is diagnosed between the ages of 10 and 30 years, significant retinopathy may arise within 6 years [2]. Puberty can accelerate the progression of retinopathy. Thus, the initial ophthalmic evaluation is recommended within 3 to 5 years of diagnosis, once the patient is aged 10 years or older [15,23]. The onset of puberty is occurring progressively earlier, and consequently the timing of initial evaluation of children is under periodic review. Diabetic retinopathy also can become particularly aggressive during pregnancy in women with diabetes [24]. Ideally, patients with diabetes who are planning pregnancy should have an eye examination within 1 year of conception. Pregnant women should have a comprehensive eye examination in the first trimester of pregnancy. Close follow-up throughout pregnancy is indicated, with subsequent examinations determined by the findings present at the first trimester examination. This guideline does not apply to women who develop gestational diabetes because they are not at increased risk of developing diabetic retinopathy. (*Adapted from* Aiello *et al.* [15].)

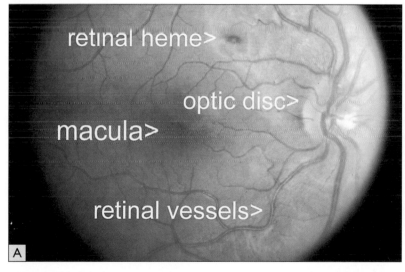

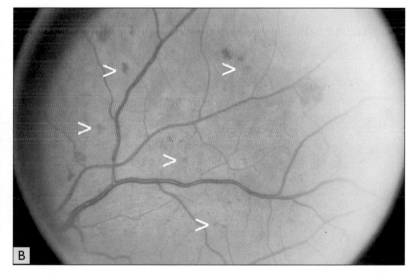

FIGURE 13-8. Characteristic findings in nonproliferative diabetic retinopathy (NPDR). The classic findings associated with NPDR are demonstrated. **A,** The central region of the human retina is called the macula and is responsible for detailed vision. This patient's right eye has minimal diabetic retinopathy, and the retina is normal except for a single retinal hemorrhage (retinal heme). The optic disc is located nasal to the macula, and the retinal vessels emanate from the optic disc and surround the macula. **B,** Retinal blot hemorrhages (*arrows*) and microaneurysms, which are saccular dilations of the vessel wall. These lesions often are two of the earliest clinically observed abnormalities. The patient has severe NPDR when hemorrhages and microaneurysms of this extent or greater in all four quadrants of the retina are observed.

(Continued on next page)

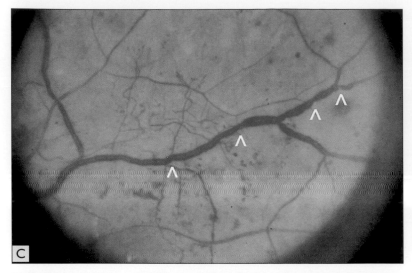

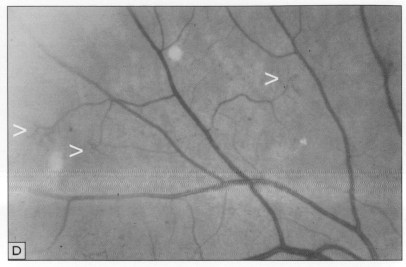

FIGURE 13-8. *(Continued)* **C,** Venous caliber changes referred to as venous beading. This finding often represents more advanced retinopathy, as is evident in this photograph (*arrows*). Two or more retinal quadrants of any venous beading (not necessarily as pronounced as shown) signify severe NPDR. **D,** *Arrows* show intraretinal microvascular abnormalities (IRMAs). IRMAs are abnormalities within the retina and may be a harbinger of early retinal neovascularization. IRMAs often are associated with more advanced NPDR, and only one or more retinal quadrants of IRMAs of this or greater extent represent severe NPDR. Note that the clinical findings associated with severe NPDR therefore may be quite subtle. Any two or more of the findings associated with severe NPDR place the patient in the very severe category of NPDR. (*Panels B–D from* the Early Treatment Diabetic Retinopathy Study Research Group [25]; with permission.)

Proliferative Diabetic Retinopathy and Macular Edema

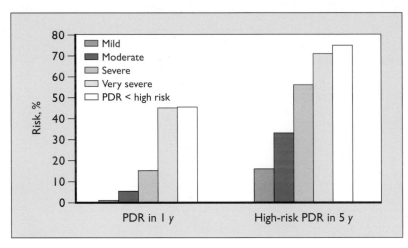

FIGURE 13-9. Progression to high-risk proliferative diabetic retinopathy (PDR) becomes more likely as the severity of nonproliferative diabetic retinopathy (NPDR) increases. Demonstrated is the likelihood of developing high-risk PDR (*see* Fig. 13-10) within 1 or 5 years for patients with mild, moderate, severe, and very severe levels of NPDR or PDR with less than high-risk characteristics. High-risk PDR is associated with the greatest incidence of severe and irreversible visual loss. Each increase in NPDR severity level is associated with an increase in progression to the sight-threatening proliferative stage of the disease. The known progression rates permit determination of appropriate intervals between follow-up ocular evaluations for patients with differing levels of diabetic retinopathy. Typically, follow-up ocular evaluations are performed as follows: annually for no retinopathy, every 6 to 12 months for mild to moderate NPDR, every 3 to 4 months for severe to very severe NPDR, and every 2 to 3 months for PDR that is less than high risk [15]. (*Adapted from* the Early Treatment Diabetic Retinopathy Study Research Group [26].)

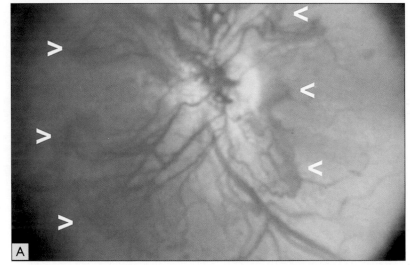

FIGURE 13-10. Characteristic clinical manifestations of proliferative diabetic retinopathy (PDR). When any neovascularization is present, diabetic retinopathy is termed proliferative diabetic retinopathy. The extent and location of neovascularization determine whether the PDR is considered to be high risk or less than high risk. Neovascularization at the optic disc (NVD), larger areas of vessels, and the presence of concurrent vitreous hemorrhages are the critical findings. Without laser photocoagulation, patients with high-risk PDR have a 28% risk of severe visual loss (< 5/200 maintained for at least four months, which is worse than legally blind) within 2 years. This risk compares with a 7% risk of severe visual loss after 2 years for patients with PDR without the high-risk characteristics [27,28]. **A,** Extensive NVD.

(Continued on next page)

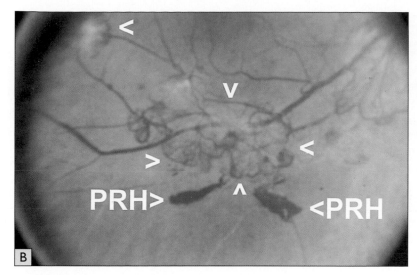

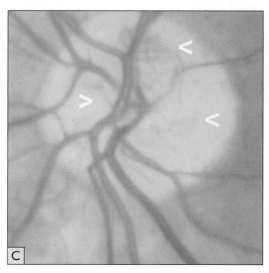

FIGURE 13-10. *(Continued)* **B,** Extensive neovascularization at an area remote (> 1500 m) from the optic disc, referred to as neovascularization elsewhere (NVE). Pre-retinal hemorrhage (PRH) also is present. **C,** NVD approximately equal to one third to one fourth of the disc area. The following are the risk factors: presence of any neovascularization within the eye, NVD, pre-retinal (or vitreous) hemorrhage, and large areas of neovascularization. NVD equal to or greater than that shown in panel C is considered large. NVE greater than or equal to half of the disc area is considered large. When three or more of the risk factors listed previously are present, the patient has PDR with high-risk characteristics (PDR-HRC). Thus, the patient in *panel A* has PDR-HRC because neovascularization is present, located at the disc, and large in extent. The patient in *panel B* also has PDR-HRC because neovascularization is present, the extent of NVE is large, and pre-retinal hemorrhage is present. *Panel C* represents the minimal amount of NVD required for PDR-HRC. *(Panels B and C from* the Early Treatment Diabetic Retinopathy Study Research Group [25]; with permission.)

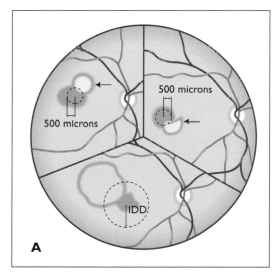

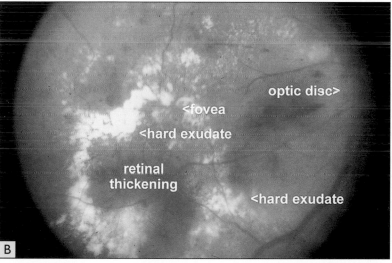

FIGURE 13-11. Clinical manifestations of diabetic macular edema. Increased permeability of the retinal microvasculature can result in transudation of serum and other blood components into the substance of the retina, often with deposition of lipid in the form of hard exudates. Retinal edema and thickening result. Macular edema may be present at any level of diabetic retinopathy and is defined as retinal thickening within 3000 mm of the center of the macula (fovea). Macular edema that threatens the center of vision is termed *clinically significant macular edema* (CSME) [26,29]. **A,** Situations in which macular edema *(white)* is of sufficient extent and correct location to be termed CSME. Specifically, edema qualifies as CSME when it is at or within 500 mm microns of the fovea; associated with hard exudates *(arrows)* at or within 500 mm microns of the fovea; or one disc area in size, with any part of the edema at or within 1500 mm microns of the fovea. **B,** CSME owing to extensive hard exudate and thickening involving the fovea and surrounding retina. 1DD—one disk diameter. *(Panel A adapted from* Cavallerano [30].)

Complications and Causes of Visual Loss

CAUSES OF VISUAL LOSS IN DIABETIC RETINOPATHY

Complication Threatening Vision	Common Therapeutic Approach
Clinically significant macular edema	Focal and/or grid laser photocoagulation surgery, if unresponsive possible intravitreous steroid (although efficacy and side effects are currently under evaluation by clinical trial)
Macular capillary nonperfusion	No currently effective therapy
High-risk proliferative diabetic retinopathy	Scatter (panretinal) laser photocoagulation surgery (PRP)
Vitreous hemorrhage	Careful observation or vitrectomy
Traction, rhegmatogenous retinal detachment, or both	Vitrectomy
Traction distorting the macula	Careful observation or vitrectomy
Fibrovascular tissues obscuring the retina	Careful observation or vitrectomy
Neovascular glaucoma	PRP, cryotherapy plus intraocular pressure management, or both

FIGURE 13-12. Diabetic retinopathy can result in permanent visual loss by several mechanisms. Long-standing clinically significant macular edema induces moderate visual loss from edema in the foveal region (see Fig. 13-11). If extensive capillary closure occurs in the macular region, vision can be permanently affected from the loss of blood supply to the fovea (see Fig. 13-13). Untreated high-risk proliferative diabetic retinopathy (PDR) primarily causes severe visual loss either by vitreous hemorrhage or retinal traction. Vitreous hemorrhage can reduce vision markedly owing to obscuration of the visual axis by blood (see Fig. 13-13). However, because the blood itself is relatively benign, vision will be recovered (in the absence of other ocular damage) once the hemorrhage clears spontaneously or, when not resolving, after vitrectomy surgery (see Fig. 13-20). In contrast, neovascularization eventually tends to undergo a scarring process with fibrosis and contraction, resulting in retinal traction (see Fig. 13-14). Such traction can cause visual loss by distorting the macula; tearing the retina; or precipitating retinal detachment, further vitreous hemorrhage, or both. Rarely, fibrovascular tissue itself may obscure the visual axis (see Fig. 13-13). If neovascularization of the iris occurs, neovascular glaucoma may result and lead to permanent visual loss (see Fig. 13-15). (*Adapted from* Aiello *et al.* [15].)

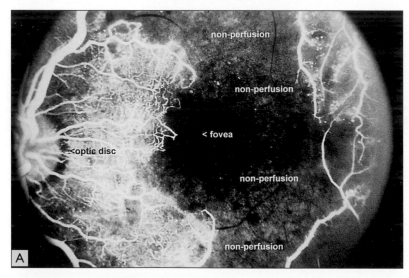

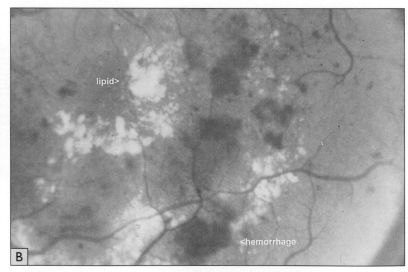

FIGURE 13-13. Ophthalmic complications associated with visual loss in diabetic retinopathy. Visual loss associated with diabetic retinopathy can arise from multiple complications of the disease. If the characteristic progressive capillary loss eventually involves a large portion of the central macula, then visual acuity is compromised. **A,** Fluorescein angiogram showing extensive macular capillary nonperfusion. Fluorescent dye (fluorescein) was injected into the patient's antecubital vein, and photographs were taken of the retina as the dye was passing through the retinal vessels. This technique, called *fluorescein angiography*, allows excellent visualization of the retinal vasculature. In this instance, the dye in the retinal vessels appears white, and the photograph shows nearly complete loss of the retinal vasculature perfusion in the macular region. These anatomic changes and their visual sequelae are irreversible. **B,** Extensive retinal vascular leakage into the macular region with retinal thickening, lipid deposits, and retinal hemorrhage. This patient has severe macular edema, with associated visual loss.

(Continued on next page)

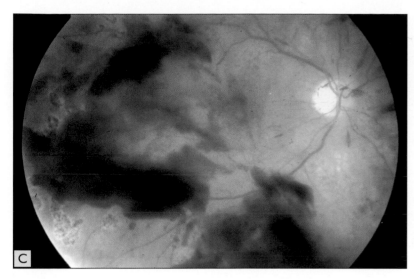

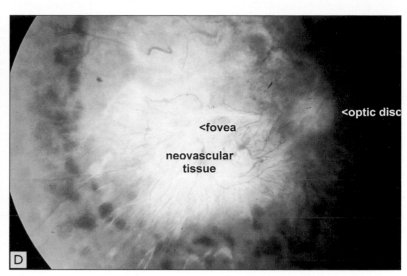

FIGURE 13-13. *(Continued)* **C**, Blood in the vitreous, a condition termed vitreous hemorrhage or pre-retinal hemorrhage. Pre-retinal hemorrhage refers specifically to blood immediately in front of the retina, whereas vitreous hemorrhage may be anywhere in the vitreous cavity. Vitreous hemorrhages are common in diabetic retinopathy owing to the fragility of new vessels and traction often exerted on these vessels by progressive retinal fibrosis. Although the hemorrhages usually clear spontaneously, surgical intervention may be required if they persist (*see* Fig. 13-20). Not only can vitreous hemorrhage obscure the patient's vision, but also the ophthalmologist's view of the retina, which may necessitate evaluation of the retinal anatomy using ultrasonography if the hemorrhage is severe (*see* Fig. 13-14). **D**, A rare form of visual loss in diabetes in which a sheet of neovascular tissue obscures the visual axis. Removal of the tissue by vitrectomy surgery often can restore useful vision (*see* Fig. 13-20). (*Panels A, B, and D courtesy of* the Wilmer Ophthalmological Institute.)

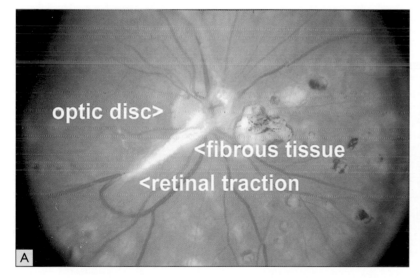

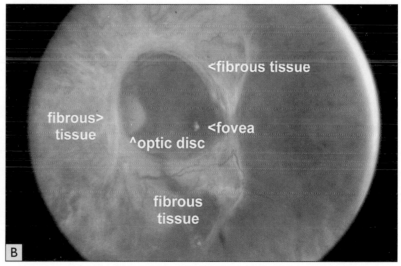

FIGURE 13-14. Ophthalmic complications associated with retinal traction in diabetic retinopathy. Some of the most severe visual losses associated with diabetic retinopathy result from the complications of traction exerted on the retina by fibrosing neovascular tissue. Initially, the traction can result in localized retinal detachment that, when distant from the critical areas of the retina, has little visual significance. **A**, A localized traction retinal detachment from the optic disc to an inferior retinal vessel. Note the elevation and distortion of the retinal vessel at the area of traction. As seen here, the detachment does not threaten the macula but should be examined carefully at regular intervals for progression toward the fovea. **B**, More extensive fibrovascular tissue and traction along the vascular arcades of the retina surrounding the macula. This configuration is typical of retinal traction in diabetic retinopathy because of the predilection for fibrovascular tissues to form along the vascular arcades. This configuration has been termed wolf-jaw owing to its apparent imminent "bite" on the macula.

(Continued on next page)

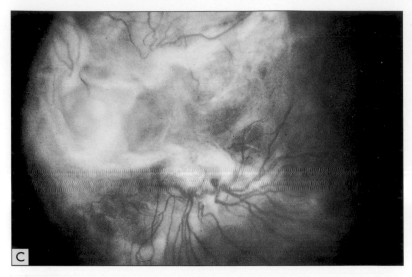

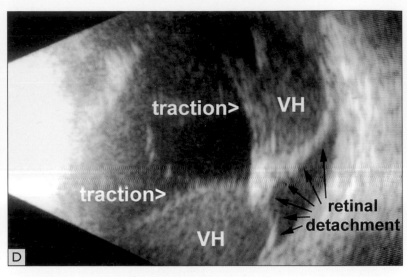

FIGURE 13-14. *(Continued)* **C,** A nearly total retinal detachment with extensive fibrovascular proliferation. Large retinal detachments also may occur when the tractional forces are sufficient to tear a hole in the retina, allowing vitreous fluid to pass into the subretinal space (rhegmatogenous detachment). If vitreous hemorrhage obscures the view of the retina, ultrasonography is indicated to monitor ocular status. **D,** Ultrasonography of vitreous hemorrhage (VH), retinal traction, and traction retinal detachment. When traction retinal detachment threatens the macula, vitrectomy surgery usually is indicated (see Fig. 13-20). *(Panel D courtesy of* R. Calderon, OD.)

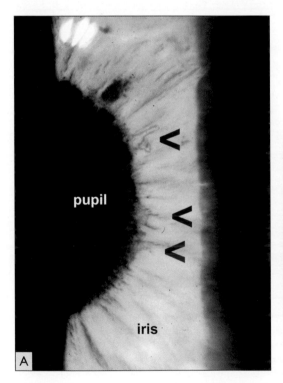

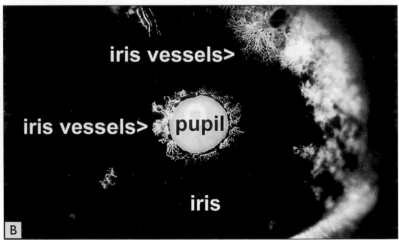

FIGURE 13-15. Neovascularization of the iris. In proliferative diabetic retinopathy, neovascularization can occur not only on the retina but also on the iris. Neovascularization of the iris sometimes is referred to as rubeosis iridis. If the neovascularization progresses to the base of the iris, the normal outflow channels for the aqueous fluid from the anterior chamber can become occluded and the intraocular pressure can increase dramatically. This condition, called neovascular glaucoma, can result in severe and permanent visual loss. Treatment involves prompt scatter laser photocoagulation as done for proliferative diabetic retinopathy (see Fig. 13-14). **A,** Neovascularization of the iris (NVI), with the iris vessels marked by arrows. **B,** Iris neovascularization using fluorescein angiography (see Fig. 13-13A). Fluorescein dye in the iris vessels (white) demonstrates the extent of the neovascularization on the iris.

Treatment

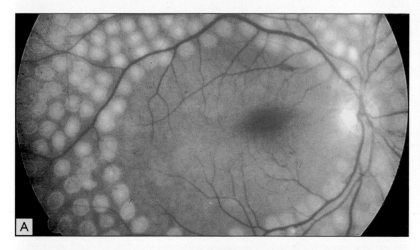

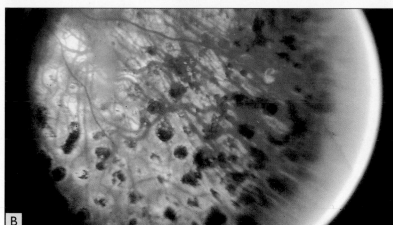

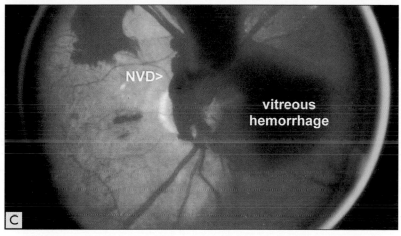

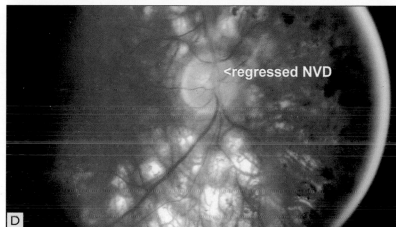

FIGURE 13-16. Panretinal laser photocoagulation for proliferative diabetic retinopathy (PDR). The primary therapy for PDR is scatter (panretinal) laser photocoagulation. However, cryotherapy or vitrectomy with endophotocoagulation may be effective when photocoagulation is not feasible. Treatment entails using a laser to place multiple burns throughout the midperiphery of the retina in an attempt to reduce the risk of visual loss. In general, prompt treatment is advised for patients with high-risk PDR. Some patients with PDR that is less than high-risk or with severe or very severe NPDR also may benefit from panretinal photocoagulation, depending on factors such as type of diabetes, medical status, access to care, compliance with follow-up, status and progression of the fellow eye, and family history [26,31]. **A,** Clinical appearance of the retina shortly after panretinal photocoagulation in PDR. The 500-mm-diameter retinal burns appear moderately white in intensity and one-half burn width apart. Laser burns are not placed over the retinal vessels, optic disc, or within the macular region. A total of 1200 to 1800 retinal burns generally are applied over two to three sessions occurring a few days to weeks apart. The procedure is done on an outpatient basis and generally requires only topical anesthesia. **B,** Panretinal photocoagulation scars as they appear months to years after their application. Note the areas of increased retinal pigmentation, atrophy, and spreading of the area of each retinal scar.

C, PDR, neovascularization of the disk, and vitreous hemorrhage before laser panretinal photocoagulation. **D,** The same patient 2 years after panretinal photocoagulation. Note the resolution of the vitreous hemorrhage and regression of the neovascularization with only a small, fibrotic, nonperfused remnant of the original neovascular frond at the optic disc. Such remnants often do not regress completely and usually do not threaten vision. NVD—neovascularization at the disk. (*Panels B–D from* The American Academy of Ophthalmology Diabetes 2000 Diabetic Retinopathy Course; with permission.)

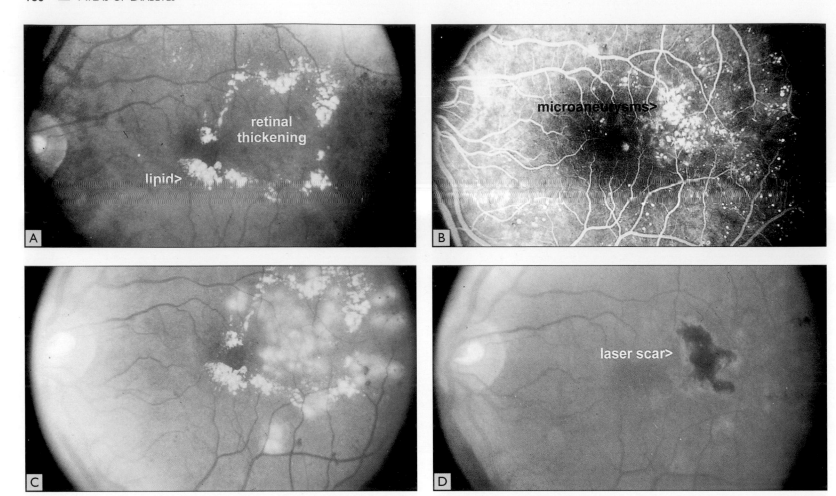

FIGURE 13-17. Focal laser photocoagulation for clinically significant diabetic macular edema. The primary therapy for clinically significant diabetic macular edema is focal laser photocoagulation. Treatment entails placing light 50- to 100-mm-diameter burns focally over leaking microaneurysms or in a grid pattern if retinal leakage is diffuse. Once the need for treatment is determined clinically, fluorescein angiography often is used to identify the type of leakage and specific microaneurysms for treatment. If treatment is successful, resolution of the macular edema may be expected 3 or more months after therapy. Treatment may be reapplied if the edema persists or recurs. **A,** Circinate lipid deposits, clinically significant macular edema, and reduced visual acuity. **B,** Fluorescein angiogram demonstrating multiple microaneurysms in the area of thickening within the circinate ring.
C, Clinical appearance of the retina immediately after focal laser photocoagulation to the leaking microaneurysms. The retinal burns applied in this case are more intense than is optimal. **D,** Clinical appearance of the eye several months after laser therapy. The lipid and edema have resolved, and no thickening of the retina is present. Likewise, visual acuity has improved. The residual scarring of the retina is heavier than desired owing to the intensity of the initial laser burns. (*From* the American Academy of Ophthalmology Diabetes 2000 Program; with permission.)

THERAPEUTIC EFFICACY IN THE TREATMENT OF DIABETIC RETINOPATHY

Indication	Treatment	Efficacy
Clinically significant macular edema	Focal laser photocoagulation	50% reduction in moderate visual loss* after 3 y
High-risk proliferative diabetic retinopathy (PDR)	Scatter photocoagulation	60% reduction in severe visual loss[†] after 3 y
Development of high-risk PDR	Scatter photocoagulation	87% reduction in severe visual loss[†] after 3 y
		97% reduction in bilateral severe visual loss[†] after 3 y
		90% reduction in legal blindness after 5 y
Severe PDR and severe vitreous hemorrhage[‡]	Vitrectomy	60% increased chance of 20/40 or better after 2 y
Severe PDR and vision 10/200 or better[‡]	Vitrectomy	34% increased chance of 20/40 or better after 2 y
No diabetic retinopathy	Intensive glycemic control	76% reduction in onset of retinopathy
Nonproliferative diabetic retinopathy	Intensive glycemic control	63% reduction in retinopathy progression
		47% reduction in severe nonproliferative diabetic retinopathy and PDR
		26% reduction in development of macular edema
		51% reduction in need for laser treatment

*Moderate visual loss is defined as at least doubling of visual angle (eg, 20/40 to 20/80)
†Severe visual loss is defined as best corrected acuity of 5/200 or worse on two consecutive visits 4 months apart.

‡For patients with type 1 diabetes only; no benefit was observed in the group having type 2 diabetes.

FIGURE 13-18. The only patient-initiated efforts proven to reduce the risk of visual loss include maintenance of optimal glycemic control and insistence on routine ophthalmologic evaluation [10,32]. Once visually significant complications of diabetes have arisen, the mainstay of therapy is laser photocoagulation. Scatter (panretinal) photocoagulation for the treatment of proliferative diabetic retinopathy is remarkably effective in preventing severe visual loss when patients at risk receive therapy in an appropriate and timely manner. Indeed, with appropriate medical and ophthalmologic care, over 95% of visual loss resulting from diabetic retinopathy can be prevented [14]. Focal photocoagulation for the treatment of clinically significant macular edema is somewhat less effective, although half of moderate visual loss can be prevented in this manner. If the application of laser photocoagulation is not possible or is ineffective, pars plana vitrectomy surgery also is useful in preventing visual impairment (see Fig. 13-20). Recently, steroids (especially triamcinolone) have been injected into the vitreous to reduced macular edema that is otherwise unresponsive to laser photocoagulation. Although many patients may have a reduction in edema following such treatment, the extent to which the edema resolves, the improvement of visual acuity, the need for reinjection and be risks of known complications including cataract and severe glaucoma have not been fully elucidated to date. Rigorous clinical trials are currently underway to address these issues and to determine the appropriate role of this therapy in treatment of patients with diabetic macular edema. (*Adapted from* Aiello et al. [15].)

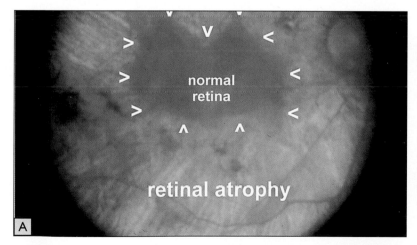 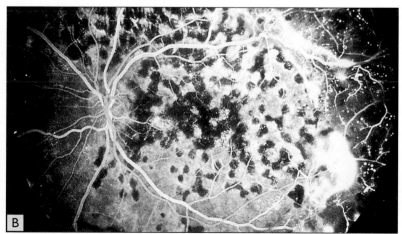

FIGURE 13-19. Side effects and complications of laser photocoagulation. Although laser photocoagulation is remarkably effective at preventing the visual loss associated with diabetic retinopathy, the therapy itself is inherently destructive. Each retinal laser burn destroys a portion of previously viable retina in an attempt to maintain better visual function than would be achieved without treatment. Thus, the therapy itself is associated with unavoidable side effects, most notably constriction of peripheral visual field and reduced night vision. These symptoms result from the selective destruction of the retinal midperiphery that subserves these functions. Unexpected complications also can arise from laser photocoagulation. **A,** Appearance of the retina several years after excessive laser panretinal photocoagulation. Note that the atrophy resulting from individual laser scars has spread to the point at which confluent loss of the peripheral retina occurs. Only the central aspect of the macula (*arrows*) remains intact. As expected, this patient has severe constriction of the visual field and significant difficulty with night vision. **B,** Fluorescein angiogram of panretinal photocoagulation mistakenly applied directly through the macula. The dark laser scars in this macular area, which is critical for detailed vision, cause permanent blind spots in the center of vision and reduced visual acuity.

(Continued on next page)

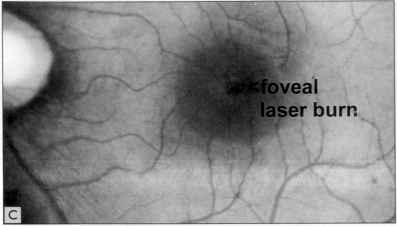

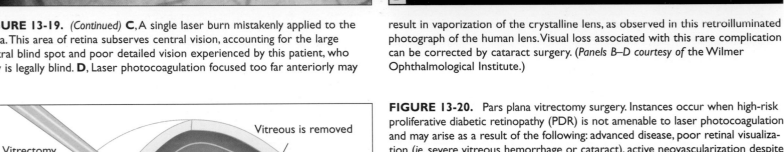

FIGURE 13-19. *(Continued)* **C,** A single laser burn mistakenly applied to the fovea. This area of retina subserves central vision, accounting for the large central blind spot and poor detailed vision experienced by this patient, who now is legally blind. **D,** Laser photocoagulation focused too far anteriorly may

result in vaporization of the crystalline lens, as observed in this retroilluminated photograph of the human lens. Visual loss associated with this rare complication can be corrected by cataract surgery. *(Panels B–D courtesy of the Wilmer Ophthalmological Institute.)*

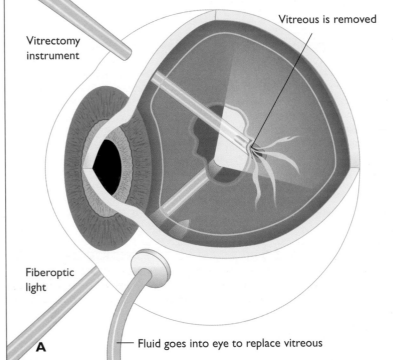

FIGURE 13-20. Pars plana vitrectomy surgery. Instances occur when high-risk proliferative diabetic retinopathy (PDR) is not amenable to laser photocoagulation and may arise as a result of the following: advanced disease, poor retinal visualization (*ie,* severe vitreous hemorrhage or cataract), active neovascularization despite complete laser treatment, traction-macular detachment, or combined traction-rhegmatogenous retinal detachment. In such cases, pars plana vitrectomy surgery may offer a therapeutic option. Vitrectomy surgery has the potential for serious complications, including profound visual loss and permanent pain and blindness. Thus, surgery should be undertaken only after careful consideration of the potential risks and benefits [33]. Vitrectomy performed by an experienced vitreoretinal surgeon, however, often can maintain vision in patients who otherwise almost certainly would have severe visual loss. **A,** Schematic representation of the pars plana vitrectomy procedure. Three openings are made from the outside of the eye into the vitreous cavity. An infusion line is placed in one opening to maintain pressure within the eye during surgery. The other two openings are used for the variety of instruments that can manipulate the vitreous and retina. Fiberoptic instruments allow for illumination, and the surgery is monitored by visualization through the pupil using an operating microscope. **B,** Proliferative diabetic retinopathy and extensive fibrovascular neovascularization before vitrectomy surgery. Note the fibrous tissue surrounding the optic disc that is exerting traction on the major superior and inferior retinal vessels, dragging them nasally. **C,** The same retina after vitrectomy surgery. Note the removal of the fibrous tissue that had surrounded the optic disc with return of the major retinal vessels to a more normal anatomic position after removal of the traction. (*Panel A from* "For my patient: retinal detachment and vitreous surgery," The Retina Research Fund; *panels B and C from* the American Academy of Ophthalmology Diabetic Retinopathy Vitrectomy Study course; with permission.)

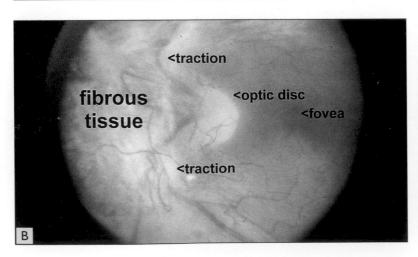

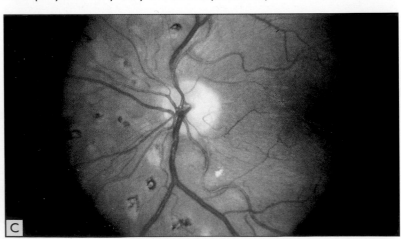

SYSTEMIC FACTORS POTENTIALLY AFFECTING DIABETIC RETINOPATHY

Glycemic control   Pregnancy
Hypertension   Smoking
Renal disease   Anemia
Dyslipidemia

FIGURE 13-21. Systemic factors affecting retinopathy. Although great emphasis is placed on the clinical evaluation of the retina and the adherence to rigorous treatment algorithms, concomitant systemic disorders can exert significant influence on the development, progression, and ultimate outcome of diabetic eye disease. Optimized control of systemic disorders can improve the visual prognosis of the patient with diabetes [11]. Such care often involves an intensive, multifaceted, health care team approach to the treatment of patients with diabetes [34]. A list of systemic disorders potentially affecting diabetic retinopathy is presented; these disorders should be managed carefully.

Growth Factors and Potential Novel Therapies

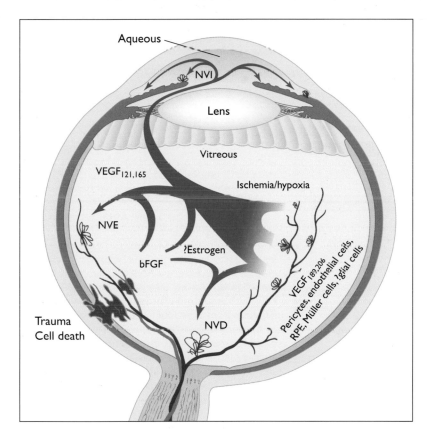

FIGURE 13-22. Model of growth factor action in diabetic retinopathy. For the past half century, investigators have recognized that numerous ischemic retinopathies result in retinal neovascularization and vascular leakage similar to that observed in diabetic retinopathy. These findings have suggested that common inciting events and mediating factors may be responsible for these complications. The potential role of growth factors in mediating retinal neovascularization was first suggested by Michaelson in 1948 and later refined by numerous investigators [35]. A schematic representation of the growth factor model of intraocular neovascularization is shown. Damage to the retinal tissues, probably caused by capillary loss and subsequent hypoxia in the case of diabetes, results in the release of growth factors from the retina. These growth factors are secreted by a variety of retinal cell types and may act locally to produce neovascularization and vascular permeability or may diffuse through the vitreous cavity to induce these complications at distant sites. The presence of two or more growth factors may actually augment the induction of neovascular activity, as is the case with basic fibroblast growth factor (bFGF) and vascular endothelial growth factor (VEGF). In addition, the growth factors may diffuse down a concentration gradient from the vitreous cavity into the aqueous cavity where they are eventually cleared through the trabecular meshwork at the base of the iris. This diffusion path would account for neovascularization observed at the iris. Numerous growth factors have been implicated in this process. Molecules that probably contribute to the neovascularization in diabetic retinopathy include VEGF, growth hormone, insulin-like growth factor-1, and bFGF. Of these, VEGF is thought to be the major mediator of intraocular neovascularization and vasopermeability, although many factors are likely to contribute to such complex processes. The relative growth factor concentrations and angiogenic potency are represented by arrow width. NVD—neovascularization at the disc; NVE—neovascularization elsewhere; NVI—neovascularization at the iris; RPE–retinal pigment epithelium. (*Adapted from* Aiello *et al.* [36].)

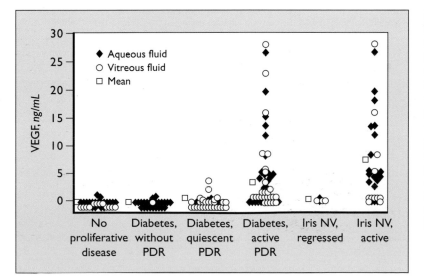

FIGURE 13-23. Angiogenic growth factors increase when neovascularization is present. For a growth factor to mediate intraocular neovascularization in diabetic retinopathy, it should be present at elevated concentrations during or shortly before the onset of active neovascularization. Demonstrated are the results of a study in which intraocular fluids were obtained from 136 patients with diabetes who were undergoing intraocular surgery. The concentration of vascular endothelial growth factor (VEGF) in the intraocular fluids was evaluated and the results plotted by extent of retinopathy. Concentrations of VEGF were low in patients who did not have diabetes or who had diabetes but no proliferative diabetic retinopathy (PDR). However, when patients had active neovascularization either of the retina or iris, concentrations of VEGF were greatly elevated. Once neovascularization had become quiescent, concentrations of vascular endothelial factor returned to baseline. The study also demonstrated the predicted concentration gradient between the vitreous and aqueous cavities and a 75% decrease in VEGF levels after successful laser panretinal photocoagulation. NV–neovascularization. (*Adapted from* Aiello *et al.* [37].)

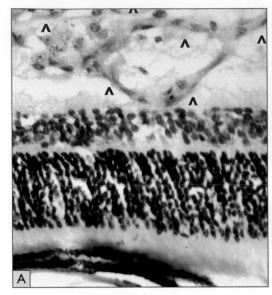
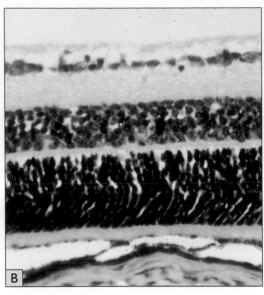

FIGURE 13-24. Inhibition of vascular endothelial growth factor (VEGF) suppresses retinal neovascularization in animals. If vascular endothelial growth factor is responsible for a significant portion of the neovascular response in ischemic retinopathies, then inhibition of this molecule should result in suppression of retinal neovascularization. Several investigators have now evaluated this causal relationship. Inhibition of VEGF using different techniques has resulted in suppression of retinal and iris neovascularization in murine

and primate models [38–40]. Demonstrated are the results from one of these studies using the chimeric receptor antagonists in a murine model of ischemia-induced retinopathy [38,41]. When these inhibitors of VEGF are injected into the neonatal eye at the time when the retinas become hypoxic, suppression of subsequent retinal neovascularization occurs in 95% to 100% of animals. The magnitude of inhibition is approximately 50%. **A**, Histologic cross-section of a neonatal mouse retina that received an intraocular injection of an inactive control compound. The *arrows* show the extensive inner retinal neovascularization. **B**, Corresponding area of retina in the contralateral eye of the same animal that received an active inhibitor of VEGF. Note the suppression of inner retinal neovascularization and normal appearance of the retina by light microscopic examination without evidence of retinal toxicity. These data suggest that growth factor inhibitors eventually may prove useful as novel therapies for diabetic retinopathy and macular edema. Such therapeutic approaches theoretically would eliminate the side effects inherent in the retinal-destructive treatments in use today (see Figs. 13-16 and 13-19). (*From* Aiello [42]; with permission.)

NOVEL THERAPEUTIC APPROACHES UNDER INVESTIGATION FOR DIABETIC NEUROPATHY

Prevention	Intervention	Restoration
Antihyperglycemics*	*Anti-permeability*	Medical approaches
ARI*	Intravitreous steroids, PKC inhibitors*, antihistamines*, anti-AGE*	Stem cell utilization
Anti-AGE*		Gene therapy
PKC inhibitors*	*Anti-angiogenesis*	Surgical approaches
Preservation of function	GH/IGF-1 inhibitors*, PKC inhibitors*, angiostatin/endostatin, ribozymes, aptamers* (eg, Macugen), antiobodies* (eg, Lucentis; Novartis, Basel, Switzerland), chimeric receptors, PEDF	Retinal transplantation
Antioxidants*		Ocular transplantation
Hemostabilization		Artificial visual prosthetics*
Neuroprotection	*Anti-proliferation*	
	Anti-integrins*, metalloproteinases*	
	*Vitreal lysis**	

Compounds in or pending clinical trials.

FIGURE 13-25. Novel therapeutic approaches for diabetic retinopathy. The possibility of preventing the visual loss from diabetes in a nondestructive manner utilizing a pharmacologic approach has become the focus of intensive investigations. Multiple approaches have been proposed, and many preclinical results have appeared promising. Several clinical trials are underway to evaluate the efficacy of these new therapeutic modalities. A partial list of approaches under investigation is presented. Anti–vascular endothelial growth factor therapy (Macugen; Pfizer, New York, NY) has been shown effective for choroidal neovascularization from age-related macular degeneration, and early clinical trials in diabetic patients suggest a possible beneficial effect for diabetic macular edema. Definitive trials are underway. In addition, intravitreous steroid appears effective in reducing macular edema, although its benefit on visual acuity and the incidence of severe side effects, such as glaucoma, await results of currently ongoing rigorous clinical trials. AGE—advanced glycation end products; ARI—aldose reductase inhibitors; IGF-1—insulin-like growth factor-1; GH—growth hormone; PEDF—pigment-epithelium derived factor; PKC—protein kinase C.

Acknowledgments

The excellent technical and editorial assistance of Jerry D. Cavallerano, OD, PhD, is gratefully acknowledged.

Portions of this chapter are adapted from Aiello *et al.* [15] and the American Academy of Ophthalmology Diabetes 2000 Diabetic Retinopathy course.

References

1. Klein R, BE Klein, Moss SE: Visual impairment in diabetes. *Ophthalmology* 1984, 91:1–9.2.

2. Klein R, Klein BE, Moss SE, Cruickshanks KJ: The Wisconsin Epidemiologic Study of Diabetic Retinopathy. XV. The long-term incidence of macular edema. *Ophthalmology* 1995, 102:7–16.

3. Javitt JC, Aiello LP, Bassi LJ, *et al.*: Detecting and treating retinopathy in patients with type 1 diabetes mellitus. Savings associated with improved implementation of current guidelines. American Academy of Ophthalmology. *Ophthalmology* 1991, 98:1565–1573.

4. Javitt JC, Aiello LP, Chiang Y, *et al.*: Preventive eye care in people with diabetes is cost-saving to the federal government. Implications for health-care reform. *Diabetes Care* 1994, 17:909–917.

5. Javitt JC, Aiello LP: Cost-effectiveness of detecting and treating diabetic retinopathy [see comments]. *Ann Intern Med* 1996, 124:164–169.

6. Javitt, JC, Canner JK, Sommer A: Cost effectiveness of current approaches to the control of retinopathy in type 1 diabetics. *Ophthalmology* 1989, 96:255–264.

7. Kahn HA, Hiller R: Blindness caused by diabetic retinopathy. *Am J Ophthalmol* 1974, 78:58–67.

8. Palmberg PF: Diabetic retinopathy. *Diabetes* 1977, 26:703–709.

9. The Diabetes Control and Complications Trial Research Group: The effect of intensive treatment of diabetes on the development and progression of long-term complications in insulin-dependent diabetes mellitus [see comments]. *N Engl J Med* 1993, 329:977–986.

10. The relationship of glycemic exposure (HbA$_{1c}$) to the risk of development and progression of retinopathy in the Diabetes Control and Complications Trial. *Diabetes* 1995, 44:968–983.

11. Retinopathy and nephropathy in patients with type 1 diabetes four years after a trial of intensive therapy. *Am J Ophthalmol* 2000, 129(5):704–705.

12. Lifetime benefits and costs of intensive therapy as practiced in the Diabetes control and complications trial. The Diabetes Control and Complications Trial Research Group [see comments]. *JAMA* 1996 276:1409–1415; published erratum, *JAMA* 1997, 278:25.

13. Resource utilization and costs of care in the Diabetes Control and Complications Trial. *Diabetes Care* 1995, 18:1468–1478.

14. Ferris FL: How effective are treatments for diabetic retinopathy? *JAMA* 1993, 269:1290–1291.

15. Aiello LP, Gardner TW, King GL, *et al.*: Diabetic retinopathy: technical review. *Diabetes Care* 1998, 21:143–156.

16. National Diabetes Data Group: *Diabetes in America*. Washington, DC: US Government Printing Office; 1995.

17. Bursell SE, Clermont AC, Kinsley BT, *et al.*: Retinal blood flow changes in patients with insulin-dependent diabetes mellitus and no diabetic retinopathy. *Am J Physiol* 1996, 270:R61–R70.

18. Wilkinson CP, Ferris FL, III, Klein RE, *et al.*: Proposed international clinical diabetic retinopathy and diabetic macular edema disease severity scales. *Ophthalmology* 2003, 110:1677–1682.

19. Chew EY: A simplified diabetic retinopathy scale. *Ophthalmology* 2003, 110:1675–1676.

20. Krolewski AS, Warram JH, Rand LI, *et al.*: Risk of proliferative diabetic retinopathy in juvenile-onset type 1 diabetes: a 40-yr follow-up study. *Diabetes Care* 1984, 9:443–452.

21. Klein R, Klein BE, Moss SE, *et al.*: The Wisconsin epidemiologic study of diabetic retinopathy. II. Prevalence and risk of diabetic retinopathy when age at diagnosis is less than 30 years. *Arch Ophthalmol* 1984, 102:520–536.

22. Klein R, Moss SE, Klein BE, *et al.*: New management concepts for timely diagnosis of diabetic retinopathy treatable by photocoagulation. *Diabetes Care* 1987, 10:633–638.

23. American Academy of Pediatrics: Screening for retinopathy in the pediatric patient with type 1 diabetes mellitus. *Pediatrics* 1998, 101:313–314.

24. Klein BE, Moss SE, Klein R: Effect of pregnancy on progression of diabetic retinopathy. *Diabetes Care* 1990, 13:34–40.

25. The Early Treatment Diabetic Retinopathy Study Research Group: Grading diabetic retinopathy from stereoscopic color fundus photographs: an extension of the modified Airlie House classification. ETDRS report number 10. *Ophthalmology* 1991, 98:786–806.

26. The Early Treatment Diabetic Retinopathy Study Research Group: Early photocoagulation for diabetic retinopathy. ETDRS report number 9. *Ophthalmology* 1991, 98:766–785.

27. The Diabetic Retinopathy Study Research Group: Photocoagulation treatment of proliferative diabetic retinopathy. Clinical application of Diabetic Retinopathy Study (DRS) findings, DRS Report Number 8. *Ophthalmology* 1981, 88:583–600.

28. The Diabetic Retinopathy Study Research Group: Indications for photocoagulation treatment of diabetic retinopathy: Diabetic Retinopathy Study Report no. 14. *Int Ophthalmol Clin* 1987, 27:239–253.

29. The Early Treatment Diabetic Retinopathy Study Research Group: Photocoagulation for diabetic macular edema. Early Treatment Diabetic Retinopathy Study report number 1. *Arch Ophthalmol* 1985, 103:1796–1806.

30. Cavallerano J: Diabetic retinopathy. *Clin Eye Vis Care* 1990, 2:4–14.

31. Ferris F: Early photocoagulation in patients with either type 1 or type 2 diabetes. *Trans Am Ophthalmol Soc* 1996, 94:505–537.

32. The Diabetes Control and Complications Trial Research Group: The effect of intensive diabetes treatment on the progression of diabetic retinopathy in insulin-dependent diabetes mellitus: the Diabetes Control and Complications Trial. *Arch Ophthalmol* 1995, 113:36–51.

33. The Diabetic Retinopathy Vitrectomy Study Research Group: Early vitrectomy for severe proliferative diabetic retinopathy in eyes with useful vision. Clinical application of results of a randomized trial: Diabetic Retinopathy Vitrectomy Study Report 4. *Ophthalmology* 1988, 95:1321–1334.

34. Aiello LP, Cahill MT, Wong JS: Systemic considerations in the management of diabetic retinopathy. *Am J Ophthalmol* 2001, 132(5):760–776.

35. Michaelson IC: The mode of development of the vascular system of the retina, with some observations on its significance for certain retinal diseases. *Trans Ophthalmol Soc UK* 1948, 68:137–180.

36. Aiello LP, Northrup JM, Keyt BA: Hypoxic regulation of vascular endothelial growth factor in retinal cells. *Arch Ophthalmol* 1995, 113:1538–1544.

37. Aiello LP, Avery RL, Arrigg PG, et al.: Vascular endothelial growth factor in ocular fluid of patients with diabetic retinopathy and other retinal disorders [see comments]. *N Engl J Med* 1994, 331:1480–1487.

38. Aiello LP, Pierce EA, Foley ED, *et al.*: Suppression of retinal neovascularization in vivo by inhibition of vascular endothelial growth factor (VEGF) using soluble VEGF-receptor chimeric proteins. *Proc Natl Acad Sci USA* 1995, 92:10457–10461.

39. Adamis AP, Shima DT, Tolentino MJ, *et al.*: Inhibition of vascular endothelial growth factor prevents retinal ischemia-associated iris neovascularization in a nonhuman primate. *Arch Ophthalmol* 1996, 114:66–71.

40. Robinson GS, Pierce EA, Rook SL, *et al.*: Oligodeoxynucleotides inhibit retinal neovascularization in a murine model of proliferative retinopathy. *Proc Natl Acad Sci USA* 1996, 93:4851–4856.

41. Smith LE, Wesolowski E, McLellan A, *et al.*: Oxygen-induced retinopathy in the mouse. *Invest Ophthalmol Vis Sci* 1994, 35:101–111.

42. Aiello LP: Vascular endothelial growth factor. 20th-century mechanisms, 21st-century therapies. *Invest Ophthalmol Vis Sci* 1997, 38:1647–1652.

DIABETES AND THE KIDNEY

Robert C. Stanton

14

Diabetic nephropathy is a serious public health concern because it has become the major cause of end-stage renal disease in the United States (*see* Fig. 14-1). It is characterized primarily by the clinical presentation of microalbuminuria, which slowly progresses to frank proteinuria, followed by a gradual decline in glomerular filtration rate, eventually leading to renal failure. Nodular sclerosis of the mesangium in the glomerular tuft is the characteristic pathologic change seen in diabetic nephropathy. A minority of patients with diabetes mellitus develop renal failure, but the number of cases of diabetic nephropathy is increasing every year, mostly because of the aging of patients with type 2 diabetes mellitus. Success in prolonging the lives of patients with types 1 and 2 diabetes mellitus has led to an increase in the numbers of patients with complications of the disease.

In the past 15 years, much has been learned about the possible causes of diabetic nephropathy. This understanding has led to the development and use of specific therapies that have been effective in slowing the progression to renal failure. Although effective, these therapies are not cures. Thus, there is an ongoing effort to further identify 1) the factors predisposing individuals to renal failure, 2) the causes of diabetic nephropathy, and 3) the factors that lead to progression to renal failure. This chapter presents an overview of the demographics, diagnosis, and natural history as well as current ideas about the pathogenesis underlying the development and progression of diabetic nephropathy. An understanding of these mechanisms has provided specific directions for the development of new, effective treatments that hold promise for the development of new clinically applicable therapies in the next 10 years. This chapter does not differentiate between the nephropathy of type 1 diabetes mellitus and the nephropathy of type 2 diabetes mellitus because recent evidence suggests that the pathogenesis and therapy for diabetic nephropathy in types 1 and 2 diabetes mellitus are similar. Although there are clear differences in susceptibility to diabetic nephropathy and there are some differences in the approach to screening and therapy, it is believed that there are more similarities than differences. Reviews by Ruggenenti and Remuzzi [1] and Ritz and Orth [2] provide more information on diabetic nephropathy in patients with type 2 diabetes mellitus.

Demographics and Prevalence

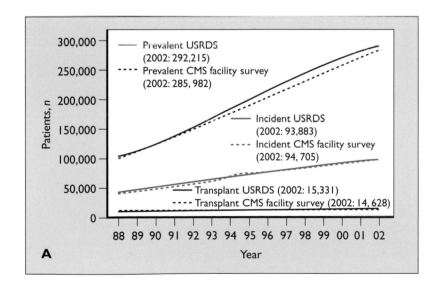

A

FIGURE 14-1. Demographics of endstage renal disease (ESRD) showing the incidence, prevalence, and transplant cases for all patients with ESRD. **A,** Diabetic nephropathy occurs In about 20% to 40% of patients with type 1 diabetes mellitus and 10% to 15% of patients with type 2 diabetes mellitus. It is a significant cause of morbidity in these patients; the appearance of nephropathy leads to a significant decrease in life expectancy and a significant increase in hospitalizations and medical care costs.

(Continued on next page)

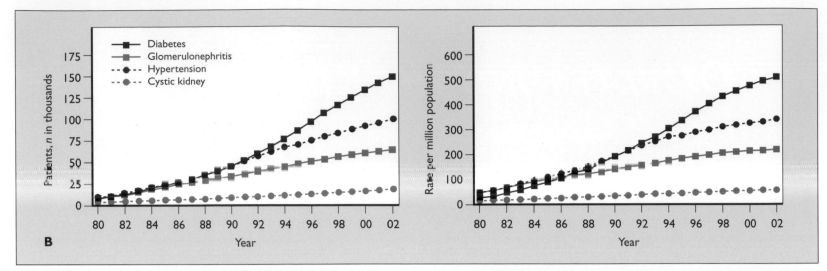

FIGURE 14-1. *(Continued)* **B,** The major causes of ESRD in the United States are diabetes, hypertension, and glomerulonephritis. Since the late 1980s, diabetes has become the leading cause [3]. The 2003 report of the US Renal Data System (USRDS) shows that over the past 10 years, the percentage of patients with ESRD has increased from 24% to 37%. This figure also shows that the rate of increase in ESRD caused by diabetes is greater than the increase for hypertension. CMS— Centers for Medicare and Medicaid Services.

PREVALENCE AND INCIDENCE OF ENDSTAGE RENAL DISEASE BY CAUSE

Cause	Prevalence	Incidence
Diabetes mellitus	149,614	42,665
Hypertension	100,472	26,617
Glomerulonephritis	65,349	7925

FIGURE 14-2. Prevalence and incidence of endstage renal disease (ESRD) by the top three causes in 2002 [3]. The prevalence shown here is the number of patients with ESRD on December 31, 2002, the incidence is the number of patients starting in ESRD in all of 2002. With present growth rates, it is expected that diabetes will surpass all other causes of ESRD combined by 2016.

Diagnosis of Diabetic Nephropathy

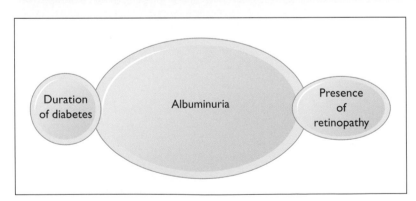

FIGURE 14-3. Diagnosis of diabetic nephropathy. The hallmark of the diagnosis of diabetic nephropathy is albuminuria. Microalbuminuria is the earliest detectable clinical sign of diabetic nephropathy. Typically, microalbuminuria progresses to frank proteinuria over a period of years. The rate of progression is based on a number of factors, which are discussed later in this chapter. In addition to microalbuminuria, patients with early diabetic nephropathy have increased glomerular filtration rates, and their kidneys undergo hypertrophy. Thus, increased creatinine clearance and increased kidney size are additional signs of early diabetic nephropathy. There are clear associations between diabetic nephropathy and two other diagnostically important factors: the duration of diabetes and preexisting retinopathy. It is unusual for diabetic nephropathy to appear in patients who have had type 1 diabetes for less than 5 years. Most patients (as many as 90%) with diabetic nephropathy also have retinopathy [4]. Thus, either a short duration of diabetes or no evidence of retinopathy in a patient with evidence of renal dysfunction should lead the clinician to consider the diagnosis of another renal disease.

REASONS TO CONSIDER OTHER RENAL DISEASES IN PATIENTS WITH DIABETES MELLITUS

Absence of albuminuria

Diabetes mellitus present for < 5 years in type 1 patients

Rapidly increasing serum creatinine

Presence of active urinary sediment

FIGURE 14-4. Reasons to consider other renal diseases in patients with diabetes mellitus. The presence of albuminuria is still considered the hallmark of diabetic nephropathy, but it has become clear recently that there are increasing numbers of patients presenting with decreased glomerular filtration rates and no albuminuria. Nevertheless, the absence of albuminuria should stimulate the physician to look for another renal disease; Other reasons to consider another kidney disease are discussed herewith. Worsening renal function in a patient with type 1 diabetes mellitus for less than 5 years should prompt the physician to consider other causes of renal failure. Typically, the decrease in glomerular filtration rate occurs over years. If a patient has a decreasing creatinine clearance or increasing serum creatinine that occurs over weeks to months, other renal diseases should be considered. The presence of an active urinary sediment (ie, the presence of such elements as erythrocytes, leukocytes, and erythrocyte casts) should lead the physician to consider other renal diseases. Although most patients with diabetic nephropathy have a relatively inactive urinary sediment, as many as 25% to 30% of patients with diabetic nephropathy may have hematuria and even erythrocyte casts [5]. The finding of an active sediment, therefore, should alert the physician to consider other causes, but by itself it may not be a reason to strongly pursue evidence for other renal diseases.

MICROALBUMINURIA AND MACROALBUMINURIA

Definition of micoralbuminuria

< 30 mg/24 h or > 20 µg/min

Albumin/creatinine ration of > 30 mg/g

Definition of frank albuminuria or macroalbuminuria

> 300 mg/24 h or > 200 µg/min

Common causes of transient increases in albuminuria

Exercise

Pregnancy

Poor glycemic control

Congestive heart failure

Hypertension

Urinary tract infection

FIGURE 14-5. Detection of albuminuria. Microalbuminuria is the hallmark of early diabetic nephropathy, so all diabetic patients should be routinely screened for the presence of microalbuminuria. Although a timed urine collection is a very effective way to determine albumin excretion accurately, it is neither convenient nor cost effective. Recent studies have shown that the albumin-to-creatinine ratio, obtained by measuring a spot urine sample for albumin and creatinine, is a highly accurate method for screening and following patients with diabetes mellitus [6]. The dipsticks used for the determination of protein in the urine are not sensitive enough to measure protein excretion less than 300 mg per 24 hours, however, so direct laboratory measurement of albumin is required to detect microalbuminuria. A spot measurement of albumin alone is affected by the urine volume, but normalizing to the amount of creatinine in the urine eliminates this concern. As shown, a value of greater than 30 mg/g is indicative of the presence of microalbuminuria.

In determining the presence of microalbuminuria, causes of transient increases in albuminuria must be considered. Macroalbuminuria reflects progressive diabetic nephropathy. Increased attention to treatment (see Fig. 14-21) should be given. Thus, repeat measurements of albumin excretion are recommended before labeling a patient with a diagnosis of early diabetic nephropathy.

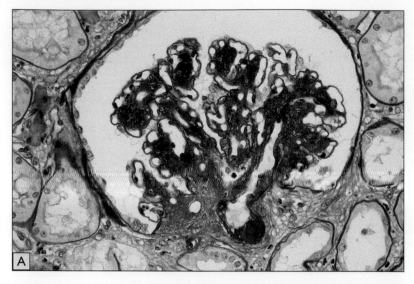

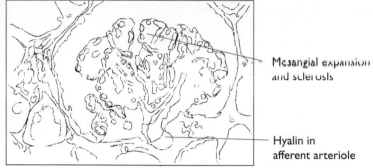

Mesangial expansion
and sclerosis

Hyalin in
afferent arteriole

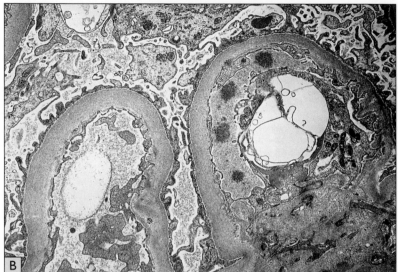

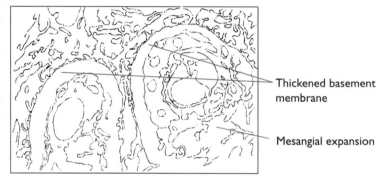

Thickened basement
membrane

Mesangial expansion

FIGURE 14-6. Pathology of diabetic nephropathy. Typical changes of diabetic nephropathy are seen in the light micrograph (**A**) and in the electron micrograph (**B**) [7]. *Panel A* shows nodular sclerosis, mesangial expansion, and hyalin deposition in the afferent arteriole. *Panel B* shows two capillary loops. The capillary loop on the right shows basement membrane thickening and mesangial expansion. Although these changes are typical of diabetic nephropathy, they are not pathognomonic. Two other diseases also must be considered in a patient with these renal biopsy findings: light chain deposition disease and amyloid. It is possible to differentiate between these diseases by specific stains and history. (*Courtesy of* Dr. Helmut Rennke, Boston, MA.)

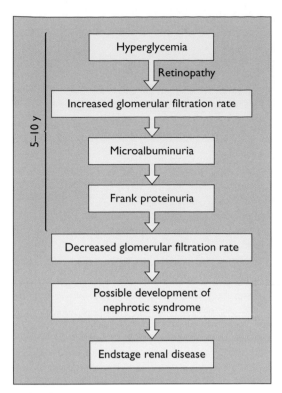

FIGURE 14-7. Natural history of diabetic nephropathy. If a patient with diabetes mellitus develops microalbuminuria, the progression to renal failure tends to be inexorable unless specific interventions are done. This schematic shows the likely progression in a hypothetical patient. As previously noted, the presence of microalbuminuria is the first easy and reliably detectable evidence of renal failure. A patient who is going to develop renal failure usually has detectable retinopathy and shows evidence of renal failure 5 to 10 years after the diagnosis of diabetes mellitus. Interestingly, if the patient has not developed proteinuria after 15 to 20 years of diabetes, the likelihood of the development of renal disease with progression to renal failure is greatly reduced [8]. The reasons for progression are multifactorial. The ensuing figures discuss the possible causes of the development of diabetic nephropathy and the reasons for the progression of diabetic nephropathy.

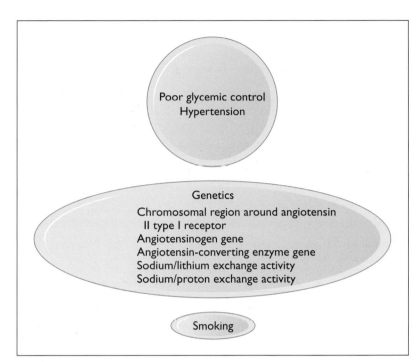

FIGURE 14-8. Risk factors for the development of diabetic nephropathy. Poor glycemic control and hypertension have been shown to increase the likelihood of developing diabetic nephropathy [9]. Both of these factors are independently correlated with the development of diabetic nephropathy. Patients with poor glycemic control are also more likely to have hypertension than are patients with good glycemic control [9]. In addition, there has been a concerted effort to detect specific genes that predispose patients to the development of diabetic nephropathy. The existence of such genes is supported by a number of findings. A family history of diabetic nephropathy increases the likelihood of developing nephropathy [10]. In addition, certain genetically similar groups are more susceptible to nephropathy than are other groups. For example, members of the Pima Indian tribe in Arizona have a high rate of development of type 2 diabetes, and in individuals in this population who are older than age 45 years, more than 60% have developed nephropathy, a percentage that is much higher than the average [11]. Specific genes listed in this figure have been suggested to be associated with the development of nephropathy. Smoking, probably because of its deleterious effects on vascular endothelial cells, has also been shown to increase the likelihood of developing diabetic nephropathy in patients with types 1 and 2 diabetes mellitus [12].

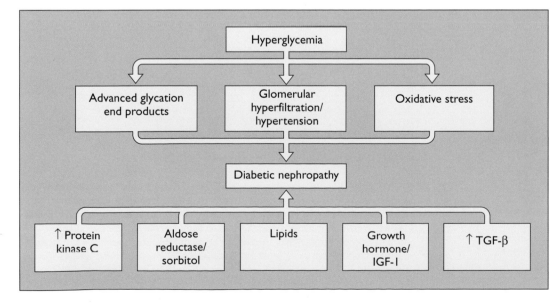

FIGURE 14-9. Suggested mechanisms underlying the development and progression of diabetic nephropathy. A number of mechanisms have been proposed to be responsible for the development of diabetic nephropathy. None of these are mutually exclusive, and it is likely that interactions of among many of these factors contribute to diabetic nephropathy. An understanding of these mechanisms is essential so that appropriate therapies may be produced to prevent the development and progression of diabetic nephropathy. A number of existing therapies, as well as treatments currently in development or in clinical trials, are based on altering one or more of the mechanisms shown in this figure. The ensuing figures provide a brief review of each of these mechanisms. IGF-1—insulin-like growth factor-1; TGF-β—transforming growth factor–β.

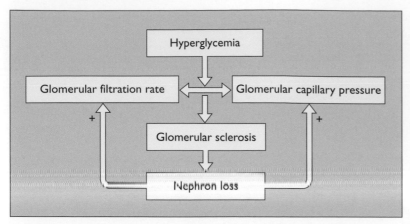

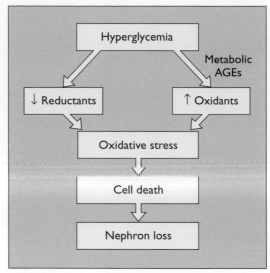

FIGURE 14-10. Glomerular hyperfiltration. Glomerular hyperfiltration is a hallmark of diabetic nephropathy. Glomerular filtration rates (GFRs) of 150 mL/min and greater are seen in patients with early diabetic nephropathy. Zatz et al. [13] were the first to show that intervention directed at decreasing hyperfiltration significantly slowed the progression of diabetic nephropathy in rats. The hypothesis is that the increased GFR is associated with increased pressure in the glomerular capillary tuft. This glomerular hypertension then leads to glomerular sclerosis and loss of functioning nephrons. Although the total GFR eventually decreases when enough nephrons undergo sclerosis, the hypothesis suggests that the filtration and, thus, the pressure in the remaining functioning glomeruli is high because the filtered load delivered to the kidney is the same as it was when there were more functioning glomeruli. Much research supports this general hypothesis. More importantly, efforts to use interventions (eg, angiotensin-converting enzyme inhibitors, angiotensin receptor blockers, and low-protein diets) that specifically lead to a reduction in glomerular capillary pressure are now mainstays of treatment for diabetic nephropathy. An extension of this hypothesis was recently suggested by Brenner and Mackenzie [14], who proposed that one predisposing factor for the progression of renal disease and possibly for the development of diabetic nephropathy is the number of glomeruli one is born with. That is, the presence of fewer glomeruli lead to relative glomerular hyperfiltration/hypertension, which slowly leads to renal failure. This hypothesis is still controversial.

FIGURE 14-11. Oxidative stress. Many studies in humans and animals have determined that patients with diabetes have evidence of increased oxidant stress [15]. Intracellular oxidants can increase as a result of intracellular production of oxidants or by exposure to extracellular oxidants. The cell carefully regulates the level of intracellular oxidants by a series of enzymes that reduce the oxidants. Defects in the actions of these enzymes also contributes to an excessive level of intracellular oxidants. Hyperglycemia alone can increase the level of intracellular oxidants. Increased oxidants can cause defects in a number of intracellular events and cause cell death. In addition, increased oxidants lead to increased activity of protein kinase C, thus linking two pathophysiologic mechanisms. A number of studies currently underway are aimed at determining whether antioxidants such as vitamin E have a therapeutic role in the treatment of diabetic nephropathy. AGE—advanced glycation end products.

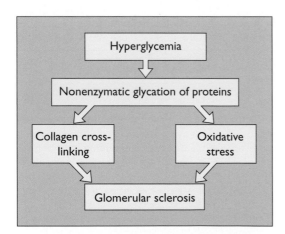

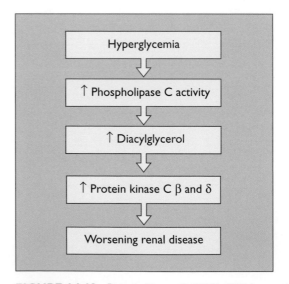

FIGURE 14-12. Advanced glycation end products (AGEs). AGEs are proteins that have reacted nonenzymatically with glucose. Although they exist normally, the number of AGEs increases significantly in patients with diabetic nephropathy. AGEs have been implicated in the development of complications of diabetes [16]. In particular, AGE production leads to increased oxidant stress. AGEs can also cause collagen crosslinking and, by binding to specific receptors, can lead to intracellular increases in oxidants. Administration of AGEs to animals can cause a number of changes that are seen in animals with diabetes, including glomerular sclerosis [17]. Accumulation of AGEs parallels the severity of diabetic nephropathy [18]. A number of trials are currently underway using an inhibitor of the formation of AGEs, aminoguanidine, to determine whether this drug can help patients with established nephropathy and help prevent diabetic nephropathy.

FIGURE 14-13. Protein kinase C (PKC). PKC is a serine/threonine kinase that has been shown to play important roles in normal cell growth, in cancerous cell growth, and in a number of other intracellular processes. Work by Koya and King [19] has shown that hyperglycemia leads to activation of PKC. More detailed work has demonstrated that specific isoforms of PKC are specifically activated by hyperglycemia. The prevention of PKC activation may reduce mesangial expansion and prevent the progression of renal disease. The deleterious effects of PKC on the kidneys may be the result of stimulation of the production of the cytokine transforming growth factor (TGF)-β (see Fig. 14-14). In particular, PKC-β has been suggested to play an important pathophysiologic role in the development of vascular, retinal, and other complications of diabetes mellitus. Ishii et al. [20] showed in diabetic rats that an inhibitor that specifically blocks PKC greatly reduced the increase in renal TGF-β and reduced the increase in other proteins associated with sclerosis. This suggests that PKC inhibitors may play an important role in future treatments for diabetic nephropathy.

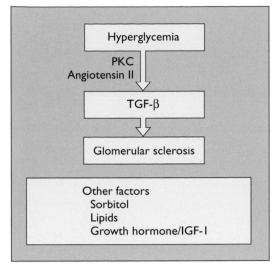

FIGURE 14-14. Transforming growth factor–β (TGF-β). TGF-β is a cytokine that can stimulate some cells to grow and inhibit the growth of other cells. Hoffman *et al.* [21] have provided a strong body of work that supports the hypothesis that TGF-β is an important mediator of the lesions seen in diabetic nephropathy. The suggestion that TGF-β plays a role in the pathogenesis of diabetic nephropathy is supported by the following evidence: 1) patients with diabetic nephropathy have increased levels of TGF-β, 2) TGF-β can cause glomerular sclerosis in animal models of diabetic nephropathy, and 3) neutralizing antibodies to TGF-β have prevented the development of diabetic nephropathy in an animal model. An interesting speculation is that increased activity of protein kinase C (PKC) leads to increased expression of TGF-β . Thus, hyperglycemia could be the initiating point that leads to increased oxidative stress, which leads to increased activity of PKC, which leads to increased expression of TGF-β. In addition, hyperglycemia leads to the production of advanced glycation end products. Thus, all of these mechanisms, separately and together, contribute to the development and progression of diabetic nephropathy.

Other factors have been implicated as well. Aldose reductase activity and the production of sorbitol have been implicated in diabetic nephropathy. Sorbitol is produced by the reduction of glucose by aldose reductase. Sorbitol is osmotically active, and, thus, increased sorbitol may lead to cell swelling and cell death. In addition, the action of aldose reductase leads to the loss of intracellular antioxidants, thereby increasing oxidative stress. Although increased aldose reductase activity appears to play a significant role in the pathogenesis of diabetic neuropathy, it remains to be shown whether it plays an important role in diabetic nephropathy. Epidemiologic studies have implicated increased lipids as possible mediators. Although it seems clear that increased lipids are associated with progression of diabetic nephropathy, the mechanism underlying this association has not been well defined. The important association of worsening vascular disease with increased lipids may be the mechanism by which lipids contribute to the progression of diabetic nephropathy. Lastly, a growing body of research suggests that growth hormone or insulin-like growth factor-1 (IGF-1) may play an important role in the pathogenesis of diabetic nephropathy. A study [21] showed a strong correlation between urinary levels of growth hormone and IGF-1 with the development of microalbuminuria and increased kidney size in patients with type 1 diabetes mellitus.

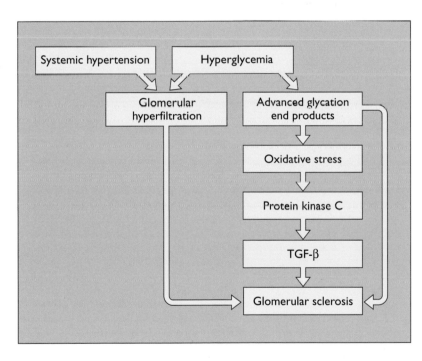

FIGURE 14-15. Possible connections between various mechanisms that may contribute to diabetic nephropathy. This model suggests that controlling the blood sugar is of paramount importance. Research from the Diabetes Control and Complications Trial (DCCT) strongly supports this idea [22]. Nevertheless, after there is evidence of diabetic nephropathy, many of these mechanisms may occur independent (to some extent) of the current blood glucose control. For example, if nephron loss has occurred, then glomerular hyperfiltration or hypertension continue even in the presence of tight control of blood sugar. Other mechanisms shown in the figure may also become somewhat autonomous after initial damage to the glomerulus is accomplished. Thus, tight control of the blood sugar, as well as other interventions that block mechanisms shown in this figure, are probably needed to prevent the progression of diabetic nephropathy. TGF-β —transforming growth factor–β.

TREATMENT FOR DIABETIC NEPHROPATHY

Mechanism	Treatment	Efficacy in Humans
Hyperglycemia	Tight control of blood sugar	Proven
Systemic hypertension	Antihypertensive agents	Proven
Glomerular hypertension	ACE inhibitors/ARB	Proven
Lipids/cholesterol	Lipid-lowering agents	Proven
Advanced glycation end products	Aminoguanidine	In trials
Oxidative stress	Antioxidants (eg, vitamin E)	In trials
Increased PKC	PKC inhibitors	In trials
TGF-β	Pirfenidone	In trials
Increased aldose reductase/sorbitol	Aldose reductase inhibitors	In trials
Growth hormone/IGF-1	No obvious therapy	Unknown

FIGURE 14-16. The efficacy in humans of various treatments for diabetic nephropathy, listed according to mechanism. As previously noted, a combined therapeutic approach probably is the most beneficial. ACE—angiotensin-converting enzyme; ARB—angiotensin receptor blocker; IGF—insulin-like growth factor; PKC—protein kinase C; TGF—transforming growth factor.

Treatment and Prevention

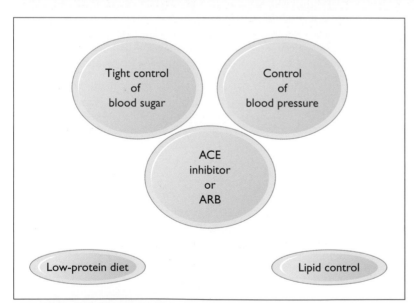

FIGURE 14-17. Treatment and prevention of diabetic nephropathy. The mainstay of prevention is tight control of the blood sugar and control of hypertension. The Diabetes Control and Complications Trial Research Group clearly showed that control of the blood sugar is very beneficial in preventing the onset and the progression of diabetic nephropathy [22]. This is entirely consistent with the information presented in Figures 14-10 through 14-15 suggesting that hyperglycemia can be the predominant mechanism that leads to the activation of the other proposed mechanisms. In addition, many studies clearly have indicated that hypertension predisposes to and worsens diabetic nephropathy [23]. Thus,

before microalbuminuria has developed, all patients should be urged to monitor their blood sugar levels closely and to control their blood pressure (BP). The current recommendation is to aim for a BP lower than 135/85 mm Hg [23]. When microalbuminuria develops, the principal therapies are those shown here. In addition to tight control of blood glucose level and control of hypertension, all patients should take an angiotensin-converting enzyme (ACE) inhibitor. The ACE inhibitors, although not a cure, clearly have been shown to slow the progression of diabetic nephropathy. These drugs reduce the levels of angiotensin II. A reduction in angiotensin II leads to a decrease in glomerular filtration and a decrease in glomerular pressure. In addition to its vasoactive properties, angiotensin II is also a growth factor. Thus, it has been proposed that ACE inhibitors also work by inhibiting the growth-promoting effects of angiotensin II [24]. Angiotensin II receptor blockers (ARBs; eg, valsartan and losartan) are now available. Studies have shown that ARBs are effective for patients with type 2 diabetic nephropathy [25–27]. The ARBs are especially useful in patients who develop a cough while taking ACE inhibitors. In addition, for unclear reasons, the hyperkalemia that can occur in patients taking ACE inhibitors is much less common in patients taking ARBs.

Other recommended treatments are adherence to a low-protein diet and control of lipids. A low-protein diet probably acts similarly to ACE inhibitors by decreasing intraglomerular pressure. In practical terms, it is somewhat difficult to achieve a low enough intake of protein because the diet is rather bland. Nevertheless, it is recommended that diet counseling be done for blood sugar control and low-protein intake so that the patients do not ingest a high-protein diet that could potentially accelerate progression of renal disease. When patients are nearing endstage renal disease, it is important for protein intake to be liberalized because at this point there is little benefit to a low-protein diet, and the risk of malnutrition is significant.

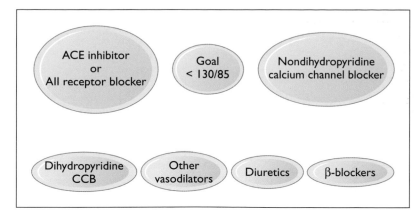

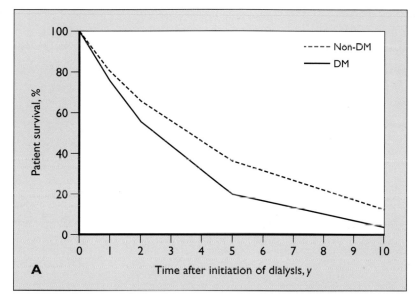

FIGURE 14-18. Antihypertensive agents. In addition to diet modifications and angiotensin-converting enzyme (ACE) inhibitors, other antihypertensive agents play important roles in the treatment of patients with hypertension in diabetic nephropathy. Of particular interest are the calcium channel blockers (CCBs). Specifically, the nondihydropyridine CCBs (eg, diltiazem and verapamil) offer benefits in reducing blood pressure and slowing the progression of renal disease that are similar to those provided by ACE inhibitors [28]. Dihydropyridine CCBs (eg, nifedipine and amlodipine) are also useful in treating hypertension, but, alone, they do not offer the same effects on the slowing of progression of renal disease that is observed with the ACE inhibitors and the nondihydropyridines. Various combinations of antihypertensive agents have also been evaluated and may offer further benefits. A combination of nondihydropyridine and ACE inhibitors may be more effective than either drug type alone in slowing the progression of diabetic nephropathy [29]. Other antihypertensive agents (eg, diuretics, β-blockers, vasodilators) can also be used in patients with diabetic nephropathy, but when they are used alone, they do not have the same effects on diabetic nephropathy as do ACE inhibitors and nondihydropyridines. AII—angiotensin II.

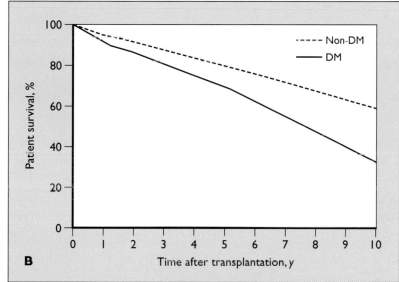

FIGURE 14-19. Survival estimates for patients on dialysis. As noted in Figure 14-1, diabetic nephropathy is the leading cause of endstage renal disease (ESRD) in the United States. In addition, the rate of increase in ESRD resulting from diabetes mellitus (DM) is significantly greater than that for the other leading causes of renal failure. Most of this increase reflects an aging population in which type 2 DM is prevalent. A review covers the general issues of ESRD in the diabetic population [30]. Probably because of the many comorbid conditions that are present in diabetic patients, diabetic patients on dialysis (**A**) or after transplantation (**B**) have a lower rate of survival than do nondiabetic ESRD patients [30]. It is not clear whether the mode of dialysis has any effects, positive or negative, on morbidity or mortality, although most ESRD diabetic patients are treated by hemodialysis [30]. The decision to use hemodialysis versus peritoneal dialysis should be made while considering such factors as lifestyle, overall health of the patient, and comorbid conditions (eg, vision impairment). The use of peritoneal dialysis may simplify or complicate glucose management.

Because peritoneal dialysate contains varying concentrations of glucose (1.5%, 2.5%, and 4.25%), glucose control can be significantly affected when dialysate exchanges occur. This problem is minimized by injecting insulin directly into the dialysate solution. This insulin delivery method can be used not only to counteract the effects of the acute exposure to the high glucose concentrations but also as a way of providing a constant level of insulin that may help in maintaining a reasonably stable blood glucose level throughout the day. This method of insulin delivery is effective for overall blood glucose maintenance only for patients who do fluid exchanges during the day. Many patients prefer to do peritoneal dialysis by repeated nighttime exchanges using a machine that cycles the fluid in and out of the abdomen. During the day, these patients have no fluid exchanges. The insulin injected in each bag at night is dosed to maintain a steady glucose concentration through the night, and the patient follows a standard schedule of subcutaneous injections throughout the day. (*Data from* US Renal Data System [31].)

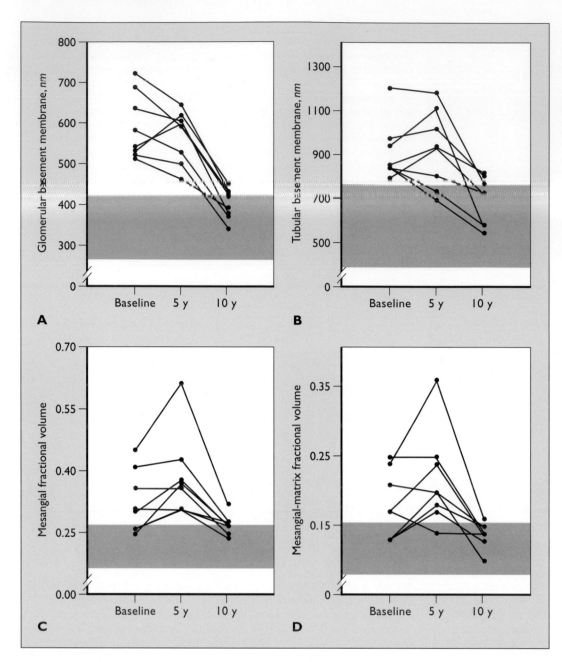

FIGURE 14-20. Kidney and pancreas transplantation. Kidney or kidney and pancreas transplantation are generally believed to be the preferred therapy for patients with endstage renal disease. Survival rates after transplantation are higher than those for patients who remain on dialysis (*see* Fig. 14-19). Diabetic nephropathy recurs in most kidney transplant recipients, although it is usually many years before diabetic nephropathy is severe enough to cause loss of the transplant (**A–D**). Loss of the transplant because of the recurrence of diabetic nephropathy is rare, therefore. Pancreas transplantation is usually done only in conjunction with a kidney transplant. It has been believed that because blood glucose levels can be controlled with insulin, pancreas transplantation offers too many risks compared with its benefits. The biggest risks relate to immunosuppression and the increased risk of life-threatening infections. In addition, there has been little evidence showing that early pancreas transplantation would affect the progression of diabetic nephropathy. An intriguing study by Fioretto *et al.* [32] shows, however, that pancreas transplantation alone can cause actual reversal in the lesions of diabetic nephropathy that become evident only after 5 years of normoglycemia. This finding may increase interest in pancreas transplantation as a way of preventing the development of diabetic nephropathy. (*Adapted from* Fioretto *et al.* [32].)

JOSLIN DIABETES CENTER SCREENING AND TREATMENT RECOMMENDATIONS FOR MICROPROTEINURIA AND MACROPROTEINURIA

Screening

Screen for microalbuminuria by checking for albumin/creatinine (A/C) ratio:

Annually in patients 10–65 years of age

As clinically indicated for patients > 65 years of age

Continue use of routine urinalysis as clinically indicated

Treatment

If A/C ratio < 20 µg/mg (30 mg/24 h)

Recheck in 1 year

If A/C ratio is 20–300 µg/mg (30–300 mg/24 h)

Confirm presence of microalbuminuria with at least two positive collections done within 3–6 mo; in the process, rule out confounding factors that cause false-positive results, eg, urinary tract infection, pregnancy, excessive exercise

Once confirmed

Initiate/modify use of ACE inhibitor; consider use for type 2 diabetes. If side effects to ACE inhibitor occur, consider angiotensin II receptor antagonist treatment

Initiate/modify hypertension treatment with a goal blood pressure under 130/80 mm Hg or MAP < 90

Encourage home blood pressure monitoring

Refer to diabetes education

Refer to registered dietitian for dietary management

Strive to improve glycemic control with an optimal goal of HbA_{1C} < 8% or as otherwise clinically indicated

Monitor serum creatinine and potassium, and treat appropriately

Repeat A/C ratio testing at least every 12 mo; consider testing more often when changes in medication are made

If A/C ratio > 300 µg/mg (> 300 mg/24 h) or overt proteinuria:

Follow all guidelines as stated for A/C ratio 20–300 µg/mg

Consider consultation with nephrology team when:

A/C ratio is > 300 µg/mg

Rapid rise in creatinine (eg, 0.8 to 1.4 in 12 mo); presence of hematuria, or sudden increase in proteinuria

Questioning etiology of nephropathy

For refinement of treatment program to prevent further decline in renal function

Refer to renal team for collaborative care when:

Creatinine is elevated (> 1.8 in women; > 2.0 in men)

Problems with ACE inhibitors, difficulties in management of hypertension or hyperkalemia

FIGURE 14-21. Screening and treatment recommendations for proteinuria. The current recommendations for treatment for proteinuria at the Joslin Diabetes Center in Boston, Massachusetts, are based on the level of proteinuria. The physicians at the Joslin Diabetes Center believe that a collaborative model of care is best for patients with diabetes. Thus, patients with early diabetic nephropathy are primarily cared for by an endocrinologist in consultation with a nephrologist. When patients near endstage renal disease, much of the care of the patient transfers to the nephrologist, but the other caregivers (eg, endocrinologist, ophthalmologist, dietitian) continue to work collaboratively to care for the patient. ACE—angiotensin-converting enzyme; HbA_{1C}—hemoglobin 1C; MAP—mean arterial pressure.

References

1. Ruggenenti P, Remuzzi G: Nephropathy of type 2 diabetes mellitus. *J Am Soc Nephrol* 1998, 9:2157–2169.

2. Ritz E, Orth SR: Nephropathy in patients with type 2 diabetes mellitus. *N Engl J Med* 1999, 341:1127–1133.

3. Agodoa LY: US Renal Data System. Available at: http;//www.usrds.org.

4. Stephenson JM, Fuller JH, Viberti GC, *et al*.: EURODIAB IDDM complications study group. Blood pressure, retinopathy, and urinary albumin excretion in IDDM. *Diabetologia* 1995, 38:599–603.

5. Chihara J, Takebayashi S, Takashi T, *et al*.: Glomerulonephritis in diabetic patients and its effect on the prognosis. *Nephron* 1986, 43:45–49.

6. Warram JH, Krolewski AS: Use of the albumin/creatinine ratio in patient care and clinical studies. In *The Kidney and Hypertension in Diabetes Mellitus*. Edited by Mogensen CE. London: Kluwer Academic Publishers; 1998:85–96

7. Tisher CC, Hostetter TH: Diabetic nephropathy. In *Renal Pathology*, edn 2. Edited by Tisher CC, Brenner BM. Philadelphia: JB Lippincott; 1994:1387–1412.

8. Parving HH, Hommel E, Mathiesen E, *et al*.: Prevalence of microalbuminuria, arterial hypertension, retinopathy, and neuropathy in patients with insulin dependent diabetes. *Br Med J* 1988, 296:156–160.

9. Krolewski AS, Fogarty DG, Warram JH: Hypertension and nephropathy in diabetes mellitus: what is inherited and what is acquired? *Diab Res Clin Practice* 1998, 39(suppl):S1–S14.

10. Quinn M, Angelico MC, Warram JH, *et al*.: Familial factors determine the development of diabetic nephropathy in patients with IDDM. *Diabetologia* 1996, 39:940–945.

11. Nelson RG, Newman JM, Knowler WC, *et al*.: Incidence of end stage renal disease in type 2 (non–insulin-dependent) diabetes mellitus in Pima Indians. *Diabetologia* 1988, 31:730–736.

12. Biesenbach G, Grafinger P, Janko O, *et al*.: Influence of cigarette smoking on the progression of clinical diabetic nephropathy in type 2 diabetic patients. *Clin Nephrol* 1997, 48:146–150.

13. Zatz R, Rentz DB, Meyer TW, *et al*.: Prevention of diabetic glomerulopathy by pharmacological amelioration of glomerular capillary hypertension. *J Clin Invest* 1986, 77:1925–1930.

14. Brenner B, Mackenzie HS: Nephron mass as risk factor for the progression of renal disease. *Kidney Int* 1997, 63(suppl):S124–S127.

15. Giugliano D, Ceriello A, Paolissa G: Oxidative stress and diabetic vascular complications. *Diabetes Care* 1996, 19:257–267.

16. Bierhaus A, Hofmann MA, Ziegler R, *et al*.: AGEs and their interaction with AGE-receptors in vascular disease and diabetes mellitus. I. The AGE concept. *Cardiovasc Res* 1998, 37:586–600.

17. Vlassara H, Striker LJ, Teichberg S, *et al*.: Advanced glycation end products induce glomerular sclerosis and albuminuria in normal rats. *Proc Natl Acad Sci U S A* 1994, 91:11704–11708.

18. Makita Z, Radoff S, Rayfield EJ, *et al*.: Advanced glycation end products in patients with diabetic nephropathy. *N Engl J Med* 1991, 325:836–842.

19. Koya D, King GL: Protein kinase C activation and the development of diabetic complications. *Diabetes* 1998, 47:859–866.

20. Ishii H, Jirousek MR, Koya D, *et al*.: Ameliorations of vascular dysfunctions in diabetic rats by an oral PKC beta inhibitor. *Science* 1996, 272:728–731.

21. Hoffman BB, Sharma K, Ziyadeh FN: Potential role of TGF-b in diabetic nephropathy. *Min Electrol Metab* 1998, 24:190–196.

22. The Diabetes Control and Complications Trial Research Group: The effect of intensive treatment of diabetes on the development and progression of long-term complications in insulin-dependent diabetes mellitus. *N Engl J Med* 1993, 329:977–986.

23. Bakris GL: Progression of diabetic nephropathy. A focus on arterial pressure level and methods of reduction. *Diab Res Clin Prac* 1998, 39(suppl):S35–S42.

24. Wolf G, Ziyadeh FN: The role of angiotensin II in diabetic nephropathy: emphasis on nonhemodynamic mechanisms. *Am J Kidney Dis* 1997, 29:153–163.

25. Lewis EJ, Hunsicker LG, Clarke WR, *et al*.: Renoprotective effect of the angiotensin-receptor antagonist irbesartan in patients with nephropathy due to type 2 diabetes. *N Engl J Med* 2001, 345:851–860.

26. Brenner BM, Cooper ME, de Zeeuw D, *et al*.: Effects of losartan on renal and cardiovascular outcomes in patients with type 2 diabetes and nephropathy. *N Engl J Med* 2001, 345:861–869.

27. Parving HH, Lehnert H, Brochner-Mortensen J, *et al*.: The effect of irbesartan on the development of diabetic nephropathy in patients with type 2 diabetes. *N Engl J Med* 2001, 345:870–878.

28. Slataper R, Vicknair N, Sadler R, *et al*.: Comparative effects of different antihypertensive treatments on progression of diabetic renal disease. *Arch Intern Med* 1993, 153:973–979.

29. Bakris GL, Weir MR, DeQuattro V, *et al*.: Effects of an ACE inhibitor/ calcium antagonist combination on proteinuria in diabetic nephropathy. *Kidney Int* 1998, 54:1283–1289.

30. Williams ME: The diabetic patient with end stage renal disease. In *Therapy in Nephrology and Hypertension*. Edited by Brady HR, Wilcox CS. Philadelphia: WB Saunders; 1999:249–255.

31. US Renal Data System: *USRDS 1996 Annual Data Report*. Bethesda, MD: National Institutes of Health, National Institute of Diabetes and Digestive and Kidney Diseases; April 1996.

32. Fioretto P, Steffes MW, Sutherland DER, *et al*.: Reversal of lesions of diabetic nephropathy after pancreas transplantation. *N Engl J Med* 1998, 339:69–75.

DIABETIC NEUROPATHIES

Aaron I. Vinik

15

Diabetic neuropathy is not a single entity but rather a number of different syndromes, each with a range of clinical and subclinical manifestations. According to the San Antonio Conference [1], the main groups of neurologic disturbance in diabetes mellitus include subclinical neuropathy determined by abnormalities in electrodiagnostic and quantitative sensory testing, diffuse clinical neuropathy with distal symmetric sensorimotor and autonomic syndromes, and focal syndromes. There is reason to add proximal neuropathy as a separate entity based on the nature of the pathology and response to treatment. However, we have found it more appropriate to classify neuropathy into different clinical syndromes based on their pathogenesis because this is what ultimately determines the choice of treatment. We classify neuropathies into somatic and autonomic. There are two types of somatic neuropathy: focal and diffuse. The focal neuropathies include mononeuritis and entrapment

syndromes. The diffuse neuropathies include proximal neuropathies and large- and small-fiber distal symmetric polyneuropathies.

Estimates of the prevalence of diabetic neuropathy range from 10% to 90% of the diabetic population, depending on the criteria used to define neuropathy [1–6]. Neurologic complications occur equally in patients with type 1 and type 2 diabetes mellitus, as well as various forms of acquired diabetes.

In this pictorial overview, clinical presentations and therapeutic approaches to common forms of neuropathy are presented and discussed, including distal symmetric, proximal motor, and autonomic neuropathies. Also provided are algorithms for recognition and management of common pain and entrapment syndromes. A global approach is used for recognition of syndromes requiring specialized treatments based on our improved understanding of their etiopathogenesis.

Distal Neuropathy

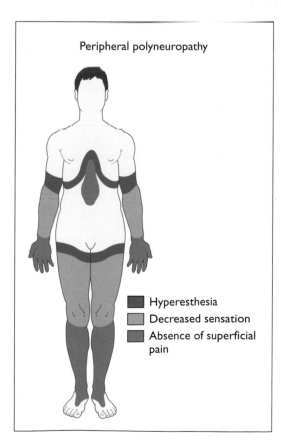

Peripheral polyneuropathy

■ Hyperesthesia
■ Decreased sensation
■ Absence of superficial pain

FIGURE 15-1. Peripheral polyneuropathy. The spectra of clinical neuropathic syndromes described in patients with diabetes mellitus include dysfunction of almost every segment of the somatic peripheral and autonomic nervous systems [7]. Each syndrome can be distinguished by its pathophysiologic, therapeutic, and prognostic features. Initial neurologic evaluation should be directed toward detection of the specific part of the nervous system affected by diabetes. Diabetes may damage small fibers, large fibers, or both. Small nerve fiber dysfunction usually, but not always, occurs early and often is present before objective signs or electrophysiologic evidence of nerve damage is found [8–10]. Small nerve fiber dysfunction is manifested first in the lower limbs by pain and hyperalgesia. Loss of thermal sensitivity follows, with reduced light touch and pinprick sensation. Large fiber neuropathies may involve sensory or motor nerves, or both. The neuropathies are manifested by reduced vibration (often the first objective evidence of neuropathy) and position sense, weakness, muscle wasting, and depressed tendon reflexes. Most patients with distal sensory polyneuropathy have a mixed variety, with both large and small nerve fiber involvement. In the case of distal sensory polyneuropathy, a "glove and stocking" distribution of sensory loss is almost universal [7]. Early in the course of the neuropathic process, multifocal sensory loss may also be found.

Diabetic peripheral symmetric polyneuropathy is thought to be a dying-back disorder, with prevailing effects on the axons and consequent demyelination. There is an early functional phase in which metabolic abnormalities are responsible for the clinical symptoms and signs. Later structural changes occur in the nerves so that treatment strategies have been to arrest or slow the rate of progression. When neuronal cell death occurs, little can be done to induce recovery. Clearly, all attempts at treating neuropathy should be oriented toward the reversible phase of the disorder.

Cutaneous Nerve Components

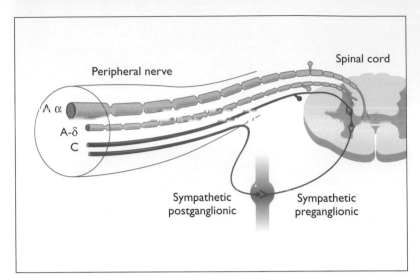

FIGURE 15-2. Cutaneous nerve components. Peripheral nerves are composed of several different types of nerve fibers, each with their own function. The large myelinated α fibers conduct rapidly and subserve motor power and proprioception and coordination. The thinner yet myelinated A-δ fibers subserve cold thermal detection and deep-seated pain. The thin unmyelinated fibers are responsible for warm detection threshold, heat pain, part of touch sensation, and sympathetic nerve supply to the skin.

Large Fiber Neuropathy

CLINICAL PRESENTATION AND MANAGEMENT OF LARGE FIBER NEUROPATHY

Presentation

Impaired vibration perception

Pain of A-δ type: deep-seated, gnawing

Ataxia

Wasting of small muscles, intrinsic minus feet with hammer toes

Weakness

Increased blood flow (the hot foot)

  Risk of Charcot neuroarthropathy

Management

  Proper shoes

  Orthotics

  Tendon lengthening

  Foot reconstruction

FIGURE 15-3. Clinical presentation and management of large fiber neuropathy.

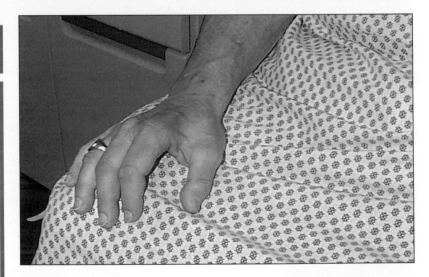

FIGURE 15-4. Wasting of the small muscle of the hand in large fiber neuropathies. This must not be mistaken for ulnar entrapment, which is amenable to treatment. In large fiber neuropathies all peripheral nerves are affected equally and the sensory disturbance is of the "glove and stocking" variety not confined to the nerve distribution. In ulnar entrapment the sensory loss involves the ring and little fingers.

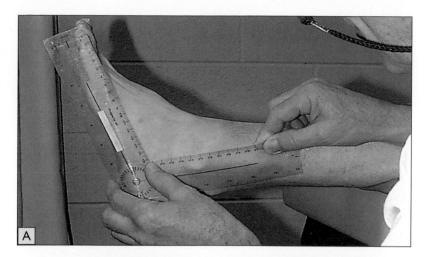

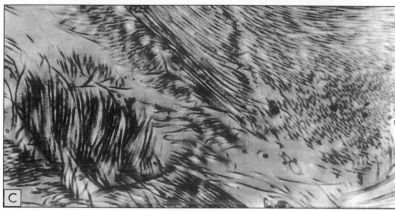

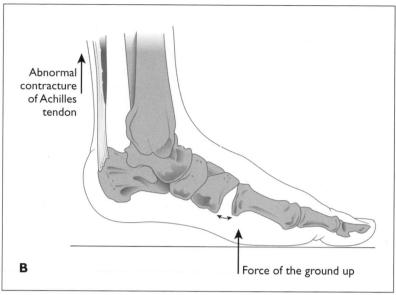

FIGURE 15-5. In large fiber neuropathies there is wasting of the small muscles of the feet: intrinsic minus feet as well as talipes equinovarus owing to shortening of the Achilles tendon. **A,** Measurement of the angle of the ankle in full flexion. Using a goniometer, the flexion should be at least 90°. **B,** Greater than 100° indicates tendo-achilles shortening, with its impact on increasing midfoot pressure and breakdown of Lisfranc's joint in the midfoot. **C,** Electron micrograph of disrupted collagen fibers in the Achilles tendon in a patient with large nerve neuropathy.

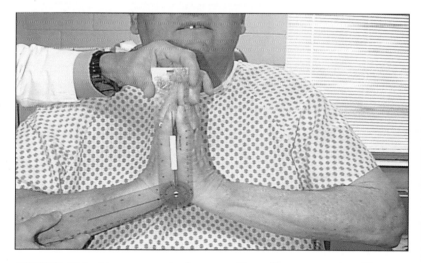

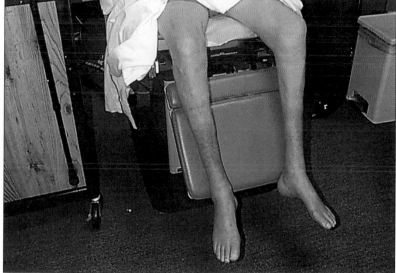

FIGURE 15-6. Upper extremity features of large fiber neuropathies. This patient is unable to extend his hands at the wrist to beyond 90°, as shown using the goniometer. Note the separation of the small fingers, creating a diamond-shaped open space indicative of cheiroarthropathy. These features accompany large fiber neuropathies as well as entrapment syndromes. This is not universal, and the two conditions may well have different causes.

FIGURE 15-7. Lower extremity features of large fiber neuropathies. This patient shows a combination of severe muscle wasting of the lower limbs resembling that seen in Charcot-Marie-Tooth disease, the equinus of the feet owing to shortening of the Achilles tendon, and wasting of the proximal muscles of the thigh owing to a combination of a proximal neuropathy and a distal large fiber neuropathy.

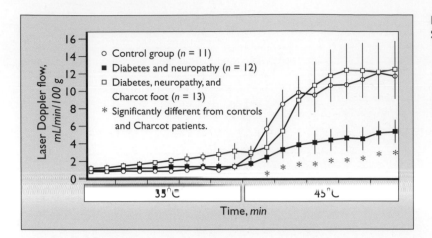

FIGURE 15-8. Neurovascular dysfunction in neuropathy. (*Adapted from* Shapiro *et al.* [11].)

C-Fiber Dysfunction in Small Fiber Neuropathy

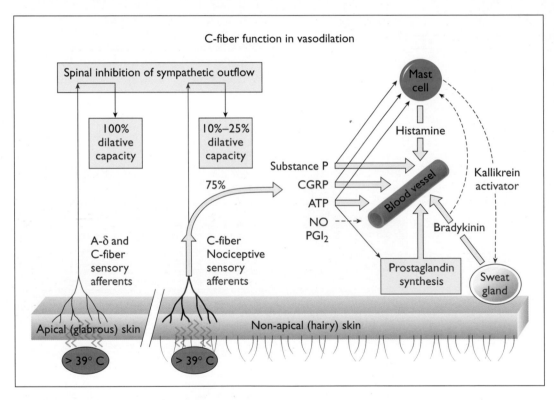

FIGURE 15-9. Vasodilation and C-fiber function. Factors controlling vasodilation in glabrous skin such as that found on the pads and soles and hairy skin found on the dorsum of the feet and hands. In glabrous skin, vasodilation is for the most part a consequence of relaxation of the sympathetic tone. In hairy skin, C fibers are essential for vasodilation, a process mediated by a variety of neurotransmitters including the neuropeptides, substance P, and calcitonin gene-related peptide (CGRP) as well as bradykinin. Defective trophic support for skin with reduced levels of neuronal growth factor results in decreased substance P and CGRP, thereby impairing the ability to dilate in response to noxious stimuli and heat. Thus nutrient delivery is compromised and there is susceptibility to ulceration. ATP—adenosine triphosphate. (*Adapted from* Burnstock and Ralevic [12]; *modified by* Vinik *et al.* [13,14].)

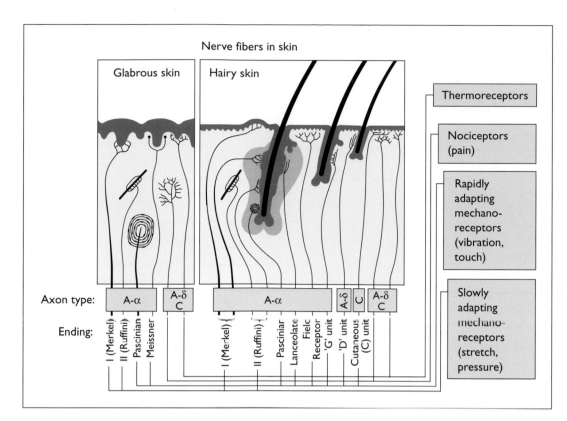

Nerve fibers in skin

FIGURE 15-10. Different nerve fibers in skin and their different roles in sensory perception and mechanoreceptor function. C-fiber type pain generally is described as throbbing, shooting, stabbing, sharp, hot, burning, and tender. Touch is misinterpreted as pain, ie, allodynia, and patients cannot bear contact with bedclothes or other objects. In contrast, A-δ pain often is described as cramping, gnawing, aching, heavy, splitting, tiring and exhausting, sickening, fearful, and punishing and cruel. A patient may say, "I have a toothache in my foot," "there is a dog gnawing at the bones of my feet," or "my feet feel as if they are encased in concrete." These pains derive from different fibers and have a different mechanism of production. The scheme is based on this information, which proves helpful in the management of patients with neuropathic pain.

Pain disappears when a loss of C-fibers occurs, and the loss heralds the phase of hypoalgesia, and hypesthesia, with impairment of warm thermal perception and insensitivity to heat pain. These symptoms are particularly dangerous and are the forerunners of repeated minor injury and subsequent loss of toes and feet.

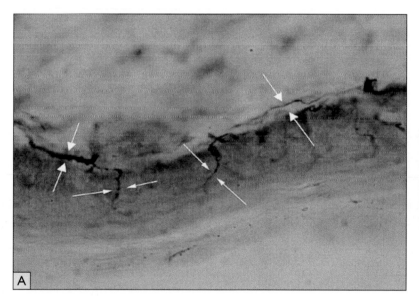

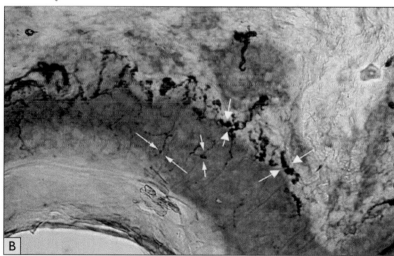

FIGURE 15-11. Photomicrographs of 50-μm sections from skin biopsy specimens taken from the upper thigh of a control subject (**A**) and a neuropathic patient (**B**). The sections were stained with antibody to PCP 9.5 and neuronal antigen and were evaluated by immunocytochemistry to reveal peripheral small unmyelinated neurons. **A** shows straight, uninterrupted unmyelinated nerve fibers running between the dermis and epidermis in normal skin (*broad arrows*). In addition, there are numerous single, relatively straight fibers projecting into the epidermis (*narrow arrows*) of normal skin. **B** demonstrates the changes observed in neuropathic skin, including malformation of the fibers running between dermis and epidermis, with multiple, irregular swelling (*broad arrows*). The fibers in the epidermis of neuropathic skin are reduced in number compared with normal skin. These changes in skin are characteristic of small fiber neuropathies and may occur in the absence of any other clinical or laboratory evidence of neuropathy [15].

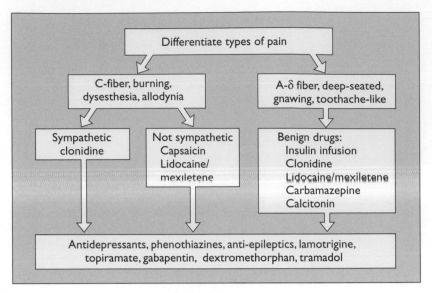

FIGURE 15-12. Managing painful diabetic neuropathy.

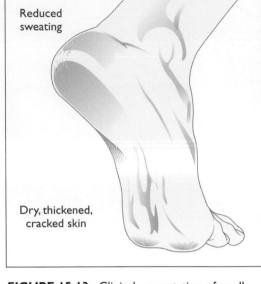

FIGURE 15-13. Clinical presentation of small fiber neuropathy. The signs of this disorder include pain (C-fiber type, burning and superficial), late hypoalgesia, hypoesthesia, impaired warm thermal perception, decreased sweating, and impaired cutaneous blood flow (the cold foot). The risks are foot ulcers, gangrene, and amputations.

MANAGEMENT OF C-FIBER DYSFUNCTION

Patients must be instructed on foot care with daily foot inspection (they must have a mirror in the bathroom for inspection of the soles of the feet)

Patients should be provided with a monofilament for self-testing

All diabetic patients should wear padded socks

Shoes must fit well with adequate support and must be inspected for the presence of foreign bodies (eg, nails, pins, teeth) before wearing

Patients must exercise care with exposure to heat (eg, avoid falling asleep in front of the fireplace)

Emollient creams should be used for the drying and cracking of skin

After bathing, feet should be thoroughly dried and powdered between the toes

Nails should be cut transversely, preferably by a podiatrist

FIGURE 15-14. Management of C-fiber dysfunction.

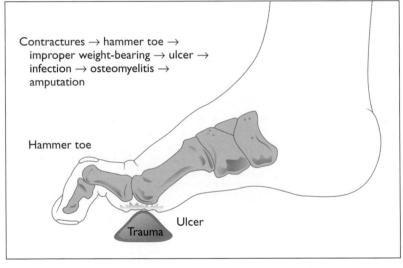

FIGURE 15-15. Management of small fiber neuropathies. In the United States, 65,000 amputations are performed each year. Half of these are attributable to diabetes, and small fiber neuropathy is implicated in 87% of cases. The combination of decreased pain perception with decreased warm thermal perception and the resulting hammer toe deformity that follows intrinsic minus feet leads to blisters on the top of the knuckles of the toes or ulcers over the heads of the metatarsals. These high-pressure points are easily recognized by forced gate analysis scans of the feet. With correct shoes, padded socks and orthotics, the likelihood of amputation can be reduced by half. Patients should be instructed to protect their feet with padded socks, wear shoes that have adequate support, regularly inspect their feet and shoes, be careful of exposure to heat, and use emollient creams for sympathetic dysfunction.

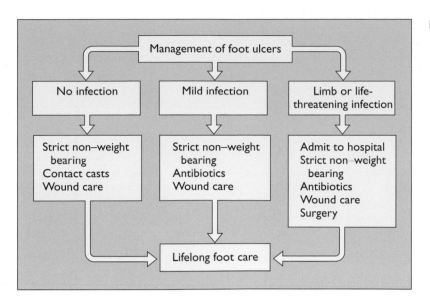

FIGURE 15-16. Management of foot ulcers.

Neuroarthropathy

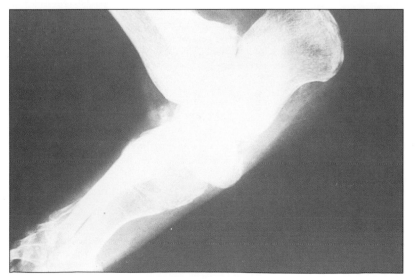

FIGURE 15-17. (See Color Plate) The hot foot of Charcot neuroarthropathy showing the end result of large fiber neuropathy. Note the red inflamed foot that is easily mistaken for infection and the collapse of the midfoot.

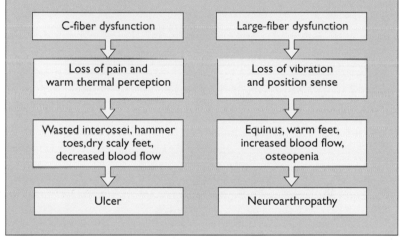

FIGURE 15-18. Prediction of foot ulcers versus neuroarthropathy.

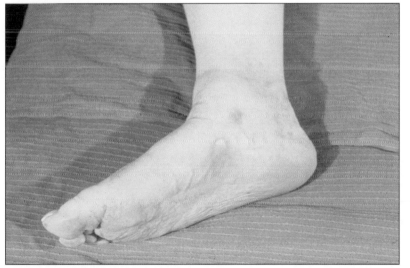

FIGURE 15-19. Radiograph of the foot shown in Figure 15-17. Note the rarefaction and osteopenia of the calcaneus with collapse of the midfoot and loss of architecture of the foot. These results of large fiber neuropathy and increased blood flow could have been prevented if recognized early.

Autonomic Neuropathy

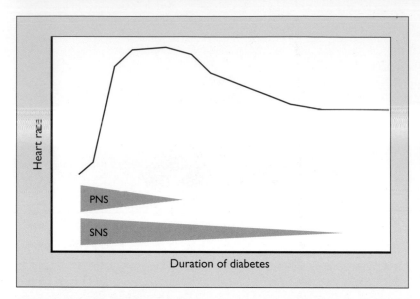

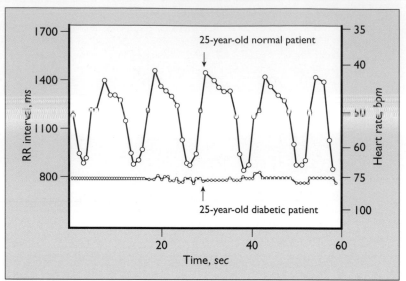

FIGURE 15-20. Model of the effects of autonomic neuropathy on heart rate. The rule in diabetic neuropathy is that the longest fibers are affected early and more severely. In the autonomic nervous system, the longest fibers are those in the vagus (parasympathetic nervous system [PNS]) nerves. Thus, the earliest observations in people with autonomic neuropathy of the cardiovascular system is an increase in heart rate.

Later, as the short efferent fibers of the sympathetic nervous system (SNS) become involved, the heart rate slows down but not to normal. It is indeed a denervated heart. With loss of the afferent fibers there also is loss of pain perception, accounting for the high incidence of painless myocardial infarctions in patients with diabetic neuropathy [16]. (*Adapted from* Ewing *et al.* [17].)

FIGURE 15-21. Respiratory rate (RR) intervals and effects of cardiac autonomic dysfunction. The most sensitive indicator of cardiac autonomic neuropathy is the loss of the normal sinus arrhythmia with breathing. This loss can be measured on an electrocardiogram as loss of the change in the RR interval with deep breathing at six breaths per minute and reflects almost entirely damage to the parasympathetic nervous system. With more sophisticated approaches, computerized spectral analysis of the electrocardiogram tracing allows one to infer the status of the sympathetic nervous system as well. Late in the course of cardiac autonomic neuropathy the advent of *orthostasis* (a decrease in blood pressure of > 30 mm Hg when arising from a lying position) reflects sympathetic nerve damage. Peripheral measures of autonomic function are described in Figures 15-8 to 15-9 on blood flow in the diabetic foot.

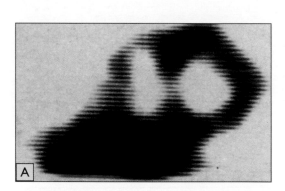

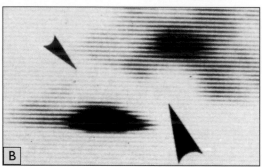

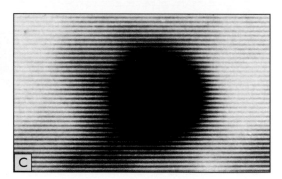

FIGURE 15-22. Segmental loss of sympathetic nerve fibers in the heart, demonstrable using multiple gated acquisition (MUGA) (**A**), meta-iodobenzyl-guanidine (**B**), and thallium scans (**C**), does not demonstrate ventricular wall defects. It is now thought that this imbalance in the sympathetic nerve supply of the myocardium is what leads to the irritable foci, leading to arrhythmia and possibly accounting for sudden death in diabetic patients with autonomic neuropathy. This mechanism also is thought to operate in people who have had a myocardial infarction and may be the reason for the effectiveness of β-blockade in reducing mortality in patients who have had a myocardial infarction. (*From* Kahn *et al.* [18]; with permission.)

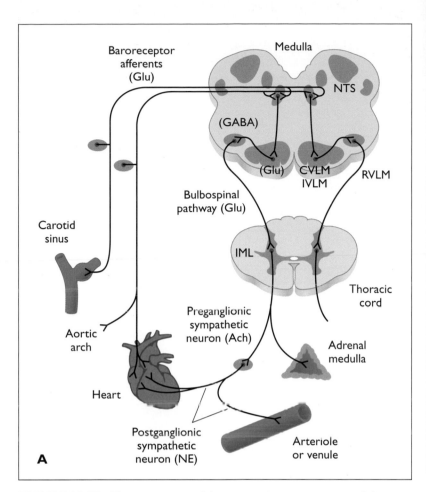

A

<table>
<tr><th colspan="2">B. ORGANIZATION OF THE AUTONOMIC
NERVOUS SYSTEM OF THE HEART</th></tr>
</table>

Eye
  Abnormal pupillary reaction, with night blindness
Cardiovascular
  Sudden death, silent myocardial infarction
  Orthostasis
  Impaired peripheral vascular reflexes
Respiratory
  Failure of hypoxia-induced respiration
Gut
  Gustatory sweating
  Gastroparesis
  Diarrhea
  Constipation
  Loss of anal sphincter tone and incontinence
Metabolic
  Hypoglycemia unawareness
  Hypoglycemia unresponsiveness
  Hypoglycemia-associated autonomic failure
Genitourinary
  Overflow incontinence
Sexual
  Males, erectile dysfunction
  Females, decreased vaginal lubrication

FIGURE 15-23. The organization of the autonomic nervous system of the heart (**A**). Note that diabetes affects the afferent and efferent components of the sympathetic and parasympathetic nervous systems and has diffuse effects throughout the body (**B**). CVLM and IVLM—paraventricular nuclei of vasomotor center; GABA—γ-aminobutyric acid; IML—intermediolateral nucleus; NTS—solitary tract nucleus; RVLM—motor nucleus of vagus.

Gastropathy

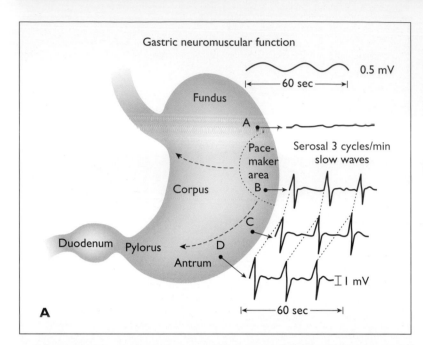

Gastric neuromuscular function

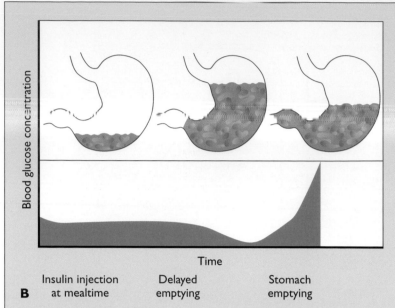

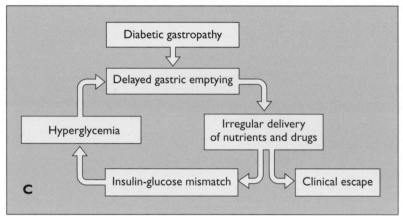

FIGURE 15-24. Gastropathy. **A** and **B,** Gastric neuromuscular function. The stomach is a complex neuromuscular organ. It has a pacemaker that discharges rhythmic electrical impulses that initiate propulsive contractions. It is sensitive to volume, viscosity, osmolarity, caloric density, and the nature of the fuel within. Functional disturbances may occur such as arrhythmias, tachygastria and bradygastria, pylorospasm, and hypomotility. Organic lesions include gastroparesis, antral dilation and obstruction, inflammation, ulceration, and bezoar formation. Gastric dysfunction should be suspected in patients with type I and type II diabetes; who have had diabetes for over 20 years; who display evidence of distal symmetric polyneuropathy and autonomic neuropathy; observations of brittle diabetes in patients with previously well-controlled symptoms; and symptoms of early satiety, bloating, and a succussion splash. Anorexia, nausea, vomiting, and dyspepsia are nonspecific and herald other conditions.

C, Clinical presentation of gastropathy. Many more patients with gastropathy present with brittle diabetes than do those who present with gastric symptoms. In fact, it has been shown that many of the gastrointestinal symptoms of gastropathy can be nonspecific and do not reflect an abnormality in gastric emptying. The most fertile soil for discovery of those with gastric dysfunction are patients with "difficult to control diabetes." The stomach can be regarded as the coarse regulator of blood glucose concentrations, releasing fuel to the small bowel at its own predetermined rate. Any dysfunction in the bowel therefore would result in a mismatch of fuel delivery and either endogenous or exogenous insulin, thereby creating the apparent pattern of insulin resistance or brittle diabetes. Of interest is that the irregular pattern of delivery applies to drugs used in the treatment of diabetes and may confound the problem. Similar concern applies to other drugs that may fail to reach their absorptive site in the small bowel leading to clinical escape from the condition being treated. Overzealous adjustment of the insulin dose may result because the real cause may be easily overlooked.

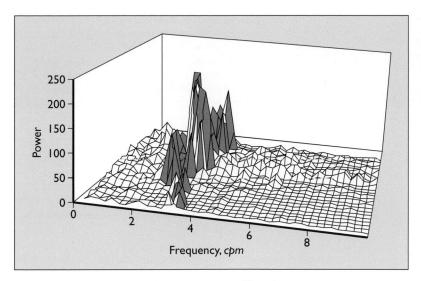

FIGURE 15-25. Normal electrogastrogram. This electrogastrogram was obtained in a normal patient. Note the predominant frequency of 3 to 6 cpm.

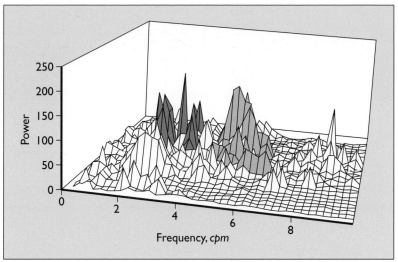

FIGURE 15-26. Electrogastrogram showing hyperglycemia-induced tachygastria. Note two peaks of activity, one at the usual frequency of 3 to 6 cpm and the major peak at over 6 cpm. Thus, hyperglycemia *per se* can markedly affect gastric function; many have made the costly error of carrying out gastric-emptying studies when the blood glucose is over 400 mg/dL. Not only does this induce tachygastria, but it may inhibit the interdigestive myoelectric complex and thus give the erroneous impression of gastroparesis. Gastric pacemaking is being added to the therapeutic armamentarium for severe gastroparesis. New drugs with prokinetic properties and Zelnorm (Novartis, East Hanover, NJ) may be appropriate for functional abnormalities [19].

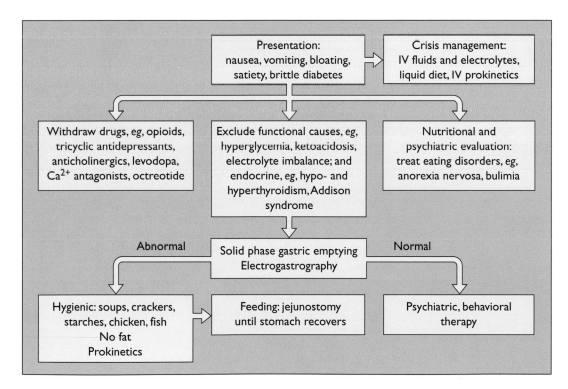

FIGURE 15-27. Algorithm for the management of gastropathy in patients with diabetes. Prokinetic agents include metoclopramide, erythromycin, and tegaserod [19]. IV—intravenous.

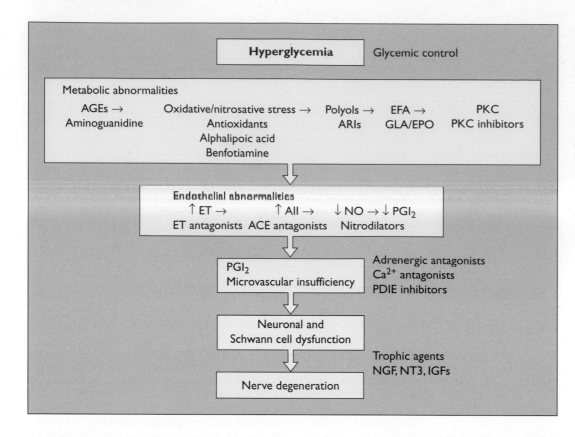

FIGURE 15-28. Specific interventions in diabetic neuropathy designed to target the major defect. Many of these interventions already have been tested in animal models and currently are in phase 2 and 3 clinical trials in the United States and elsewhere. Some of these interventions are further along and may well be in clinical trials shortly. ACE—angiotensin-converting enzyme; AGEs—advanced glycation end products; AII—angiotensin II; ARIs—aldose-reductose inhibitors; Ca^{2+}—calcium ion; EFA—essential fatty acid; EPO—evening primrose oil; ET—endothelin; GLA—γ-linolenic acid; IGF—insulin like growth factor; NGF—neuronal growth factor; NO—nitric oxide; NT3—neurotropin 3; PDIE—phosphodiesterase; PGI_2—prostaglandin I_2; PKC—protein kinase C.

References

1. American Diabetes Association, American Academy of Neurology: Consensus statement: report and recommendations of the San Antonio Conference on Diabetic Neuropathy. *Diabetes Care* 1988, 11:592–597.

2. Vinik AI, Mitchell BD, Leichter SB, *et al.*: Epidemiology of the complications of diabetes. In *Diabetes: Clinical Science and Practice,* Edited by Leslie RDG, Robbins DC. Cambridge: Cambridge University Press; 1995:15,221.

3. Kjiturnan M, Welborn T, McCann V, *et al.*: Prevalence of diabetic complications in relation to risk factors. *Diabetes* 1986, 35:1332–1339.

4. Young MJ, Boulton AJ, MacLeod AF, *et al.*: A multicenter study of the prevalence of diabetic neuropathy in the United Kingdom hospital clinic population. *Diabetologia* 1993, 36:150–154.

5. Feldman JN, Hirsch SR, Bever BS, *et al.*: Prevalence of diabetic nephropathy at time of treatment for diabetic retinopathy. In *Diabetic Renal-Retinal Syndrome.* Edited by Friedman L'Esperance FA. London: Grune & Stratton; 1982:9.

6. Dyck PJ, Kratz KM, Karnes MS, *et al.*: The prevalence by staged severity of various types of diabetic neuropathy, retinopathy, and nephropathy in a population based cohort: The Rochester Diabetic Neuropathy Study. *Neurology* 1993, 43:817–824.

7. Vinik AI, Holland MT, LeBeau JM, *et al.*: Diabetic neuropathies. *Diabetes Care* 1992, 15:1926–1975.

8. Hanson PH, Schumaker P, Debugne T, Clerin M: Evaluation of somatic and autonomic small fibers neuropathy in diabetes. *Am J Phys Med Rehabil* 1992, 71:44–47.

9. Dyck PJ: Small-fiber neuropathy determination. *Muscle Nerve* 1988, 11:998–999.

10. Jarnal GA, Hansen S, Weir AI, Ballantyne JP: The neurophysiologic investigation of small fiber neuropathies. *Muscle Nerve* 1987, 10:537–545.

11. Shapiro SA, Stansberry KB, Hill MA, *et al.*: Normal blood flow response and vasomotion in the diabetic Charcot foot. *J Diabetes Complications* 1998, 12:147–153.

12. Burnstock G, Ralevic V: New insights into the local regulation of blood flow by perivascular nerves and endothelium. *Br J Plastic Surg* 1994, 47:527–543.

13. Vinik AI, Erbas T, Park T, *et al.*: Methods for evaluation of peripheral neurovascular dysfunction. *Diabetes Technol Ther* 2001, 3:29–50.

14. Vinik AI, Erbas T, Park T, *et al.*: Dermal neurovascular dysfunction in type 2 diabetes. *Diabetes Care* 2001, 24:1468–1475.

15. Pittenger G, Ray M, Burcus N, *et al.*: Intraepidermal nerve fibers are indicators of small fiber neuropathy in both diabetic and non-diabetic patients. *Diabetes Care* 2004, 27:1974–1979.

16. Vinik AI, Maser R, Mitchell B, Freeman R: Autonomic neuropathy. *Diabetes Care* 2003, 26:1553–1579.

17. Ewing J, Campbell IW, Clarke BF, *et al.*: Heart rate changes in diabetes mellitus. *Lancet* 1981, 1:183–186.

18. Kahn J, Ida B, Vinik A: Stress and cardiovascular function in diabetes. *Diabetes Care* 1985, 12:3–5.

19. Vinik AI, Mehrabyan A, Johnson D: Gastrointestinal disturbances. In *Therapy for Diabetes Mellitus and Related Disorders*, edn 4. Alexandria: American Diabetes Association; 2004:424–439.

OBESITY
Eleftheria Maratos-Flier

16

Obesity, generally defined as weight exceeding 20% of ideal body weight or a body mass index (BMI) greater than 30, is a complex problem. In the United States, the prevalence of clinically significant obesity is more than 25%. Obesity is associated with excess mortality because of the elevated risk for such diseases as diabetes, hypertension, lipid disorders, and coronary artery disease and increased rates of endometrial and colon carcinoma. Despite the magnitude of the problem, the cause of obesity is poorly understood, and effective weight loss is difficult to achieve.

Recent work in mouse models has increased our understanding of the molecular mechanisms that may lead to obesity. The identification of leptin has provided insight into peripheral signals important in mediating eating behavior. Leptin, the product of the obesity gene, is predominantly expressed in white fat tissue and signals information about peripheral energy stores to the central nervous system. In ob/ob mice, a premature stop codon prevents transcription of the mature leptin peptide and leads to a severe obesity syndrome. Leptin interacts with two leptin receptor variants, the long and short forms. Severe obesity is seen in db/db mice, which do not make the long form of the leptin receptor, are leptin resistant, and have high circulating leptin levels. In ob/ob animals, exogenous leptin leads to weight reduction; restoration of fertility; and correction of abnormal physiologic measures, including hyperglycemia, hyperinsulinemia, and hypercortisolemia. Leptin administration also reduces hypothalamic neuropeptide Y messenger RNA.

Attention has recently focused on a number of neuropeptides known to affect feeding behavior in mice. For example, ablation of the melanocortin-4 (MC4-R) receptor leads to rodent obesity and has brought to the fore the importance of the melanocortin pathway. Similarly, ablation of melanin-concentrating hormone (MCH) leads to a model of rodent leanness, indicating that MCH is a significant contributor to feeding.

The findings of single gene defects in rodents focused attention on certain peptides and receptors and led to a search for single gene defects in humans. Thus far, humans with obesity secondary to leptin deficiency, leptin-receptor deficiency, preproopiomelanocortin abnormalities, MC4-R abnormalities, prohormone convertase-1 abnormalities, and abnormalities of peroxisome proliferator-activated receptor-κ have been identified.

The neuropeptides that regulate body weight and eating probably interact at several levels in the central nervous system; however, the anatomic and functional basis for this interaction has not been defined. In addition, the molecular basis by which signals from the lateral hypothalamus might be integrated into systems involved in weight regulation has only recently been explored.

Understanding the molecular mechanisms of obesity in the general population will improve as our understanding of the regulators of eating behavior improves. Most human obesity is likely caused by dysregulation of several factors. Although current treatments are limited, the potential for new specific treatments based on the identification of specific molecular targets has increased.

Prevalence of Obesity

PREVALENCE OF OBESITY IN THE US POPULATION

Preobesity: BMI 25.0–25.9
  Constant rate over past 3–4 decades; prevalence has remained
  constant at 32%
Obesity: BMI > 30
  Prevalence is increasing
  ~ 13% in 1960
  ~ 23% in 1994
More than half the adult US population has a BMI that exceeds the
  healthy range

FIGURE 16-1. Prevalence of obesity. In the United States, the prevalence of obesity has increased over the past 4 decades. In some populations, such as non-Hispanic white men 50 to 59 years of age, the prevalence of overweight and obesity (body mass index [BMI] > 25) is 72.9%. The prevalence in non-Hispanic black women of the same age is 78.1% [1].

Obesity and the Risk for Other Diseases

DISEASES FOR WHICH OBESITY IS A RISK FACTOR

Diabetes
Cardiovascular disease
Hypertension
Sleep apnea
Endometrial cancer
Breast cancer
Colon cancer
Gallbladder disease

FIGURE 16-2. Obesity increases the risk for many diseases [2].

EXAMPLES OF INCREASED RISK RELATED TO OBESITY

Relative risk in persons 20–44 years of age:
Diabetes, 3.8
Hypertension, 5.6
Hypercholesterolemia, 2.1

FIGURE 16-3. Obesity is associated with a substantially increased risk for diabetes and cardiovascular disease, even in young persons.

OBESITY AND TYPE 2 DIABETES

80% to 90% of patients with type 2 diabetes are obese
Weight loss (as little as 10–20 pounds) can be adequate treatment
Most people (> 90%) cannot lose weight successfully.
Patients with type 2 diabetes are at risk for usual complications, including
cardiovascular disease, retinopathy, neuropathy, and nephropathy

FIGURE 16-4. Obesity and type 2 diabetes. Type 2 diabetes typically occurs in obese persons and has a significant component of insulin resistance. Even modest weight loss can lead to normalization of glucose control or to improved control with any given dose of oral medication. However, successful weight loss is unusual.

REGIONAL FAT DEPOSITS

Visceral	Subcutaneous
Mesenteric	Superficial
Omental	Deep
Retroperitoneal	
Perirena	

FIGURE 16-5. Regional fat deposits. Visceral fat deposits include mesenteric, omental, retroperitoneal, and perirenal deposits. According to location, fat deposits have different metabolic characteristics and thus pose different levels of risk for the complications of obesity. Central fat can be assessed by computed tomography, but a fairly good estimate can also be obtained by determining the waist-to-hip ratio. The abdominal circumference halfway between the lower rib and the iliac crest is compared with the circumference at the level of the greater trochanter [3]. Consideration of the waist-to-hip ratio augments evaluation of the risks of obesity. Data from a study by Goodpaster *et al.* [4] indicate that in men, for any given body mass index, increased waist-to-hip ratio confers additional risk. This increase is also seen in women. (*See* Fig. 16-38 for relative risk.) Recent data from mouse models suggest that the enzyme 11-β hydroxysteroid dehydrogenase may contribute to visceral obesity. This enzyme, which is expressed in fat, activates glucocorticoids. Mice overexpressing this enzyme in adipose tissue develop a syndrome of central obesity that mimics the metabolic syndrome [5].

Role of Molecular Mechanisms

REQUIREMENT FOR STABLE WEIGHT

Calories In	Calories Out
Can only equal what one eats	Basal metabolic rate
	Thermogenesis
	Activity

FIGURE 16-6. Requirements for stable weight. Stable weight requires a match between calories consumed and calories expended. Fat-free mass is a major determinant of resting energy expenditure [6]. Weight gain leads to an increase in both fat and fat-free mass; thus, the basal metabolic rate of obese persons is higher than that of lean persons of the same height [7]. Obesity results from chronic excess of calories ingested over calories expended. Calories expended include the resting metabolic rate, the thermic effects of food and exercise, and adaptive thermogenesis. Body fat is not significantly influenced by resting energy expenditure or the thermic effect of food [8], but changes in energy expenditure resulting from physical activity influence weight and body composition [9].

VIEWS OF ENERGY HOMEOSTASIS

Very old view
  Obesity is the result of excess calories and inactivity; voluntary overeating and laziness indicate moral fault
Old view
  Obesity is the result of excess calories, but some lucky people can eat more because they have a "faster metabolism"
New view
  Obesity is the result of interactions between factors that regulate appetite and total energy expenditure

FIGURE 16-7. Energy homeostasis. For many years, obesity was considered to be the consequence of a moral fault. Eating was considered a process entirely under voluntary control, and decreased energy expenditure was ascribed to inactivity. Over time, various studies revealed that thermogenesis varied among people and that when placed on diets consisting of equal calories, people might gain, maintain, or even lose weight. The discovery of leptin in 1994 revolutionized the understanding of the pathophysiologic basis of obesity. It is now clear that multiple factors regulate appetite and total energy expenditure. The demonstration that single gene defects can lead to obesity has also proven that excessive eating is a process that is not always amenable to conscious control.

HYPOTHALAMIC ORGANIZATION

Lateral hypothalamus—eating center (1951)

  Stimulates eating behavior

  Triggers feeding

  Ablative lesions cause aphagia, adipsia, and weight loss

Medial hypothalamus—satiety center (1940)

  Inhibits eating behavior

  Electrical stimulation of ventromedial hypothalamus inhibits eating

  Ablative lesions (surgical and goldthioglucose) cause hyperphagia
  and obesity

FIGURE 16-8. Hypothalamic organization. The role of the hypothalamus in the regulation of eating behavior was initially defined decades ago in studies of electrical stimulation and anatomical lesions. The role of the lateral hypothalamus in mediating eating was first considered in 1951 [10]. In 1940, experimental hypothalamic lesions of the ventromedial hypothalamus were reported to produce obesity [11].

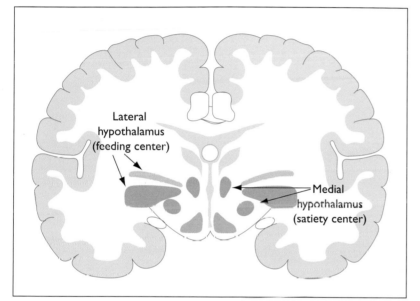

FIGURE 16-9. Hypothalamic areas implicated in eating behavior. The lateral hypothalamus is on the left (the *lighter* area indicates the zona incerta). Melanin-concentrating hormone [12] and orexin [13] localize to this area and stimulate feeding. The medial hypothalamus (ventral medial and dorsal medial) is on the right. and the paraventricular nucleus is *green*. The arcuate nucleus, in which cell bodies making neuropeptide Y, preproopiomelanocortin (the precursor to melanocyte-stimulating hormone [MSH]), agouti-related peptide (AgRP), and cocaine- and amphetamine-regulated transcript (CART) are localized, is *light green*. Neuropeptide Y and AgRP stimulate eating, and MSH and CART inhibit eating. Monoamines also play a role in appetite regulation. In experimental animals, administration of norepinephrine leads to an acute increase in food intake, and chronic administration leads to weight gain. This effect appears to be dependent on the receptor stimulated because whereas a2 agonists increase food intake, a1 and b2 agonists lead to decreased food intake [14–16]. Dopamine plays an important role in regulating food intake; however, effects are dependent on where it is released. Administration of dopamine in the lateral hypothalamus leads to decreased meal size [17], and release in the nucleus accumbens increases food intake [18]. Serotonin also affects food intake; however, the effects are complex and vary depending on the anatomic area of the brain targeted and the receptor activated.

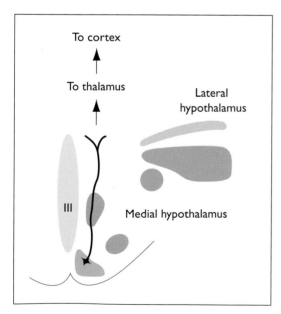

FIGURE 16-10. Neuropeptide Y. Neuropeptide Y (NPY) is made in neurons in the arcuate nucleus. The role of NPY in eating is attributed to direct projections of NPY to the paraventricular nucleus [19]. Repetitive injection of NPY into the hypothalamus induces hyperphagia and obesity [20]. NPY also alters energy metabolism. After repetitive injections of NPY, brown fat thermogenic activity is decreased and white fat lipoprotein lipase activity is decreased [21]. This finding suggests that the neuropeptides that regulate appetite may have multiple roles. One action of leptin is the suppression of NPY synthesis in the arcuate nucleus. This peptide appears to function as an important central regulator in eating behavior. Injection of NPY into rat lateral ventricles leads to a marked increase in eating; NPY-treated animals eat six- to 10-fold more than control animals over the ensuing 24-hour period. Repetitive injections over several days cause weight gain. NPY also suppresses energy expenditure through actions on the sympathetic nervous system. Although NPY is diffusely expressed, it is the NPY-synthesizing neurons in the arcuate nucleus that project to paraventricular nucleus, and the dorsal medial hypothalamus that is responsible for mediating eating behavior. In ob/ob mice, messenger RNA (mRNA) levels in the arcuate nucleus are two- to threefold higher than mRNA levels in control mice; peptide levels are also increased in ob/ob mice. Similar results are seen in the Zucker fatty rat.

Both central intracerebroventricular and peripheral leptin treatment of ob/ob animals reduced NPY messages in the arcuate nucleus, suggesting that NPY is a leptin target. In normal animals, peripheral administration of leptin significantly inhibits the increase in the arcuate NPY mRNA levels seen with starvation. Although NPY may normally mediate eating behavior, NPY knockout mice lacking NPY in all tissues have no demonstrable changes in eating behavior. Crossbreeding of the NPY knockout mice with ob/ob mice revealed that the double-knockout offspring mice had an attenuated obesity phenotype. These data indicate that NPY is an important but not exclusive regulator of eating behavior and energy expenditure.

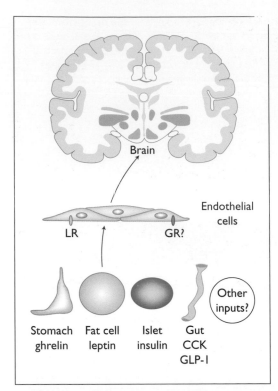

FIGURE 16-11. A number of peripheral factors that contribute to appetite may act on the brain [22]. Ghrelin, which is synthesized in the stomach, has been found to play a role in meal initiation, possibly through actions on target neurons in the hypothalamus [23,24]. Peptide YY is synthesized in the gut and has an orexigenic effect through action in the brain [25]. Anorectic agents may also be produced by the gut. Glucagon-like peptide 1 (GLP-1) is synthesized in the gut and acts to suppress appetite in animals and humans [26]. Cholecystokinin (CCK), which is made in enteroendocrine cells, also acts to inhibit appetite [27]. Finally, insulin, which is made in the pancreas in response to meals, may also act on the brain to regulate food intake and energy expenditure [28]. GR—ghrelin receptor; LR—leptin receptor.

Role of Monogenic Mechanisms

MONOGENIC CAUSES OF RODENT OBESITY

Spontaneous
   Leptin deficiency (ob/ob)
   Absence of long form of leptin receptor (db/db)
   Ectopic agouti expression (Ay mouse)
   Fat (fa/fa)
   Tub
Engineered
   Serotonin 2C-receptor knockout
   Melanocortin-4 receptor knockout
   AgRP overexpression
   NPY 1 and NPY 5 receptor knockouts
   CRH overexpression
   B-3 receptor knockout
   Bombesin B-3 receptor knockout
   Glut-4 overexpression in fat

FIGURE 16-12. Monogenic causes of rodent obesity. The identification of spontaneously occurring monogenic causes of obesity provide significant clues to understanding regulation of body weight. Identification of the fat hormone leptin [29] provided a mechanism by which fat can signal the status of peripheral energy stores to the brain [30]. Leptin is also important in regulating physiologic responses to fasting [31]. Analysis of other models of obesity, such as Ay mice, provided significant insight into pathways that are important in regulating body weight. Engineered models have been important in confirming the importance of the pathways and in identifying the roles of different peptides. AgRP—agouti-related peptide; CRH—corticotrophin-releasing hormone; NPY—neuropeptide Y.

MONOGENIC CAUSES OF HUMAN OBESITY

Leptin deficiency	Mutations
Leptin-receptor deficiency	PC-1 mutations
POMC gene mutations	PPARγ2 mutations
Melanocortin-4 receptor mutations	

FIGURE 16-13. Monogenic causes of human obesity. Key peptides identified in mice led to the pursuit of patients with similar defects. These studies were done in patients with morbid obesity of very early onset. In many cases (eg, leptin deficiency, leptin-receptor deficiency, melanocortin-receptor abnormalities, and PC-1 mutations), the human phenotype is similar to the rodent phenotype. Some mutations, however, such as POMC gene mutations and PPARγ2 mutations, have been described only in humans.

MONOGENIC CAUSES OF RODENT LEANNESS

Uncoupling protein overexpression in white fat and brown fat tissue
Glut-4 gene ablation
Dopamine D_1 receptor knockout
Melanin-concentrating hormone knockout
Protein kinase A knockout
Hepatic leptin overexpression
Mahogany mutation

FIGURE 16-14. Monogenic causes of rodent leanness. Most monogenic causes of rodent leanness have been specifically engineered lesions. The mechanism by which some of these manipulations cause leanness is understood, as in hepatic leptin over-expression and melanin-concentrating hormone deficiency [32]. In other cases, however, such as protein kinase A knockout, the mechanism of leanness is not understood. Of note, ablation of the neuropeptide Y (NPY) gene in rodents did not cause leanness or any change in the eating phenotype [33]. However, absence of NPY led to an attenuation of the obesity seen in Lepob/Lepob mice [34]. Monogenic causes of human leanness have not been identified because the pursuit of such mutations would be complicated. Setting criteria for screening appropriate families would be difficult because weights, although reduced, might still be in the normal range.

PEPTIDES THAT REGULATE EATING

Increase Feeding	Decrease Feeding
Neuropeptide Y	Leptin
Melanin-concentrating hormone	α-Melanocyte-stimulating hormone
Agouti-related peptide	Glucagon-like peptide-1
Galanin	Neurotensin
Orexin A and B (?)	Corticotrophin-releasing hormone
Dynorphin	Urocortin
β-Endorphin	CART
	Bombesin
	Cholecystokinin
	Enterostatin

FIGURE 16-15. Partial listing of peptides that regulate eating. Several peptides are known to stimulate eating, and more are known to suppress eating. In addition, eating is regulated by monoamines (not discussed here). CART—cocaine- and amphetamine-regulated transcript.

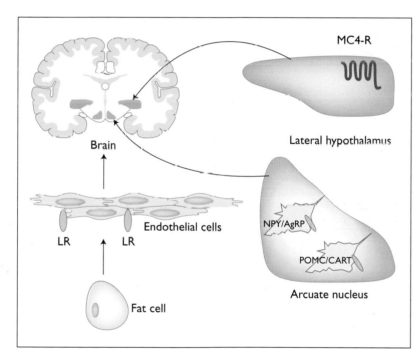

FIGURE 16-16. Sites of single gene lesions that lead to human obesity. The relationship among peptides involved in the regulation of eating is complex. This figure summarizes some of the known interactions. Leptin is synthesized by adipocytes and released into the circulation. Leptin transport across the blood–brain barrier is mediated by the short form of the leptin receptor (LR). In the brain, leptin targets long-form receptors [35] in both the arcuate and the dorsal medial hypothalamus (not shown). In the arcuate hypothalamus, leptin regulates cell bodies that coexpress agouti-related peptide (AgRP) and neuropeptide Y (NPY) (peptides that stimulate eating) and cells that coexpress preproopiomelanocortin (POMC, the melanocyte-stimulating hormone precursor) and cocaine- and amphetamine-regulated transcript (CART) (peptides that inhibit eating). Cells from the arcuate project to several areas, including the lateral hypothalamus [36], where the melanocortin-4 receptor (MC4-R) [37], which responds to POMC and AgRP, is expressed. This receptor may be present on neurons expressing orexin or melanin-concentrating hormone, although this localization has not yet been confirmed.

FEATURES OF CONGENITAL LEPTIN DEFICIENCY

Homozygous frameshift mutation of leptin gene to synthesis of an unsecreted truncated lyk species
Normal birthweight, early severe obesity
  Patient 1: 82 kg, age 8 y
  Patient 2: 30 kg, age 2 y
HPA axis normal, normal glycemic control, slightly elevated TSH level
Parents of both patients are heterozygotes

FIGURE 16-17. Leptin deficiency causes of the syndrome of obesity seen in ob/ob mice. These mice develop early obesity associated with hyperphagia and insulin resistance. Leptin deficiency has been described in two related children. Both had normal birth weights but were markedly obese during infancy. The hypothalamus-pituitary-adrenal (HPA) axis was normal in these children, although the thyroid-stimulating hormone (TSH) level was slightly elevated. In both children, glycemic control was normal; this finding differs from the severe insulin resistance seen in mice. Both sets of parents were of normal weight. Analysis of the leptin gene revealed that parents were heterozygotes and that the children were homozygous for a frameshift mutation that led to synthesis of a truncated, unsecreted species [38].

CLINICAL FEATURES OF HUMAN LEPTIN RECEPTOR MUTATION*

Age, y	Gender	Weight, kg	BMI	Genotype	Leptin level, mg/mL
12	Male	37	16	wt/wt	5.6
13	Female	159	71.5	m/m	670
16	Male	87	30	wt/m	212
17	Female	102	34	wt/wt	88
19	Female	166	65.5	m/m	600
19	Female	133	52.5	?	526
22	Female	76	27.5	m/wt	240
24	Female	67.8	26.5	m/wt	294

*Additional features: growth delay; no overnight burst of growth hormone; poor response of growth hormone to stimulation tests; low IgF levels; low TSH; sustained TSH response to thyroid-releasing hormone; hypothalamus-pituitary-adrenal axis grossly normal.

FIGURE 16-18. Human leptin receptor mutation. Leptin-receptor deficiency has been described in a large family [39]. The proband presented with significant obesity and hypogonadotrophic hypogonadism. Affected homozygotes have 100-fold increased leptin levels (body mass index [BMI]) in excess of fat content. Affected heterozygotes had BMIs in the preobese or minimally obese range and leptin levels of approximately 200 mg/mL. TSH—thyroid-stimulating hormone.

THE STRANGE LINK BETWEEN EATING AND PIGMENTATION

Agouti

Melanocortin-4 receptor

Melanocyte-stimulating hormone

Agouti-related peptide

Melanin-concentrating hormone

FIGURE 16-19. Peptides involved in regulating eating behavior and pigmentation. The intriguing connection between pigmentation and eating was first suggested by the finding that spontaneously mutant yellow mice (Ay), known as agouti mice, were also markedly obese. Agouti (normally expressed in the skin) acts on melanocytes as a paracrine factor to inhibit the conversion of phycomelanin (yellow) to eumelanin (black). Most mice are brown because of variable mixtures of these two pigments. Ay mice express agouti in all tissues and in an unregulated form. These findings suggested that melanocortin receptors have a role in mediating eating behavior. Agouti protein is expressed in the skin and regulates skin coloration, acting through the melanocortin 1 receptor, where it inhibits the action of melanocyte-stimulating hormone (MSH); when expressed ubiquitously, it leads to yellow pigmentation (inhibiting melanocortin-1 receptor) and obesity by inhibiting centrally expressed melanocortin-4 receptors. These receptors are expressed in the central nervous system; when activated by MSH, they mediate inhibition of eating behavior [40]. Melanin-concentrating hormone regulates skin pigmentation in fish, where it is made in the pituitary and released into the circulation and acts on melanophores (cells containing pigment granules) to cause granule aggregation and skin darkening. It has no known role in pigmentation in mammals, but in mammals, it is made in the lateral hypothalamus and stimulates eating behavior through a still-unidentified receptor. A potential endogenous antagonist ligand for the hypothalamic melanocortin receptors is agouti-related protein (AgRP), a recently cloned homologue of agouti. This protein is expressed in the arcuate nucleus of the hypothalamus, and its messenger RNA is upregulated in ob/ob and db/db mice. AgRP appears to inhibit the melanocortin receptor in a manner similar to that of agouti.

THE AY MOUSE

Homozygous lethal

Heterozygote is obese, macrosomic, insulin-resistant

Heterozygote has mustard yellow color

Syndrome results from ectopic expression of agouti in all organs

Why is the mouse yellow?

Why is the mouse obese?

FIGURE 16-20. Ay mice, in which normal agouti protein is expressed ectopically, are yellow and obese [41].

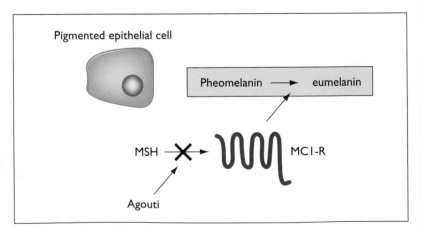

FIGURE 16-21. Agouti protein. Agouti protein is normally expressed in hair follicles in the skin and regulates pigmentation of skin and fur. Agouti protein expressed peripherally inhibits the melanocortin-1 receptor (MC1-R) and prevents the melanocyte-stimulating hormone (MSH)–mediated conversion of yellow pigment to black pigment [42]. If MSH is made in the pituitary, it regulates pigmentation; if it is made in the hypothalamus, it regulates feeding.

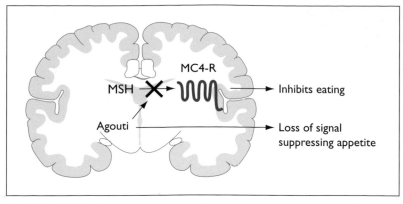

FIGURE 16-22. Agouti protein. Agouti (Ay) protein expressed centrally acts on the melanocortin-4 receptor (MC4-R) [43] and inhibits melanocyte-stimulating hormone (MSH)—mediated inhibition of eating. The obesity syndrome could be mimicked by genetically engineering a mouse that lacked MC4-R [44]; this capability demonstrates the importance of this receptor. In Ay mice, agouti is expressed in the brain. Agouti blocks MC4-R, one of two brain melanocortin receptors. The MC4-R cannot respond to α-MSH. The inhibitory effects of α-MSH on feeding are lost; thus, Ay mice are obese.

EXPRESSION OF AGOUTI AND AGRP

Agouti is not expressed in brain of normal animals

A related peptide, AgRP, is expressed in the brain

AgRP is found exclusively in arcuate neurons, which are leptin-responsive and co-express neuropeptide Y

FIGURE 16-23. Expression of agouti and agouti-related peptide (AgRP). Because agouti is not normally expressed in the central nervous system (CNS), the finding of the agouti effect on centrally expressed melanocortin receptors led to a search for agouti-like peptides in the CNS. AgRP [45,46] is expressed in the arcuate nucleus and is one of the CNS peptides regulating the melanocortin-4 receptor (MC4-R). In addition, attention has focused on α-melanocyte–stimulating hormone (MSH), a product of preproopiomelanocortin in the arcuate, and on the role of α-MSH in the regulation of eating by acting as an agonist on MC4-R.

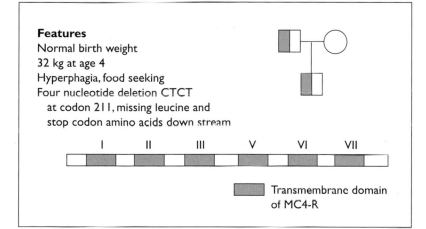

FIGURE 16-24. Mutations in melanocortin-4 receptor (MC4-R). A cohort of severely obese children was screened for mutations in MC4-R by using direct nucleotide sequencing [47]. One patient was heterozygous for a four-base pair deletion at codon 211 of the MC4-R. This mutation resulted in a stop codon in the region encoding for the fifth transmembrane domain. Residues at the fifth and sixth transmembrane domain are important for MC4-R signaling, so this mutation results in a nonfunctional receptor. The proband's mother is normal weight, but the father is obese (body mass index, 41). The same mutation was identified in the father.

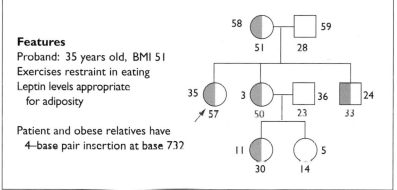

FIGURE 16-25. Melanocortin-4 receptor (MC4-R) frameshift mutations and dominantly inherited human obesity. A French population was screened by selecting persons with a history of obesity in infancy and highest lifetime body mass index (BMI) at any given age [48]. The entire single exon of MC4-R was evaluated by using five primer pairs. Direct sequencing identified a proband in which a heterozygous frameshift mutation resulted in a nonfunctional truncated receptor. The proband's family was screened, and additional relatives with the mutation were identified. All of these relatives had similar levels of adiposity. Individuals' ages are indicated to the side of the symbols, and their BMIs are shown below the symbols.

OBESITY, ADRENAL INSUFFICIENCY, AND RED HAIR PIGMENTATION ASSOCIATED WITH *POMC* MUTATIONS

Patient 1

Obesity of very early onset, red hair, ACTH deficiency; ACTH deficiency led to clinical presentation

Two mutations in exon 3

  Paternal allele

    G T at nt 7013 leads to premature stop codon 79 (complete absence of ACTH, α-MSH,

      β endorphin)

  Maternal allele

    1–base pair deletion nt 7133 leads to a frameshift-disrupting binding motif of ACTH and α-MSH

Patient 2

Obesity of very early onset, red hair, ACTH deficiency; ACTH deficiency led to clinical presentation

Homozygous C A transversion at nt 3804 leads to out-of-frame start codon

Abolishment of translation of wild-type protein

FIGURE 16-26. Preproopiomelanocortin (POMC) mutations. Mutations in the POMC gene lead to a syndrome of adrenal insufficiency, red hair pigmentation, and obesity. POMC is the precursor for many peptides, including adrenocorticotropin hormone (ACTH), melanocyte-stimulating hormone (MSH), and β-endorphin. In patient 1, two different POMC mutations led to interference with appropriate synthesis of ACTH and MSH. The adrenal insufficiency results from the absence of ACTH. Red hair results from the absence of MSH regulation of pigmentation in the hair follicle, which would be mediated by the melanocortin-1 receptor. Obesity results from the absence of centrally acting MSH, which would regulate eating through the melanocortin-4 receptor [41]. A syndrome of obesity, adrenal insufficiency, and red hair pigmentation was seen in another patient described by Krude et al. [49]. This patient was homozygous for a mutation that abolished POMC translation.

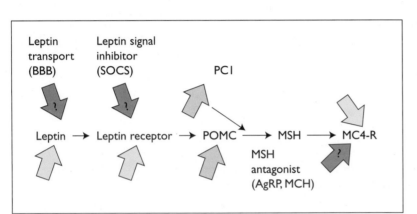

FIGURE 16-27. Summary of mutations in central nervous system pathways that may be associated with obesity in humans. *Pink arrows* point to mutations that have been identified. *Red arrows* with question marks point to sites where mutations may occur but that have not yet been confirmed. AgRP—agouti-releasing peptide; BBB—blood–brain barrier; MC4-R—melanocortin-4 receptor; MCH—melanin-concentrating hormone; MSH—melanocyte-stimulating hormone; PC-1—prohormone convertase-1; POMC—preproopiomelanocortin; SOCS—suppressors of cytokine signaling.

PROHORMONE CONVERTASE 1 GENE AND OBESITY

Extreme childhood obesity

Abnormal glucose homeostasis, hypogonadotropic hypogonadism, hypocortisolism, elevated plasma proinsulin level, low insulin level, elevated POMC level

Compound heterozygote in PC-1

  Gly Arg 483 prevents processing of prepro PC-1 and retention in endoplasmic reticulum

  A C + 4 intron 5-splice site, skipping of exon 5, loss of 26 residues, frameshift, and premature stop codon

Similarity in genetic abnormality and phenotype to fat/fat mouse

FIGURE 16-28. Prohormone convertase 1 (PC-1) gene and obesity. At least one severely obese patient with a *PC-1* mutation has been described. The patient was a compound heterozygote for the *PC-1* gene [50]. This patient's clinical syndrome was very similar to that seen in fa/fa ratS. POMC—preproopiomelanocortin.

PPAR-γ2

358 unrelated German patients

121 were obese (BMI > 29)

Examined for mutations at or near serine phosphorylation site at amino acid 114. This site negatively regulates transcriptional activity of the protein

Mutation identified: praline glutamine at position 115

  4 of 121 obese patients had this mutation

  0 of 237 nonobese patients had this mutation

Overexpression of the mutant gene in fibroblasts led to synthesis of a phosphorylation defective protein and accelerated differentiation of cells into adipocytes

FIGURE 16-29. Peroxisome proliferator-activated receptor γ2 (PPARγ2). PPARγ2 is an important regulator of adipocyte differentiation. In a large study [51] of German patients, four obese patients with a missense mutation in PPARγ2 were identified. This mutation resulted in the conversion of proline at position 115 to a glutamine. Overexpression of the mutant gene in mouse fibroblasts revealed that the mutant protein is defective in phosphorylating a serine in position 114. Fibroblasts expressing the mutant gene showed accelerated differentiation into adipocytes. BMI—body mass index.

Treatment of Obesity

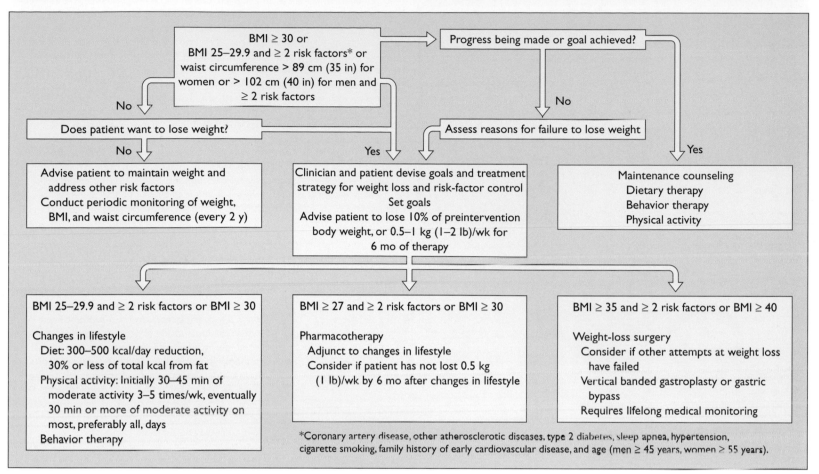

FIGURE 16-30. Evidence-based algorithm for the treatment of obesity. BMI body mass index. (*Adapted from* the National Heart, Lung, and Blood Institute [52].)

NATIONAL INSTITUTES OF HEALTH ASSESSMENT CONFERENCE: METHODS OF VOLUNTARY WEIGHT LOSS AND CONTROL, BETHESDA, MARYLAND, 1992

40% of women and 24% of men attempt weight loss at any time

Most people can lose 10% of initial weight

One third to one half regain weight within 1 year, and most regain weight within 5 years

For many overweight persons, achieving and maintaining a healthy weight is a lifelong challenge

FIGURE 16-31. Voluntary weight control. The treatment of obesity poses major challenges. A large proportion of the U.S. population is trying to lose weight at any given time. Although most persons lose a modest amount of weight, weight loss is not usually maintained.

RATIONALE FOR LONG-TERM USE OF OBESITY MEDICATIONS

Obesity is a chronic disease with morbid consequences

If medications are effective at weight loss, affect morbid consequences, and are safe, they should be used

Precise cut-off point for use of therapy must be determined through clinical trials, as is the case with therapies for other conditions (eg, hypertension, diabetes, hyperlipidemia)

FIGURE 16-32. Long-term use of obesity medications. Obesity is a chronic illness associated with complications. Some chronic illnesses, such as hypertension, may respond to dietary maneuvers (eg, reduction in salt intake). However, patients may be unable to make the necessary changes, or the response may be inadequate. Safe medications that help obese individuals achieve sustained weight loss would substantially affect the morbidity and mortality associated with obesity.

RECENT AND FUTURE APPROACHES TO WEIGHT LOSS

Sibutramine—novel serotonin and norepinephrine reuptake inhibitor

Orlistat—inhibitor of intestinal fat absorption

Old standbys—phentermine, diethylpropion, mazindol

β-3 adrenergic agonists

Leptin or leptin analogues/mimics

Centrally acting agents based on new discoveries

Antagonists of melanin-concentrating hormone, orexin, neuropeptide Y, galanin

Agonists of melanocortin-4 receptor, corticotropin-releasing hormone receptors

Inhibitors of leptin resistance

FIGURE 16-33. Pharmacologic approaches to weight loss. Many potential medications are available for the treatment of obese patients. The odds of successful pharmacologic therapy are increased when drug therapy is combined with a behavior modification program. Commercial programs may be as effective as hospital-based programs. Sibutramine [53] leads to effective weight loss in a subset of motivated patients; its effectiveness appears to be similar to that of phentermine used as a sole agent. The Food and Drug Administration has recently approved orlistat. One-year trials of orlistat with doses of 120 mg three times daily revealed that in the treatment group, weight loss at 1 year was approximately 50% greater than that in the control group (10.3 kg compared with 6.1 kg) [54]. Although the drug was effective in large clinical trials, its effectiveness in patients seen in a standard office practice has not yet been evaluated. Novel therapies, such as β-3 adrenergic agonists, leptin mimetics, and agents based on neuropeptide regulation, are the subject of intense investigation. Another potential class of medications is cannabinoid receptor (CB) antagonists. Rimonabant, an antagonist for the CB1 receptor, is in use in clinical trials, and early reports indicate that it may be effective in producing weight loss. However, assessment of overall effectiveness will require assessment of its effectiveness in the general population [55].

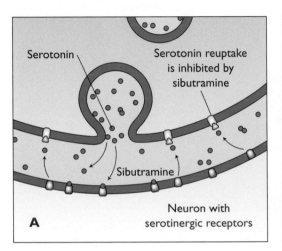

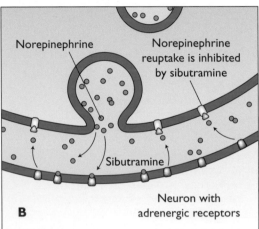

FIGURE 16-34. Mechanisms of action of sibutramine. Sibutramine acts to inhibit reuptake of norepinephrine, serotonin, and dopamine. Treatment is associated with modest degrees of weight loss of about 5% over placebo over a 6-month period. Hypertension is a side effect that may limit the usefulness of sibutramine in obese patients with the metabolic syndrome. In the presynaptic neuron, sibutramine and its active metabolites inhibit the reuptake of serotonin (**A**) and norepinephrine (**B**), thereby prolonging the actions of these neurotransmitters at their postsynaptic receptors. (*Adapted from* Yanovski and Yanovski [56].)

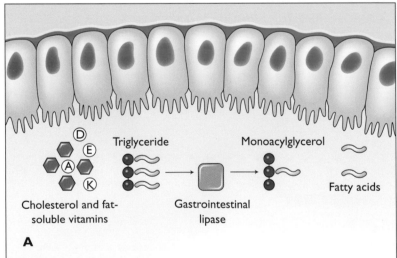

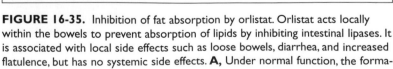

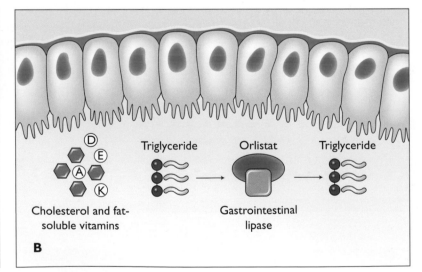

FIGURE 16-35. Inhibition of fat absorption by orlistat. Orlistat acts locally within the bowels to prevent absorption of lipids by inhibiting intestinal lipases. It is associated with local side effects such as loose bowels, diarrhea, and increased flatulence, but has no systemic side effects. **A,** Under normal function, the formation of micelles in the intestinal lumen allows absorption of approximately 90% of dietary triglycerides as monoacylglycerol and fatty acids; cholesterol and fat-soluble vitamins are absorbed with lipids. **B,** With orlistat, approximately one third of dietary triglycerides are excreted unchanged in the stools.

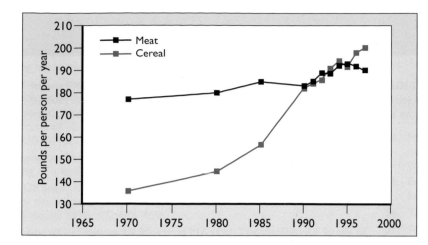

FIGURE 16-36. Paradoxically, the increase in rates of obesity occurred at a time when low-fat diets were recommended as a means for avoiding weight gain based on the concept that high-fat diets were less satiating [57]. Because many high-fat diets are high in saturated fat, they also contribute to heart disease; low-fat diets have been recommended as a way of lowering saturated fat and cholesterol [58]. However, the recommendation for low-fat diets was not strongly associated with a recommendation in portion control. In the past few decades, although per capita fat consumption remained relatively constant, portion size

increased significantly [59]. Although the consumption of high-fat meats has declined, the consumption of salty snacks, candy, and soft drinks has increased, leading to an overall increase of per capita calorie consumption of almost 200 calories per day [60]. Furthermore, the increase in obesity occurred at a time when the percent of calories of energy from fat declined [61].

The inexorable increase in rates of obesity has led to a reevaluation of the wisdom of recommending low-fat diets as well as an interest in alternative diets for both weight loss and prevention of weight gain. Increasingly, it is recognized that dietary fat is not a determinant of body fat, and consumption of diets in which fat contributes between 18% and 40% of the energy has little effect on obesity [62]. Attention has focused on low–glycemic index diets, which may act to enhance satiety and prolong intermeal intervals by reducing both peak postmeal glucose levels, insulin responses to meals, and subsequent increases in counterregulatory hormones [63–68]. The effect of very low-carbohydrate diets on weight loss is also of interest. Although popularized by Atkins and in common lay use for more than 2 decades, these diets have received little evaluation. However several reports examining very low carbohydrate diets have recently appeared and indicate that these diets are modestly more effective at causing weight loss than are low-fat diets, and they have no adverse effects on glucose, insulin, lipids, or blood pressure [69–71]. A recent study [72] in overweight adults showed that patients on low-carbohydrate, calorie-restricted diets are more likely to complete the study than are those on low-fat, calorie-restricted diets, lose more weight, and have greater improvements in serum lipid profiles. Similar results have also been reported in adolescents [73]. Hence, reports indicate that low-carbohydrate, calorie-restricted diets are safe and probably more effective than low-fat diets in the short term.

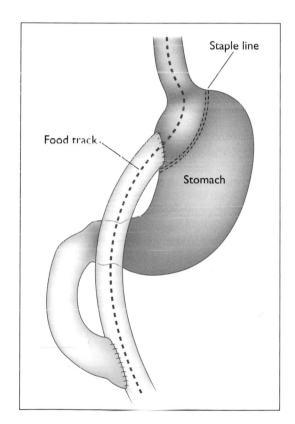

FIGURE 16-37. One of the few effective treatments for morbid obesity is surgical therapy. Although a number of surgical procedures can be performed, the most widely performed surgical procedure is the Roux-en-Y gastric bypass. This achieves permanent (longer than 14 years) and significant weight loss and has a relatively low incidence of side effects. When patients are screened appropriately, 90% of patients lose 50% or more of excess body weight. Successful surgery is associated with marked improvements in many of the comorbidities associated with obesity, including glucose homeostasis, high blood pressure, and lipid profiles [74].

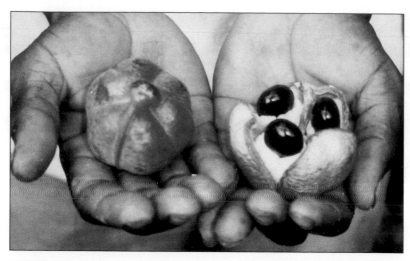

FIGURE 17-6. The ackee fruit in its unripe form (*left*) and ripe form (*right*). The ackee tree, indigenous to west Africa, was introduced to Jamaica in 1778 by Thomas Clarke. In Jamaica it is considered a dietary staple. It is well known in west Africa and Jamaica that the fruit may be poisonous during certain stages in its development.

Outbreaks of a disorder commonly called Jamaica vomiting sickness tend to occur during the colder months of the year, when other food is scarce and the fruit is still unripe. The major clinical features of this disorder, caused by ingestion of an unripe ackee fruit, include the sudden onset of vomiting and violent retching, which is preceded by generalized epigastric discomfort lasting 2 hours to 3 days. After a period of prostration averaging 10 hours, the second bout of vomiting may occur, followed by convulsions and sometimes death. The most striking finding is marked hypoglycemia. Well-nourished people may never develop manifestations of the disease, whereas those with chronic malnutrition, especially children between 2 and 5 years of age, are much more likely to become symptomatic. Hypoglycins A and B mediate the illness: they inhibit transport of long-chain fatty acids into the mitochondria, thereby suppressing their oxidation and resulting in depression of gluconeogenesis [3].

PROTOCOL FOR PROLONGED SUPERVISED FAST

1. Date the onset of the fast as of the last ingestion of calories. Discontinue use of all nonessential medications

2. Allow the patient to drink calorie-free and caffeine-free beverages

3. Ensure that the patient is active during waking hours

4. Measure plasma levels of glucose, insulin, C-peptide, and proinsulin in the same specimen: repeat measurements every 6 hours until the plasma glucose level is < 60 mg/dL. At this point, the interval should be reduced to every 1 to 2 hours

5. End the fast when the plasma glucose level is < 45 mg/dL and the patient has symptoms or signs of hypoglycemia or < 55 mg/dL if Whipple's triad previously demonstrated

6. At the end of the fast, measure plasma levels of glucose, insulin, C-peptide, proinsulin, β-hydroxybutyrate, and sulfonylurea in the same specimen. Then inject 1 mg of glucagon intravenously and measure plasma glucose level after 10, 20, and 30 minutes. At this point the patient can be fed

FIGURE 17-7. Protocol for prolonged 72-hour fast. There are two endpoints for the 72-hour fast: 1) establish Whipple's triad and roles of β-cell polypeptides; or 2) establish role of β-cell polypeptides in patients previously shown to satisfy Whipple's triad.

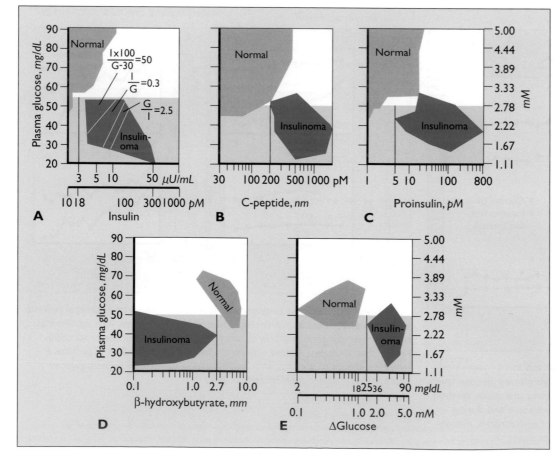

FIGURE 17-8. Limits of plasma levels of insulin (**A**), C-peptide (**B**), proinsulin (**C**), and β-hydroxybutyrate (**D**), and changes in plasma glucose levels (**E**) in response to intravenous glucagon, according to 1) plasma glucose levels at the end of a 72-hour fast in 25 control patients and 2) the point at which the features of Whipple's triad were noted in 40 patients with histologically confirmed insulinomas. The shaded areas represent plasma glucose levels (50 mg/dL [2.8 mmol/L]). The vertical lines represent the diagnostic criteria for insulinoma: insulin level of at least 3 microunits per mL (18 pmol/L), C-peptide level of at least 200 pmol/L, proinsulin level of at least 5 pmol/L, β-hydroxybutyrate level of 2.7 mmol/L or less, and change in glucose level of at least 25 mg/dL (1.4 mmol/L). The ratios of glucose and insulin have no diagostic utility.

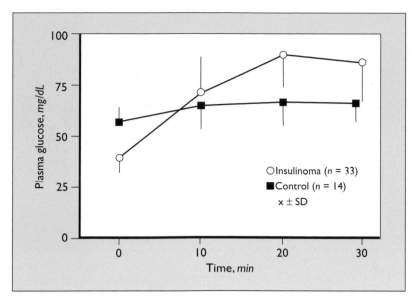

FIGURE 17-9. Plasma glucose responses to glucagon, 1 mg, administered intravenously at the end of the prolonged fast (0 minutes). These responses are greater in patients with insulinoma than in control patients. The rationale for this procedure is that insulin is glycogenic and antiglycogenolytic and therefore results in persistence of hepatic glycogen despite fasting. Patients with insulin-mediated hypoglycemia have a maximum increment of at least 25 mg/dL above the terminal fasting plasma glucose levels, whereas others (control patients or those with non–insulin-mediated hypoglycemia whose hepatic glycogen has been depleted by fasting) have lower increments [7]. Error bars represent the standard deviation. (*Adapted from* Service and Nelson [5].)

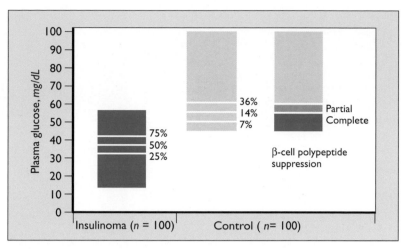

FIGURE 17-10. Plasma glucose levels at the end of a 72-hour fast. The *grey panel* depicts the range (57 to 44 mg/dL) at the termination of the prolonged 72-hour fast (Whipple's triad) in 100 patients with insulinoma (the fast was terminated well before the 72-hour point because of the occurrence of symptomatic hypoglycemia confirmed biochemically). The 75th percentile (42 mg/dL), 50th percentile (38 mg/dL), and 25th percentile (33 mg/dL) are also shown. The *red panel* shows the plasma glucose levels at the 72-hour point in 100 control patients who underwent the 72-hour fast. Thirty-six percent of patients had a plasma glucose level of 60 mg/dL or less, 14% had a level of 55 mg/dL or less, and 7% had a level of 50 mg/dL or less. Two patients had terminal plasma glucose levels of 44 mg/dL. The *darker panel* depicts suppression of β-cell polypeptides in normal persons at the end of the 72-hour fast. One or two of the three β-cell polypeptides (insulin, C-peptide, and proinsulin) were suppressed below our diagnostic criteria for hyperinsulinemia in the range of 60 to 55 mg/dL, and all three were suppressed when the plasma glucose level was 55 mg/dL or lower.

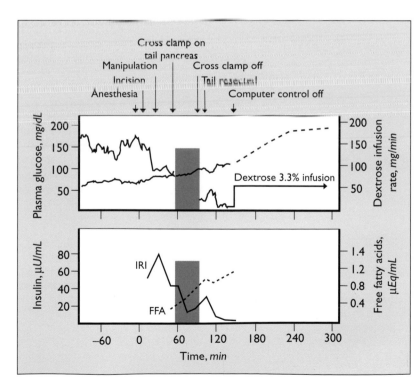

FIGURE 17-11. Artificial pancreas. The Biostator (Life Science Instruments, Elkhart, IN) has been used by some practitioners to maintain euglycemia in the preoperative and intraoperative period. A reduction in the glucose infusion rate after removal of the insulinoma indicates that all hyperfunctioning tissue has been removed. An alternate approach is to conduct frequent serial measurements of plasma glucose levels in the operating room. Patients are taken to the operating room without glucose running, and the plasma glucose level is permitted to decrease to a modestly hypoglycemic range. After tumor removal, an increase in the plasma glucose level can be expected within 30 minutes in most patients. In some patients, the plasma glucose level is increasing as a result of stress before tumor removal. Also after removal of the tumor, the slope of the elevation in the glucose level increases distinctly. FFA—free fatty acids; IRI—insulin resistance index. (*Adapted from* Kudlow et al. [8].)

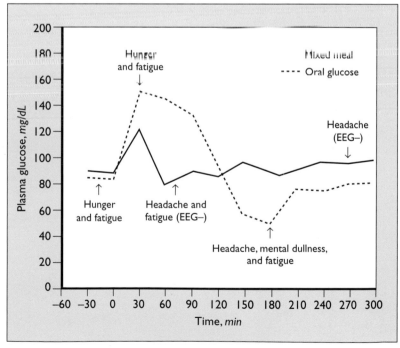

FIGURE 17-12. The oral glucose tolerance test. This test has been used to evaluate patients with suspected reactive hypoglycemia. Unfortunately, this test is of no use because a high percentage of normal persons have a post–oral glucose testing nadir of 50 mg/dL or less. The preferred assessment is a mixed-meal test. As shown in this figure, individual symptoms occurred throughout the oral glucose tolerance test, both at the nadir and at the apogee. In addition, symptoms were present during the mixed-meal test when no evidence of hypoglycemia was noted. These observations provide strong evidence that symptoms could not be ascribed to hypoglycemia. EEG—electroencephalogram. (*Adapted from* Service [3].)

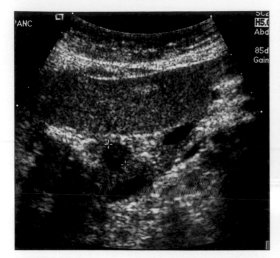

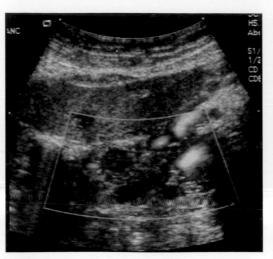

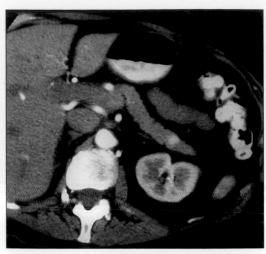

FIGURE 17-13. Hypoechogenicity of insulinomas. The ultrasonographic characteristic of insulinoma is hypoechogenicity. The insulinoma is marked with white crosses and is distinctly hypoechogenic in contrast to surrounding tissue.

FIGURE 17-14. (See Color Plate) Hypoechogenicity of insulinomas. Color Doppler analysis shows the hypervascularity of the insulinoma noted in Figure 17-13.

FIGURE 17-15. Insulinoma. A 0.8-cm insulinoma is seen in the arterial phase of the spiral CT scan, which was obtained by using triple-phase agent.

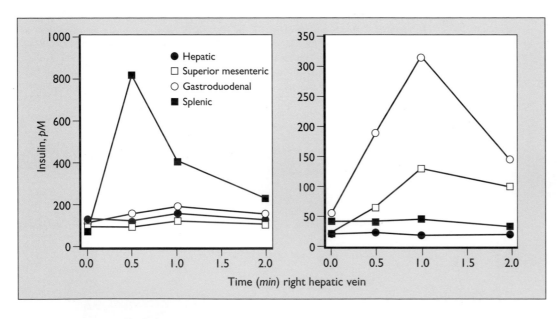

FIGURE 17-16. The selective arterial calcium stimulation test. This is both a localization (actually a regionalization) procedure and a dynamic test. The principle of this procedure is that hyperfunctioning β cells release insulin in response to the injection of a small dose of calcium intra-arterially, whereas normal β cells do not. During this procedure, the insulin level is measured before and at fixed time sequences after the injection of 0.025 mEq of calcium per kg of body weight sequentially into the splenic, gastroduodenal, and superior mesenteric arteries. A two- to threefold increment in the level of insulin in the right hepatic vein indicates hyperfunctioning β cells—either insulinoma or hypertrophic islets—in the arterial distribution of the injected artery. In the left panel, the positive response after injection into the splenic artery indicates that hyperfunctioning β cells (presumably an insulinoma) are present in the tail of the pancreas. In the right panel, the positive responses to injections into the superior mesenteric and gastroduodenal arteries suggest that the insulinoma is likely to be in the head of the pancreas. (*Adapted from* Doppman et al. [9].)

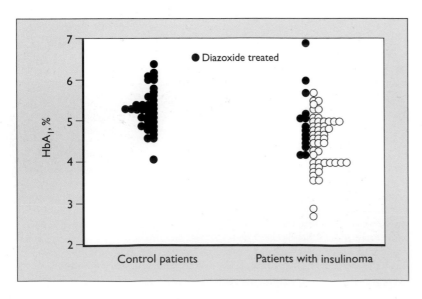

FIGURE 17-17. Glycated hemoglobin values (measured by affinity chromatography) for control patients evaluated for potential hypoglycemic disorder and insulinomas, some of whom had been treated with diazoxide. Although glycated hemoglobin values are lower in patients with insulinoma than in control patients, the values overlap too much to allow a diagnostic level to be established. Twenty-five percent of the patients with insulinoma had glycated hemoglobin values of 4.1% or less; this was at the lower limit of values observed in control patients. (*Adapted from* Hassoun et al. [10].)

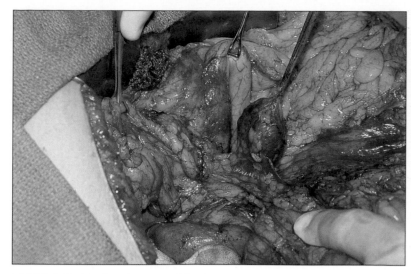

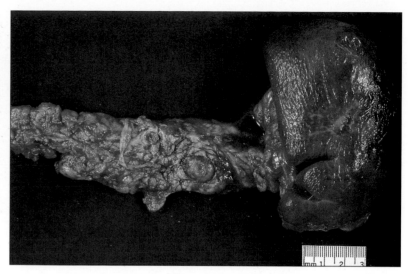

FIGURE 17-18. (See Color Plate) Insulinomas. Insulinomas vary in size, from a few millimeters to several centimeters. The median is 1.5 cm. This figure shows a 4-cm tumor. In a large series of patients (*n* = 224) observed at the Mayo Clinic from 1927 to 1986 [11], 86.6% of patients had a single benign tumor, 5.9% had malignant tumors, 8.9% had multiple tumors, and 7.6% had multiple endocrine neoplasia type syndrome. The estimated incidence in the northern European population is 4 cases per 1 million patient-years. The median age in the Mayo Clinic series was 47 years (range, 8 to 82 years), and 59% of patients were women. During the study period, one patient had islet hyperplasia.

FIGURE 17-19. (See Color Plate) Removal of the distal pancreas and spleen in a patient with multiple islet cell tumors as part of the multiple endocrine neoplasia (MEN) I syndrome. Insulinoma constitutes the second most common pancreatic tumor in the MEN I syndrome. In a study from the Mayo Clinic [11], more than 50% of patients with insulinoma as part of MEN I syndrome had multiple tumors. The associated endocrinopathies have primarily been hyperparathyroidism, prolactinoma, gastrinoma, and Cushing disease. The standard operative approach is to enucleate tumors in the head of the pancreas and, if tumors are present in the rest of the pancreas, to conduct a partial pancreatectomy.

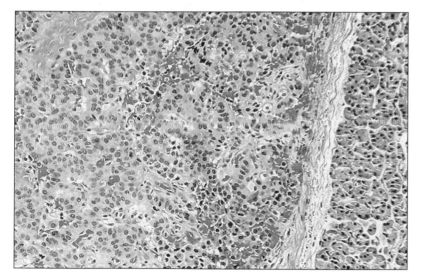

FIGURE 17-20. Pancreatic tissue showing normal exocrine pancreas on the right side of the figure. The left side of the figure shows an islet cell tumor composed of uniform cells with round nuclei and eosinophilic cytoplasm. The tumor is highly vascular, and small clusters of red blood cells are present throughout the neoplasm. Mitotic figures are not identified, and there is no invasive growth of the neoplasm. These findings suggest that this tumor is probably benign. (Hematoxylin and eosin; original magnification, ×6.)

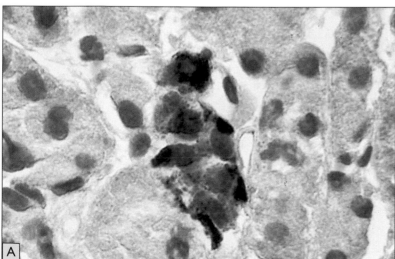

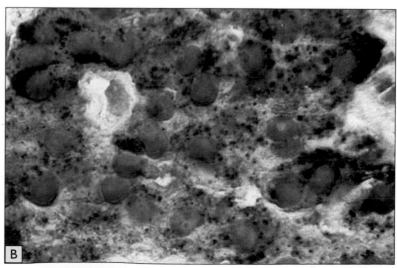

FIGURE 17-21. (See Color Plate) Higher magnification of an insulin-producing islet cell tumor after immunostaining. **A,** Normal exocrine and endocrine pancreatic tissues. An islet cell staining positively for insulin is present in the middle of the pancreatic exocrine tissue.

B, An insulinoma with strong diffuse positive immunoreactivity after staining with an insulin antibody. The tumor cells reveal diffuse granular cytoplasmic staining. The blue staining of the nuclei is from the hematoxylin counterstain (×40).

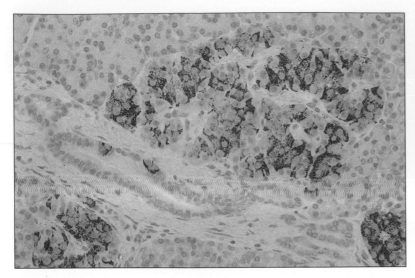

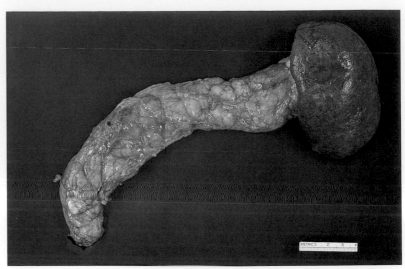

FIGURE 17-22. Islet hyperplasia/nesidioblastosis, a rare cause of hyperinsulinemic hypoglycemia in adults. This slide shows large islets immunostained with insulin, as well as two β cells budding from the acinar duct. The latter is the characteristic of nesidioblastosis (×150) [12].

FIGURE 17-23. (See Color Plate) Islet hyperplasia/nesidioblastosis. When hyperinsulinemic hypoglycemia in an adult is suspected to be due to islet hyperplasia/nesidioblastosis and an insulinoma cannot be identified by intraoperative ultrasonography or complete mobilization and palpation of the pancreas, gradient-guided partial pancreatectomy is indicated. In this patient, a selective arterial calcium stimulation test indicated hyperfunctioning β cells in the region of the splenic and gastroduodenal arteries. As a result, resection was performed to the right of the superior mesenteric vein [12].

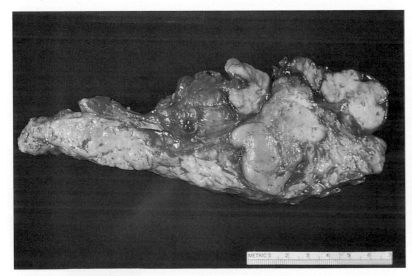

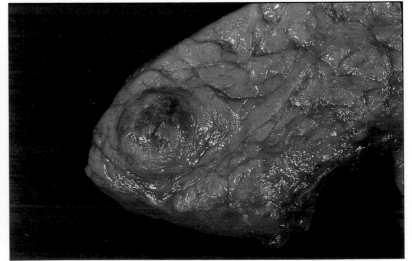

FIGURE 17-24. (See Color Plate) Islet-cell carcinoma in the body of the pancreas. The tail of the pancreas is to the right. The tumor has a paler appearance than the surrounding pancreas. In addition, the tumor involves adjacent nodes shown on the inferior portion of the resected tissue. In general, islet-cell carcinomas are larger than benign tumors and metastasize regionally to nodes. The life expectancy of patients with islet-cell carcinoma is considerably longer than that of patients with acinar-cell pancreatic carcinoma [11].

FIGURE 17-25. (See Color Plate) Solitary insulinoma slightly less than 2 cm in diameter embedded in the tail of the pancreas. The pancreatic duct is adjacent to the tumor, and the proximity of the tumor to the duct mandated distal pancreatectomy. Insulinomas are reddish-brown or gray, which distinguishes them from normal pancreatic tissue. In this case, the tumor is reddish-brown. These tumors also have a firmer consistency than normal pancreatic tissue.

Survival Rates and Recurrence

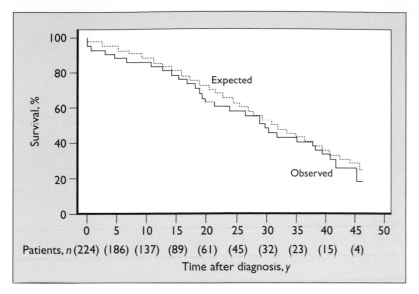

FIGURE 17-26. Survival after diagnosis of insulinoma (Mayo Clinic patients: 1927–1986). Among 224 patients whose initial surgery resulted in removal of an insulinoma at the Mayo Clinic, the overall survival rate (including the small number of patients with malignant insulinoma) was no different from the rate expected for the general population. (*Adapted from* Service *et al.* [11].)

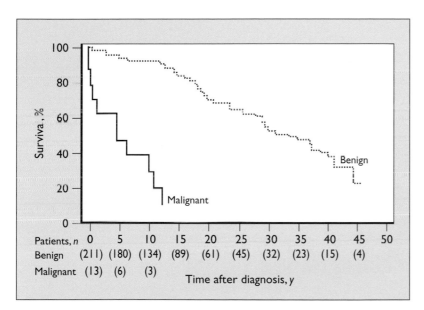

FIGURE 17-27. Survival rates for malignant insulinoma diagnosed on the basis of the presence of metastases at the time of pancreatic exploration (Mayo Clinic patients: 1927–1986). The 10-year rate was approximately 40%. Although this is far less than the survival rate seen in patients with benign insulinoma, it does exceed the rate associated with acinar-cell pancreatic carcinoma. (*Adapted from* Service *et al.* [11].)

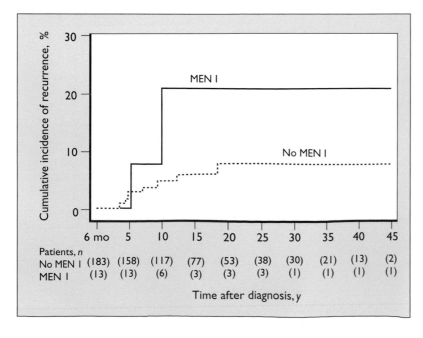

FIGURE 17-28. Recurrence rates in 224 patients whose initial surgery resulted in the removal of an insulinoma at the Mayo Clinic observed over a 60-year period (1927 to 1986) and followed for 45 years. Insulinomas did not recur within the first 4 years of follow-up, indicating that subsequent hyperinsulinemic hypoglycemia was not caused by persistent insulinoma. The recurrence rates were 7% for patients without multiple endocrine neoplasia (MEN) I syndrome and 21% for those with MEN I syndrome. No patient had a documented recurrence 20 years after the initial surgery. (*Adapted from* Service *et al.* [11].)

References

1. Service FJ: Hypoglycemic disorders. *N Engl J Med* 1995, 332:1144–1152.

2. Service FJ: Clinical presentations and laboratory evaluation of hypoglycemic disorders in adults. In *Hypoglycemic Disorder: Pathogenesis, Diagnosis and Treatment.* Edited by Service FJ. Boston: GK Hall; 1983:73–95.

3. Service FJ: Hypoglycemias. In *Cecil's Textbook of Medicine, Update 4.* Edited by Smith LH Jr. Philadelphia: WB Saunders; 1989.

4. Cryer PE: Glucose counter regulation: the physiological mechanisms that prevent or correct hypoglycemia. In *Hypoglycaemia and Diabetes: Clinical and Physiological Aspects.* Edited by Frier BM, Fisher BM. London: Edward Arnold; 1993:34–55.

5. Service FJ, Nelson RL: Insulinoma. *Compr Ther* 1980, 6:70–74.

6. Rizza RA, Haymond MW, Verdonk CA, *et al.*: Pathogenesis of hypoglycemia in insulinoma patients: suppression of hepatic glucose production by insulin. *Diabetes* 1981, 30:377–381.

7. O'Brien T, O'Brien PC, Service FJ: Insulin surrogates in insulinoma. *J Clin Endocrinol Metab* 1993, 77:448–451.

8. Kudlow JE, Albisser AM, Angel A, *et al.*: Insulinoma resection facilitated by the artificial endocrine pancreas. *Diabetes* 1978, 27:774–777.

9. Doppman JL, Chang R, Fraker DL, *et al.*: Localization of insulinomas to regions of the pancreas by intra-arterial stimulation with calcium. *Ann Intern Med* 1995, 123:269–273.

10. Hassoun AAK, Service FJ, O'Brien PC. Glycated hemoglobin in insulinoma. *Endocr Pract* 1998, 4:181–183.

11. Service FJ, O'Brien PC, Kao PC, *et al.*: C-peptide suppression test: effects of gender, age and body mass index. Implications for the diagnosis of insulinoma. *J Clin Endocrinol Metab* 1992, 74:204–210.

12. Service FJ, Natt N, Thompson GB, *et al.*: Non-insulinoma pancreatogenous hypoglycemia: a novel syndrome of hyperinsulinemic hypoglycemia in adults independent of mutations in Kir6.2 and SURI genes. *J Clin Endocrin Metab* 1999, 84(5):1582–1589.

SECONDARY FORMS OF DIABETES

18

Veronica M. Catanese

Primary forms of diabetes mellitus include type 1, or insulin-dependent diabetes mellitus, and type 2, or non–insulin-dependent diabetes mellitus. Secondary forms of diabetes and glucose intolerance may occur in association with a variety of disorders of both endocrinologic and nonendocrinologic origin [1].

Most endocrine diseases associated with glucose intolerance produce the metabolic abnormality through excessive production of insulin counterregulatory hormones, such as growth hormone, glucocorticoids, glucagon, and catecholamines. These hormones affect both glucose production (through glycogenolysis and gluconeogenesis) and glucose utilization (through insulin secretion and insulin action) to varying degrees. In these diseases, the secondary diabetes is usually reversible with successful treatment of the underlying disorder, and the risk for ketoacidosis is low.

Nonendocrine conditions associated with abnormal glucose tolerance may be grouped into three major categories: diseases affecting pancreatic function (pancreatoprivic); drug-induced glucose intolerance; and complex genetic syndromes that affect multiple aspects of hepatic, renal, and musculoskeletal function. Pancreatitis, pancreatectomy, and hemochromatosis are the main components of the pancreatoprivic group. As expected, these conditions are associated with variable amounts of insulin deficiency and at least the potential for ketoacidosis. Pharmacologic agents can alter glucose tolerance by affecting insulin secretion, insulin action, or both. Genetic syndromes producing diabetes have multiple mechanisms, but in most cases, the exact cause still remains poorly understood.

Microangiopathic complications of diabetes are uncommon in patients with glucose intolerance secondary to diseases of hormonal overproduction. This is because these diseases rarely persist in an untreated state for many years. Retinal, renal, and neurologic sequelae do occur, however, in patients whose disease has lasted a decade or more. Because duration of hyperglycemia is a critical factor in the development of microvascular complications, it is not surprising that patients with long-standing pancreatitis, exocrine, and endocrine pancreatic dysfunction secondary to pancreatic reductive surgery, hemochromatosis, and genetic syndromes that include glucose intolerance are at risk for the development of classic diabetic complications.

Therapy for all types of secondary diabetes should center on correction of the underlying disturbance when possible. If this cannot be accomplished or until this is accomplished, treatment should reflect an understanding of the pathophysiologic basis of the diabetes. If insulin secretion is impaired (for example, in patients with pheochromocytoma), then exogenous insulin therapy should be instituted promptly until the underlying source of the problem has been eliminated. Patients with preserved insulin secretion should be treated with diet or oral hypoglycemic agents given as single drugs or in combination. In these cases, insulin should also be used if necessary to achieve glycemic goals. In all cases, little evidence suggests a correlation between the need for insulin therapy during a period of secondary diabetes and the risk for permanently altered glucose tolerance after successful treatment of the underlying primary disease.

FIGURE 18-1. Secondary forms of diabetes mellitus.

SECONDARY FORMS OF DIABETES

Endocrine diseases
  Changes in balance of insulin counterregulatory hormones disrupt
    glucose homeostasis
Nonendocrine conditions
  Pancreatic functional defects
  Drug-induced glucose intolerance
  Genetic syndromes

Abnormal Glucose Homeostasis Secondary to Endocrinologic Disorders: Acromegaly

ACUTE AND DELAYED EFFECTS OF SUPRAPHYSIOLOGIC GROWTH HORMONE ON CARBOHYDRATE METABOLISM

Metabolic Variable	Short-Term GH Administration	Chronic GH Excess
Glucose uptake	↑	↓
Glucose utilization	↑	↓

FIGURE 18-2. Acute and delayed effects of supraphysiologic growth hormone (GH) on carbohydrate metabolism. Intravenous administration of GH produces insulinomimetic effects during the first 4 hours after infusion. Glucose uptake and glucose utilization by insulin-sensitive tissues are increased, and plasma glucose and free fatty acid levels decrease. These effects may result from a rapid, direct effect of GH on insulin secretion; GH-mediated increase in hepatic production of insulin-like growth factor-I; or GH-induced activation of some of the early steps in insulin receptor intracellular signaling pathways [2]. The delayed effects of GH administration, however, counter insulin action. Glucose uptake and use by insulin-sensitive tissues are impaired, resulting in hyperinsulinism and varying patterns of glucose tolerance. Free fatty acid levels increase only with concomitant fasting; this supports the concept that excess GH does not promote significant lipolysis in the presence of adequate insulin.

A. RESPONSES TO ORAL GLUCOSE TOLERANCE TESTING IN ACROMEGALY

Abnormal OGTT	Normal OGTT
↑ Glucose	→ Glucose
↑ Insulin	↑ Insulin
↑ Glucose	→ Glucose
↓ Insulin	→ Insulin

FIGURE 18-3. Spectrum of response to oral glucose tolerance testing in acromegaly. **A,** The spectrum of abnormalities in glucose homeostasis. The prevalence of glucose intolerance in patients with acromegaly is approximately 60%. Most acromegalic patients with abnormal results on oral glucose tolerance tests (OGTTs) have normal fasting plasma glucose levels but impaired handling of a glucose load associated with elevated basal or stimulated insulin levels. A small subset have low basal insulin levels and profoundly impaired insulin responses to glucose loading, and they clinically manifest severe hyperglycemia. It is not clear whether these patients represent a distinct subgroup with coincident insulin-dependent diabetes or β-cell desensitization as a consequence of prolonged hyperglycemia. Acromegalic patients with normal glucose tolerance, however, often exhibit insulin resistance as defined by elevated plasma insulin levels under basal or glucose-stimulated conditions. In these patients, glucose uptake in skeletal muscle and nonoxidative glucose metabolism are impaired in the postabsorptive state [3]. Therefore, oral glucose tolerance testing underestimates the prevalence of insulin resistance in patients with acromegaly. It is not clear, however, that progression from hyperinsulinemic euglycemia to a more severe defect manifested by hyperglycemia occurs with progressive acromegaly, such as that seen in the patient photographed over time (**B**). (Panel B from Thorner et al. [4]; with permission.)

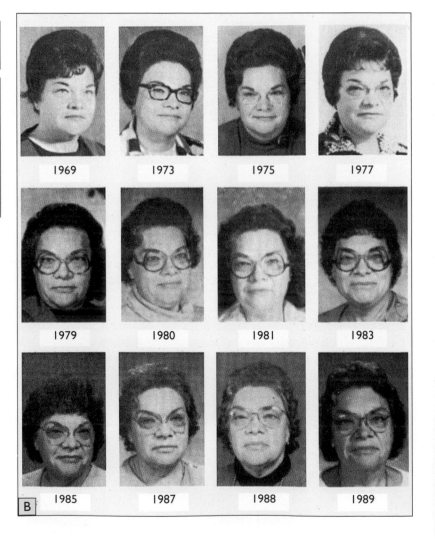

1969   1973   1975   1977

1979   1980   1981   1983

B 1985   1987   1988   1989

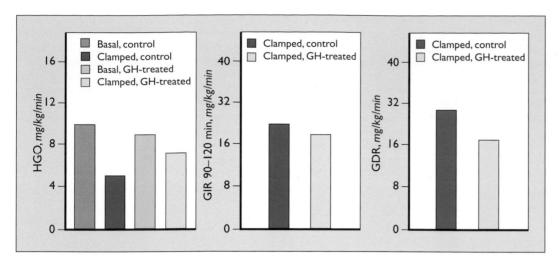

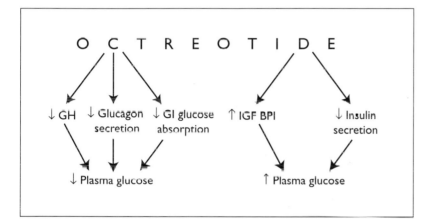

FIGURE 18-4. Growth hormone (GH)–induced hepatic and peripheral insulin resistance. Continuous administration of recombinant human GH to normal rats reduces insulin-mediated suppression of hepatic glucose output (HGO) and produces significant decreases in steady-state glucose infusion rate (GIR) and glucose disposal rate (GDR) during hyperinsulinemic glucose clamping. Similar results have been obtained in normal human patients studied under conditions of continuous GH infusion [5]. In both rats and humans, fasting plasma glucose and insulin levels during GH treatment did not differ from those in controls, providing an experimental correlate of patients with acromegaly who have evidence of impaired insulin action in the postabsorptive state. The mechanisms responsible for this insulin resistance, however, remain unclear. Impairment of early events in insulin signal transduction in liver and muscle is a likely contributing factor. Insulin receptor substrate (IRS)-1 and IRS-2 tyrosine phosphorylation and association of these substrates with phosphatidylinositol 3-kinase are reduced in the livers and muscle of rats receiving long-term GH therapy [6]. Insulin receptors substrate (IRS)-1 and IRS-2 tyrosine phosphorylation and association of these substrates with phosphatidylinositol 3-kinase are reduced in the livers and muscles of rats receiving long-term GH therapy [6] and in the livers of GH-transgenic mice [7]. In addition, GH excess promotes free fatty acid mobilization, a process that worsens insulin resistance because free fatty acids inhibit insulin-stimulated glucose oxidation [8]. (*Adapted from* Sugimoto et al. [9].)

FIGURE 18-5. Effects of octreotide on glucose homeostasis in acromegaly. Unlike other effective treatment options for acromegaly, octreotide (the synthetic, long-acting somatostatin analogue) has complex effects on several hormonal factors that affect carbohydrate metabolism. In addition to inhibiting growth hormone (GH) and insulin-like growth factor-I (IGF-I) hypersecretion, octreotide inhibits insulin and glucagon secretion, delays gastrointestinal glucose absorption, and increases production of insulin-antagonistic IGF-binding protein 1 (BPI) [10]. The interplay of these pharmacologic effects may lead to concomitant improvement in glucose tolerance with control of the GH hypersecretion; however, it may also cause worsened glucose tolerance upon institution of octreotide therapy, particularly if GH secretory profiles remain abnormal [11]. GI—gastrointestinal

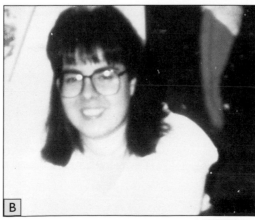

Cushing Syndrome

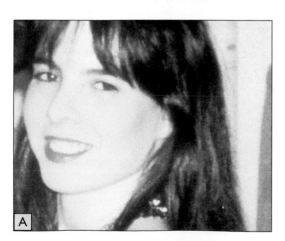

FIGURE 18-6. Cushing syndrome. Cushing syndrome is a common endocrine cause of secondary glucose intolerance and diabetes. Abnormal glucose homeostasis may result from exogenous daily or alternate-day administration of glucocorticoids or as a consequence of chronic endogenous excess of glucocorticoids due to pituitary hypersecretion of adrenocorticotropic hormone (ACTH), paraneoplastic production of ACTH by tumor cells, or autonomous adrenal cortical hyperfunction. The latter affected this patient, photographed (**A**) before and (**B**) after presentation with phenotypic Cushing syndrome. The patient was found to have an adrenal cortical adenoma.

Although fasting hyperglycemia occurs in approximately 5% of patients with Cushing syndrome, insulin resistance with basal or stimulated hyperinsulinemia occurs in up to 90% of patients. Glucocorticoid excess directly affects hepatic glucose production (*see* Fig. 18-7), peripheral glucose utilization (*see* Fig. 18-8), and pancreatic insulin secretion (*see* Fig. 18-9). It may also exacerbate insulin resistance indirectly through the effects of circulating adipokines, particularly resistin [12] and adiponectin [13]. (*Courtesy of* Jaishree Jagirdar, New York University School of Medicine, New York.)

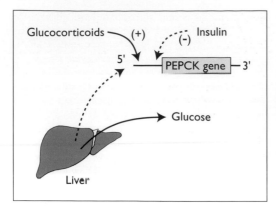

FIGURE 18-7. Glucocorticoid excess promotes hepatic glucose production. Several key enzymes controlling the production and utilization of metabolic fuels are directly regulated by glucocorticoids at the level of gene transcription. Phosphoenolpyruvate carboxykinase (PEPCK), a critical enzyme in gluconeogenesis, is positively regulated by glucocorticoids [14]. Transgenic mice overexpressing PEPCK, in fact, exhibit impaired glucose tolerance [15]. In addition, exposure of pregnant rats during late gestation to glucocorticoid excess permanently increases hepatic expression of PEPCK and glucocorticoid receptor and causes glucose intolerance in adult offspring [16]. Under normal physiologic conditions, however, insulin regulates PEPCK even more potently and dominantly in a negative manner [17]. Thus, replete insulin prevents the enhanced gluconeogenesis that would be caused by glucocorticoid excess. In the presence of insulin deficiency or impaired insulin action, however, the stimulatory effects of glucocorticoids on glucose production become apparent. Because patients with Cushing syndrome almost always have insulin resistance, the stage is set for glucocorticoid-enhanced gluconeogenesis, which contributes to glucose intolerance.

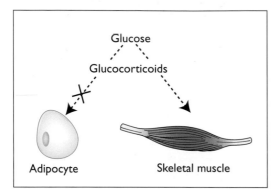

FIGURE 18-8. Glucocorticoid excess diminishes peripheral glucose utilization. Glucocorticoids induce resistance to insulin-stimulated glucose uptake in rat adipocytes [18]. This effect may be at least partly mediated by direct glucocorticoid-mediated inhibition of insulin-induced protein kinase C translocation from cytosol to plasma membrane. Glucocorticoids also inhibit activation of glucose transport in rat skeletal muscle by insulin, insulin-like growth factor-I, and hypoxia [19]. In rat soleus muscle, this effect is associated with preservation of total content of GLUT4 glucose transporters but also reduced translocation of GLUT4 transporter units to the plasma membrane [20]. In addition to these effects on GLUT4 subcellular trafficking, glucocorticoids affect early steps in insulin receptor signaling in skeletal muscle and in the liver [21]. As a result, both basal and insulin-stimulated glucose uptake and utilization are subject to modulation by excess glucocorticoids.

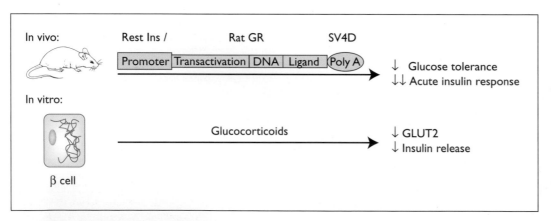

FIGURE 18-9. Glucocorticoids inhibit insulin secretion from pancreatic β cells. Insulin resistance has long been a recognized consequence of glucocorticoid excess. Effects of glucocorticoids on insulin secretion in vivo and in vitro, however, have only recently been described. Transgenic mice overexpressing the glucocorticoid receptor (GR) under the control of the insulin promoter have increased glucocorticoid sensitivity that is restricted to pancreatic β cells [22]. These animals have normal fasting and postabsorptive blood glucose levels but also have a markedly reduced insulin response and impaired glucose tolerance during intravenous glucose loading. This in vivo evidence suggesting a diabetogenic effect of glucocorticoids on pancreatic β cells is supported by in vitro evidence for dexamethasone-induced, posttranslational degradation of β cell GLUT2 glucose transporters [23] and by dexamethasone-induced inhibition of exocytotic insulin release from rodent islets in culture [24]. Diminished glucose utilization in Cushing syndrome may therefore be a composite result of deficient insulin secretion and impaired insulin action.

Glucagonoma

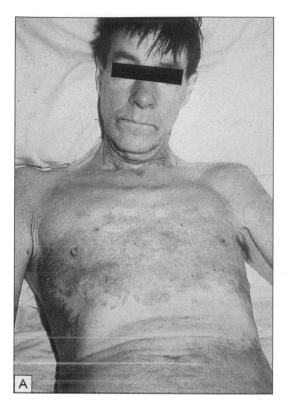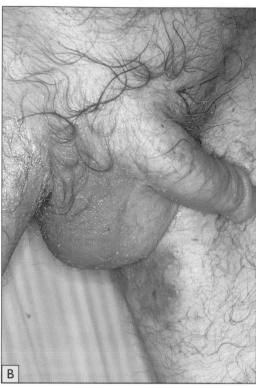

FIGURE 18-10. (See Color Plate) Glucose intolerance in the "glucagonoma syndrome." Although hyperglucagonemia may be associated with a variety of secretory islet-cell tumors and is rarely associated with multiple endocrine neoplasia type I (MEN I), the characteristic glucagonoma syndrome is most frequently seen in patients with clinically malignant, glucagon-producing tumors of pancreatic α cells. **A** and **B**, Central to the classic glucagonoma syndrome is necrolytic migratory erythema—the pathognomonic erythematous rash involving the perineum, extremities, trunk, or perioral region. This rash may be reproduced by infusion of glucagon into normal individuals and can be alleviated by infusion of parenteral amino acids, despite continued hyperglucagonemia. Thus, it is likely that amino acid deficiency produced by glucagon-induced muscle proteolysis is responsible for the rash. The incidence of glucose intolerance in patients with glucagonoma approaches 100%, with metabolic defects ranging from mild to very severe. Despite the excess production of glucagon and its potent effects on glycogenolysis and gluconeogenesis, ketoacidosis is rare. This probably reflects the stimulatory effect of glucagon on insulin secretion and the importance of the relative concentrations of insulin and glucagon to hepatic glucose production and ketogenesis. In addition, functional heterogeneity of the various circulating species of immunoreactive glucagon may titrate glucagon's biological effects. (*Courtesy of* Dr. C.R. Kahn, Joslin Diabetes Center, Boston.)

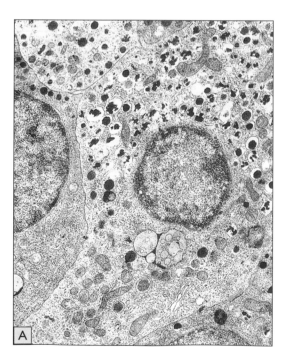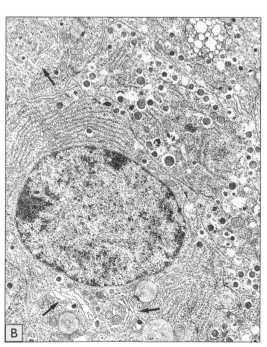

FIGURE 18-11. Effects of endogenous hyperglucagonemia on pancreatic β cells. It is unlikely that an increased glucose production rate alone could produce glucose intolerance in the absence of an absolute or relative decrease in glucose disposal rate. Decreased insulin secretion or insulin resistance could result in dimin-

ished glucose utilization. Insulin resistance has not been described clinically in patients with glucagonoma. Glucagon is a potent stimulus of epinephrine release; thus, α-adrenergic receptor– mediated inhibition of insulin secretion may diminish glucose disposal in patients with glucagonoma syndrome. Excess glucagon also has direct paracrine stimulatory effects on β-cell insulin secretion. β cells in the nontumoral endocrine pancreatic tissue of patients with glucagonoma have reduced immunoreactive insulin content and have ultrastructural features suggestive of accelerated insulin synthesis and secretion.

A, β cell from a control human pancreas, with moderate amounts of rough endoplasmic reticulum, a small Golgi apparatus, and numerous mature granules with crystal-like cores. **B,** β cell from a glucagonoma-associated pancreas. This cell contains several elongated rough endoplasmic reticulum cisternae, stacks of Golgi with adjacent progranules (*arrows*), and fewer secretory granules, which primarily contain immature rounded cores. It is therefore possible that the balance of multiple effects of hyperglucagonemia on insulin secretion may determine the degree of impairment in glucose utilization rate. (*From* Bani *et al.* [25]; with permission.)

Pancreatoprivic Diabetes: Pancreatectomy and Chronic Pancreatitis

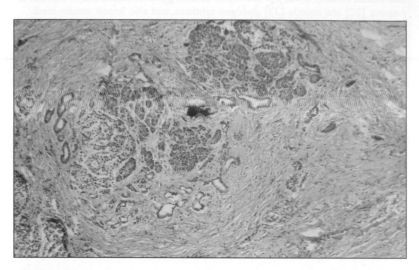

FIGURE 18-16. Reductions in pancreatic functional mass impair glucose tolerance by affecting multihormonal islet cell activity. Pancreatic exocrine and endocrine deficiency develop predictably with removal or destruction of more than 75% of pancreatic tissue. Glucose intolerance after pancreatectomy, fibrocalcific or

"J-type" tropical diabetes, and chronic pancreatitis, particularly as a result of alcoholism, share several features that distinguish them from other types of primary and secondary diabetes. Endocrine secretion from all islet cell types is reduced, resulting not only in insulin deficiency under basal or stimulated conditions, but also diminished pancreatic glucagon, somatostatin, and pancreatic polypeptide secretion. Despite preserved secretion of glucagon-like substances of duodenal origin in patients who have not undergone pancreaticoduodenectomy, reduced levels of pancreatic glucagon account for the relative resistance of these patients to ketoacidosis under conditions of insulin deficiency. In addition, iatrogenic hypoglycemia is common, and the response to spontaneous or induced hypoglycemia is delayed compared with that observed in both insulin-dependent and non–insulin-dependent diabetics. Although carbohydrate intolerance in these patients is usually attributed to reduced insulin secretion, insulin deficiency alone may not be the only factor responsible for secondary diabetes under these conditions. Hepatic resistance to insulin, accompanied by loss of sensitivity to insulin-induced hepatic glucose suppression, is a prominent feature of canine chronic pancreatitis. Deficiency of pancreatic polypeptide has been implicated as a factor in this resistance. Infusion of bovine pancreatic polypeptide improves glucose tolerance and restores suppression of hepatic glucose output by insulin in pancreatic polypeptide–deficient animals [46] and patients with chronic pancreatitis [47] (hematoxylin-eosin stain). (*Courtesy of* Dr. Howard Mizrachi, St. Luke's–Roosevelt Hospital Center, New York.)

Hemochromatosis

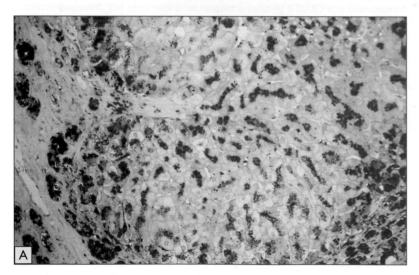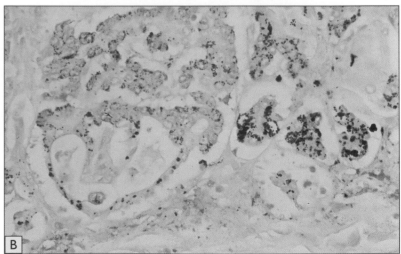

FIGURE 18-17. (See Color Plate) Hemochromatosis. Whether hereditary or secondary to iron overload, hemochromatosis is associated with abnormal glucose tolerance. Clinical diabetes or impaired glucose tolerance occurs in 75% to 90% of patients with primary hemochromatosis and in up to 65% of patients with hemochromatosis as a consequence of hemolytic anemia, multiple transfusion, or iron ingestion. Although the presence of cirrhosis increases the likelihood of abnormal glucose metabolism, hepatic iron content (shown by Prussian blue staining in **A**), serum ferritin levels, or extent of liver damage correlate poorly with the presence of impaired glucose homeostasis. A positive family history of diabetes may be the best predictor of glucose intolerance, at

least among patients with hereditary hemochromatosis [48]. Hepatic insulin resistance clearly plays an important role in patients with both varieties of hemochromatosis [49,50]. Defective first-phase insulin secretion, however, is also observed, even in the absence of significant degrees of islet iron deposition, such as that shown in **B**. Taken together, these physiologic abnormalities resemble those seen during the natural history of non–insulin-dependent diabetes. The relative importance of genetic factors versus iron overload in the pathophysiology of diabetes secondary to hemochromatosis, however, is not yet clear. (*Courtesy of* Dr. Howard Mizrachi, St. Luke's–Roosevelt Hospital Center, New York.)

Pharmacologic Effects on Glucose Homeostasis

DRUGS CAUSING DIABETES

Drugs That Affect Insulin Secretion

Anticonvulsants	Cations	Hormones	Anthelmintics
Phenytoin	Barium	Somatostatin	Pentamidine
Diuretics	Cadmium	Pesticides	Antineoplastics
Thiazides	Lithium	DDT	L-Asparaginase
Furosemide	Potassium	Fluoride	Mithramycin
Ethacrynic acid	Zinc	Pyriminil (Vacor)	

Drugs That Affect Insulin Action

Hormones
  Growth hormone

Drugs That Affect Insulin Secretion and Insulin Action

Hormones/hormone antagonists	Antihypertensives	Blocking agents	Psychopharmacologic agents
Glucagon	Clonidine	β-Adrenergic blockers	Benzodiazepines
Glucocorticoids	Diazoxide	Calcium-channel blockers	Ethanol
Octreotide	Prazosin	Histaminergic blockers	Opiates
Adrenergic compounds			Phenothiazines
Epinephrine			Olanzapine
Norepinephrine			

FIGURE 18-18. Drug-induced diabetes. The list of pharmacologic agents that can induce diabetes is long. Individual drugs may affect glucose homeostasis by interfering with insulin secretion, insulin action, or both. Whether its effect is primarily on insulin secretion or insulin action, a drug itself may mediate the effect directly, or indirectly through hormones or cations critical to the mechanisms that control insulin release or biologic effect. Glucohomeostatic effects of supraphysiologic levels of growth hormone, glucocorticoids, and catecholamines best illustrate the direct and indirect consequences of "pharmacologically" altered insulin action. As the links between altered insulin sensitivity and altered insulin secretion tighten, it becomes more and more difficult to assign an effect to a drug solely on the basis of insulin action. Clinically, these agents may uncover previously silent insulin secretory defects or insulin resistance and consequently induce glucose intolerance in a previously undiagnosed patient or worsen the diabetic state when administered to patients with antecedent diabetes mellitus. (*Adapted from* Argetsinger and Carter-Su [2].)

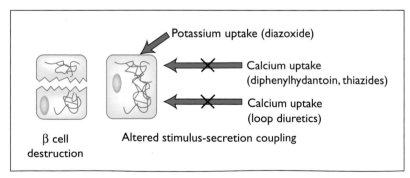

Potassium uptake (diazoxide)

Calcium uptake
(diphenylhydantoin, thiazides)

Calcium uptake
(loop diuretics)

β cell
destruction

Altered stimulus-secretion coupling

FIGURE 18-19. Prototypical pharmacologic impairment of insulin secretion: direct and indirect effects. Insulin secretion by pancreatic β cells may be impaired directly by destruction of the β cells themselves or by interference with the normal mechanism of stimulated insulin secretion. Pentamidine, a widely used anthelmintic agent active against *Pneumocystis carinii*, produces β–cell-selective necrosis and irreversibly reduces β-cell responses to glucose and nonglucose secretagogues after initially causing cytolytic release of insulin [51]. In contrast, diphenylhydantoin, at therapeutic blood levels, reversibly reduces both first and second phases of insulin release by inhibiting calcium inflow into the β cell through voltage-dependent Ca^{2+} channels [52]. Unlike diphenylhydantoin, thiazide diuretics were thought to adversely affect insulin secretion and promote glucose intolerance indirectly through production of hypokalemia [53], in a manner similar to that proposed for primary hyperaldosteronism. Although prevention or correction of hypokalemia does alleviate thiazide-induced glucose intolerance, direct effects of thiazides themselves on the β cell secretion have been described. Unlike the structurally related compound diazoxide, thiazides do not hyperpolarize β cells by opening the adenosine triphosphate–sensitive potassium channels closed by the sulfonlyureas [54]. Instead, they, like diphenylhydantoin, may affect stimulus-secretion coupling in the β cell by inhibiting calcium uptake [55]. Similarly, the loop diuretics, thought to share with the thiazides an indirect effect on β-cell secretion mediated through hypokalemia, also directly affect insulin secretion by inhibiting chloride pump function in the β-cell membrane [56].

Genetic Syndromes Associated with Impaired Glucose Tolerance

GENETIC SYNDROMES ASSOCIATED WITH IMPAIRED GLUCOSE TOLERANCE

Acute intermittent porphyria

Alström syndrome (obesity, deafness, retinitis pigmentosa)

Ataxia-telangiectasia

Cockayne's syndrome

Cystic fibrosis

Friedreich's ataxia (spinocerebellar ataxia)

Glycogen storage disease type I

Herrmann's syndrome (photomyoclonus, nerve deafness, nephropathy, cerebral dysfunction)

Huntington's chorea

Isolated growth hormone deficiency

Klinefelter's syndrome

Laurence-Moon-Biedl syndrome

Leprechaunism

Lipoatrophic diabetes

Machado-Joseph disease (ataxia, nystagmus, dysarthria, depressed tendon reflexes, distal muscle atrophy)

Myotonic dystrophy

Panhypopituitary dwarfism

Prader-Willi syndrome

Trisomy 21

Turner's syndrome

Werner's syndrome

Wolfram syndrome (hereditary optic atrophy, visual loss, neurosensory deafness)

FIGURE 18-20. Genetic syndromes associated with impaired glucose tolerance. The list of genetic syndromes that include glucose intolerance as part of their profile is extensive and growing. Among members of this list, relatively "pure" defects in insulin secretion are represented by diseases such as cystic fibrosis; leprechaunism, on the other hand, may be regarded as a prototypical syndrome of insulin resistance. It is clear, however, that multiple pathophysiologic mechanisms that affect both glucose production and glucose utilization coalesce, in most cases, to produce the full-blown syndromes and the glucose intolerance that characterize them. It is likely that advances in the molecular genetics and molecular pathophysiology of these syndromes will shed light not only on the dysregulated glucose handling in these syndromes, but also on mechanisms of altered glucose homeostasis common both to secondary and primary forms of diabetes.

References

1. Catanese VM, Kahn DR: Secondary forms of diabetes. In *Principles and Practice of Endocrinology and Metabolism, edn 3*. Edited by Becker KL, Bremner WJ, Hung W, et al. Philadelphia: JB Lippincott; 2001:1327–1336.

2. Argetsinger L, Carter-Su C: Mechanism of signaling by growth hormone receptor. *Physiol Rev* 1996, 76:1089–1107.

3. Foss MC, Saad MJ, Paccola GM, et al.: Peripheral glucose metabolism in acromegaly. *J Clin Endocrinol Metab* 1991, 72:1048–1053.

4. Thorner MO, Vance ML, Laws ER, et al.: The anterior pituitary. In *Williams Textbook of Endocrinology*, edn 9. Edited by Wilson JD, Foster DW, Kronenberg HM, Larsen PR. Philadelphia: WB Saunders; 1998: 296.

5. Orskov L, Schmitz O, Jorgensen JOL, et al.: Influence of growth hormone on glucose-induced glucose uptake in normal men as assessed by the hyperglycemic clamp technique. *J Clin Endocrinol Metab* 1989, 68:276–282.

6. Thirone ACP, Carvalho CRO, Brenelli SL, et al.: Effect of chronic growth hormone treatment on insulin signal transduction in rat tissues. *Mol Cell Endocrinol* 1997, 130:33–42.

7. Dominici FP, Cifone D, Bartke A, Turyn D: Loss of sensitivity to insulin at early events of the insulin signaling pathway in the liver of growth hormone transgenic mice. *J Endocrinol* 1999, 161:383–392.

8. Clemmons DR: Roles of insulin-like growth factor-I and growth hormone in mediating insulin resistance in acromegaly. *Pituitary* 2002, 5:181–183.

9. Sugimoto M, Takeda N, Nakashima K, et al.: Effects of troglitazone on hepatic and peripheral insulin resistance induced by growth hormone excess in rats. *Metabolism* 1998, 47:783–787.

10. Ezzat S, Ren SG, Braunstein GD, et al.: Octreotide stimulates insulin-like growth factor-binding protein-1: a potential pituitary-independent mechanism for drug action. *J Clin Endocrinol Metab* 1992, 75:1459–1463.

11. Koop BL, Harris AG, Ezzat S: Effect of octreotide on glucose tolerance in acromegaly. *Eur J Endocrinol* 1994, 130:581–586.

12. Krsek M, Silha JV, Jezkova J, et al.: Adipokine levels in Cushing's syndrome: elevated resistin levels in female patients with Cushing's syndrome. *Clin Endocrinol* 2004, 60:350–357.

13. Fallo F, Scarda A, Sonino N, et al.: Effect of glucocorticoids on adiponectin: a study in healthy subjects and in Cushing's syndrome. *Eur J Endocrinol* 2004, 150:339–344.

14. Imai E, Stromstedt PE, Quinn PG, et al.: Characterization of a complex glucocorticoid response unit in the phosphoenolpyruvate carboxykinase gene. *Mol Cell Biol* 1990, 10:4712–4719.

15. Valera A, Pujol A, Pelegrin M, et al.: Transgenic mice overexpressing phosphoenolpyruvate carboxykinase develop non-insulin-dependent diabetes. *Proc Natl Acad Sci U S A* 1994, 91:9151–9154.

16. Nyirenda MJ, Lindsay RS, Kenyon CJ, et al.: Glucocorticoid exposure in late gestation permanently programs rat hepatic phosphoenolpyruvate carboxykinase and glucocorticoid receptor expression and causes glucose intolerance in adult offspring. *J Clin Invest* 1998, 101:2174–2181.

17. O'Brien RM, Granner DK: Regulation of gene expression by insulin. *Biochem J* 1991, 278:609–619.

18. Ishizuka T, Nagashima T, Kajita K, et al.: Effect of glucocorticoid receptor antagonist RU 38486 on acute glucocorticoid-induced insulin resistance in rat adipocytes. *Metabolism* 1997, 46:997–1002.

19. Weinstein SP, Paquin T, Pritsker A, et al.: Glucocorticoid-induced insulin resistance: dexamethasone inhibits the activation of glucose transport in rat skeletal muscle by both insulin- and non–insulin-related stimuli. *Diabetes* 1995, 44:441–445.

20. Dimitriadis G, Leighton B, Parry-Billings M, et al.: Effects of glucocorticoid excess on the sensitivity of glucose transport and metabolism to insulin in rat skeletal muscle. *Biochem J* 1997, 321:707–712.

21. Saad MJA, Folli F, Kahn JA, et al.: Modulation of insulin receptor, insulin receptor substrate-1, and phosphatidylinositol 3-kinase in liver and muscle of dexamethasone-treated rats. *J Clin Invest* 1993, 92:2065–2072.

22. Delaunay F, Khan A, Cintra A, et al.: Pancreatic beta cells are important targets for the diabetogenic effects of glucocorticoids. *J Clin Invest* 1997, 100:2094–2098.

23. Gremlich S, Roduit R, Thorens B: Dexamethasone induces posttranslational degradation of GLUT2 and inhibition of insulin secretion in isolated pancreatic beta cells. *J Biol Chem* 1997, 272:3216–3222.

24. Lambillotte C, Gilon P, Henquin JC: Direct glucocorticoid inhibition of insulin secretion. *J Clin Invest* 1997, 99:414–423.

25. Bani D, Biliotti G, Sacchi TB: Morphological changes in the human endocrine pancreas induced by chronic excess of endogenous glucagon. *Virchows Archiv B Cell Pathol* 1991, 60:199–206.

26. Keiser HR: Pheochromocytoma and other diseases of the sympathetic nervous system. In *Principles and Practice of Endocrinology and Metabolism, edn 3*. Edited by Becker KL, Bremner WJ, Hung W, et al. Philadelphia: JB Lippincott; 2001:827–834.

27. Lehr S, Herbst M, Kampermann J, et al.: Adrenaline inhibits depolarization-induced increases in capacitance in the presence of elevated intracellular calcium concentration in insulin secreting cells. *FEBS Lett* 1997, 415:1–5.

28. Renstrom E, Ding WG, Bokvist K, et al.: Neurotransmitter-induced inhibition of exocytosis in insulin-secreting beta cells by activation of calcineurin. *Neuron* 1996, 17:513–522.

29. Capaldo B, Napoli R, Di Marino L, et al.: Epinephrine directly antagonizes insulin-mediated activation of glucose uptake and inhibition of free fatty acid release in forearm tissues. *Metab Clin Exp* 1992, 41:1146–1149.

30. Laakso M, Edelman SV, Brechtel G, et al.: Effects of epinephrine on insulin-mediated glucose uptake in whole body and leg muscle in humans: role of blood flow. *Am J Physiol* 1992, 263:E199–204.

31. Raz I, Katz A, Spencer MK: Epinephrine inhibits insulin-mediated glycogenesis but enhances glycolysis in human skeletal muscle. *Am J Physiol* 1991, 260:E430–435.

32. Malbon CC, Campbell R: Thyroid hormones regulate hepatic glycogen synthase. *Endocrinology* 1984, 115:681–686.

33. Dimitriadis GD, Leighton B, Vlachonikolis IG, et al.: Effects of hyperthyroidism on the sensitivity of glycolysis and glycogen synthesis to insulin in the soleus muscle of the rat. *Biochem J* 1988, 253:87–92.

34. Holness MJ, Sugden MC: Hepatic carbon flux after re-feeding: hyperthyroidism blocks glycogen synthesis and the suppression of glucose output observed in response to carbohydrate re-feeding. *Biochem J* 1987, 247:627–634.

35. Tosi F, Moghetti P, Castello R, et al.: Early changes in plasma glucagon and growth hormone response to oral glucose in experimental hyperthyroidism. *Metabolism* 1996, 45:1029–1033.

36. Fryer LG, Holness MJ, Sugden MC: Selective modification of insulin action in adipose tissue by hyperthyroidism. *J Endocrinol* 1997, 154:513–522.

37. Matthei S, Trost B, Hamann A, et al.: Effect of in vivo thyroid hormone status on insulin signalling and GLUT1 and GLUT4 glucose transport systems in rat adipocytes. *J Endocrinol* 1995, 144:347–357.

38. Gonzalo MA, Grant C, Moreno I, et al.: Glucose tolerance, insulin secretion, insulin sensitivity and glucose effectiveness in normal and overweight hyperthyroid women. *Clin Endocrinol* 1996, 45:689–697.

39. Bonadonna RC, DeFronzo RA: Glucose metabolism in obesity and type II diabetes. In *Obesity*. Edited by Bjorntorp P, Brodoff BN. Philadelphia: JB Lippincott; 1992:474–501.

40. Sorenson RL, Brejle TC, Hegre OD, et al.: Prolactin (in vitro) decreases the glucose stimulation threshold, enhances insulin secretion, and increases dye coupling among islet B cells. *Endocrinology* 1987, 121:1447–1453.

41. Brejle TC, Parsons JA, Sorenson RL: Regulation of islet beta-cell proliferation by prolactin in rat islets. *Endocrinology* 1994, 43:263–273.

42. Weinhaus AJ, Stout LE, Sorenson RL: Glucokinase, hexokinase, glucose transporter 2, and glucose metabolism in islets during pregnancy and prolactin-treated islets in vitro: mechanisms for long term up-regulation of islets. *Endocrinology* 1996, 137:1640–1649.

43. Wade GN, Schneider JE: Metabolic fuels and reproduction in female mammals. *Neurosci Biobehav Rev* 1992, 16:235–272.

44. Matsuda M, Mori T: Effect of estrogen on hyperprolactinemia-induced glucose intolerance in SHN mice. *Proc Soc Exp Biol Med* 1996, 212:243–247.

45. Reis FM, Reis AM, Coimbra CC: Effects of hyperprolactinaemia on glucose tolerance and insulin release in male and female rats. *J Endocrinol* 1997, 153:423–428.

46. Sun YS, Brunicardi FC, Druck P, et al.: Reversal of abnormal glucose metabolism in chronic pancreatitis by administration of pancreatic polypeptide. *Am J Surg* 1986, 151:130–140.

47. Brunicardi FC, Chaikcn RL, Ryan AS, et al.: Pancreatic polypeptide administration improves abnormal glucose metabolism in patients with chronic pancreatitis. *J Clin Endocrinol Metab* 1996, 81:3566–3572.

48. Hramiak IM, Finegood DT, Adams PC: Factors affecting glucose tolerance in hereditary hemochromatosis I. *Clin Invest Med* 1997, 20:110–118.

49. Stremmel W, Niederau C, Berger M, et al.: Abnormalities in estrogen, androgen, and insulin metabolism in hereditary hemochromatosis. *Ann NY Acad Sci* 1988, 526:209–223.

50. Merkel PA, Simonson DC, Amiel SA, et al.: Insulin resistance and hyperinsulinemia in patients with thalassemia major treated by hypertransfusion. *N Engl J Med* 1988, 318:809–814.

51. Shen M, Orwoll ES, Conte JE Jr, et al.: Pentamidine-induced pancreatic beta-cell dysfunction. *Am J Med* 1989, 86:726–728.

52. Siegel EG, Janjic D, Wollheim CB: Phenytoin inhibition of insulin release. Studies on the involvement of Ca^{2+} fluxes in rat pancreatic islets. *Diabetes* 1982, 31:265–269.

53. Helderman JH, Elahi D, Andersen DK, et al.: Prevention of the glucose intolerance of thiazide diuretics by maintenance of body potassium. *Diabetes* 1983, 32:106–111.

54. Tucker SJ, Gribble FM, Zhao C, et al.: Truncation of Kir6.2 produces ATP-sensitive K^+ channels in the absence of the sulphonylurea receptor. *Nature* 1997, 387:179–183.

55. Sandstrom PE: Inhibition by hydrochlorothiazide of insulin release and calcium influx in mouse pancreatic beta cells. *Br J Pharmacol* 1993, 110:1359–1362.

56. Sandstrom PE: Bumetanide reduces insulin release by a direct effect on the pancreatic beta cells. *Eur J Pharmacol* 1990, 187:377–383.

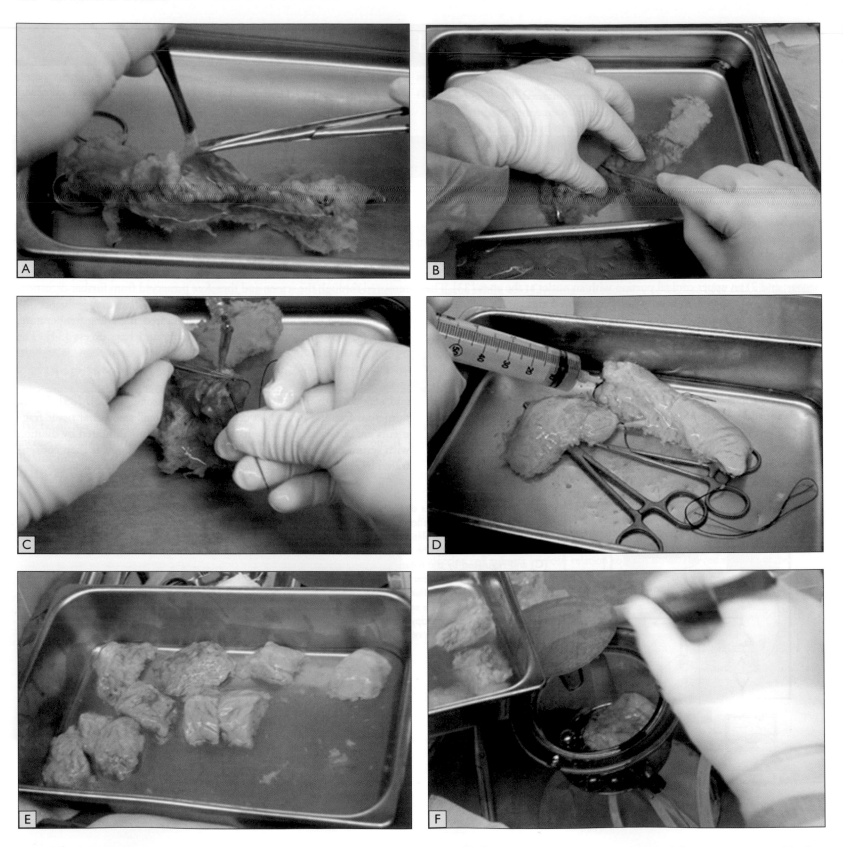

FIGURE 19-3. The pancreas is generally obtained en block with spleen and a segment of the duodenum, which are removed before on the back table before starting the isolation (**A**). Cleaning also includes the removal of the surrounding adipose and connective tissue, taking great care in preserving the pancreatic capsule integrity in order to prevent leak of the enzyme during the distension phase (**B**). The gland is cut into two portions, and the pancreatic duct of both portions is then cannulated (**C**) and injected with the enzyme solution, resulting in the distention of the gland (**D**). After distention, the gland is divided into several pieces of equal size (**E**) and transferred into the digestion chamber (**F**). The chamber *(Continued on next page)*

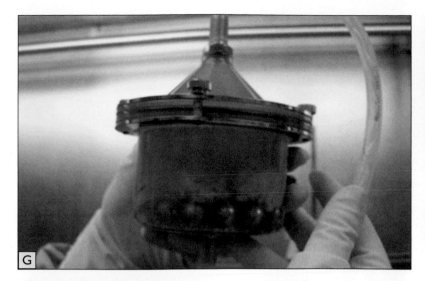

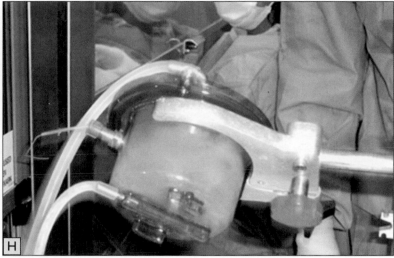

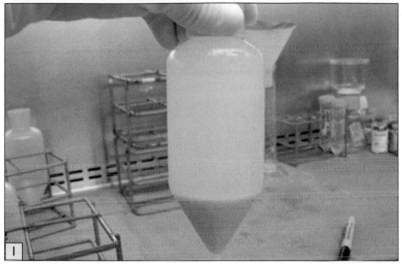

FIGURE 19-3. (Continued) (**G**) consists of a lower cylinder and an upper conical portion separated by a removable stainless steel screen, and it contains hollow stainless steel marbles. The screen retains the pancreas in the lower portion of the chamber, and the marbles enhance the mechanical disruption during a manual or automated shaking (**H**). A combination of both enzymatic and mechanical actions lead to the disruption of the tissue and progressive release of small particles, which are removed and preserved from further digestion. After digestion, the pancreatic slurry is concentrated by centrifugation (**I**) and prepared for the next purification step.

Purification of Pancreatic Islet Cells

The purification step is performed to physically separate islet cells from non-endocrine tissue. The goal of the purification step is to minimize the volume of tissue to be implanted in the recipient's portal system in order to prevent excessive ischemic insult to the liver and elevation of portal pressure, thereby decreasing the potential for procedure-related complications.

Islet cell purification is obtained by isopycnic separation, which takes advantage of the differences in density that exist between the endocrine and exocrine tissues [36,37]. Centrifugation of the pancreatic digest on density gradients allows each tissue to migrate to the gradient of equal density. Despite the fact that acinar cells have densities much higher than other cell types, swelling and edema consecutive to the dissociation procedure may alter densities and interfere with the efficiency of the separation, therefore precluding high degrees of purity [36]. The semiautomated separation method uses the COBE 2991 computerized centrifuge system, which consists of a centrifuge bowl that bears a doughnut-shaped bag in which the pellet sediments to the outside and the lower density layers to the center (*see* Fig. 19-5) [38,39]. The centrifuge has a hydraulic system that can apply uniform pressure to the separation bag, allowing for the collection of the fractions starting from the center portion of the bag.

The pancreatic digest can be resuspended in preservation solution and loaded on top of the gradient layers. Top loading allows keeping the digested pancreas in physiological medium for the longest possible time, but it may be associated with increased cell aggregation with acinar tissue migrating to the denser gradient layers dragging down islet cells from the upper interfaces [36–38]. It has been suggested that reduction of cellular swelling and edema obtained by incubating the slurry in preservation (hyperosmolar) solutions before and during the purification process can significantly improve top-loading efficiency [36–38]. The use of top loading and continuous density gradients is currently considered the gold standard because it may allow for higher yields and purity [36]. However, it is a laborious and time-consuming process because numerous fractions are collected and assessed separately. Alternatively, the pancreatic digest can be resuspended in the heaviest density gradient and loaded in the bottom of the bag, generally using discontinuous density gradients [36]. This procedure is short because only few fractions are collected and assessed, but it may allow for a lower effective cell load associated with accumulation of cells at the interfaces, which interferes with the migration producing cell aggregation [36].

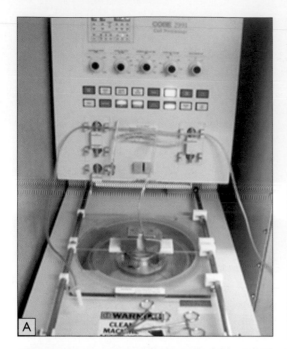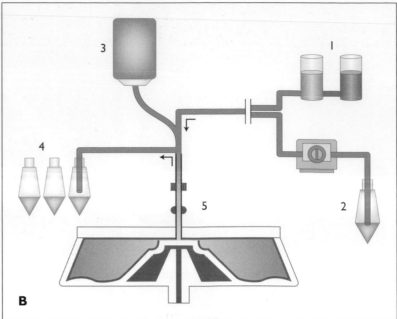

FIGURE 19-4. Islet cell isolation procedure: purification. Islet cells represent approximately 2% of the total pancreatic tissue. The digested pancreas is centrifuged on isopycnic gradients (separation according to differences in density) using the semiautomated COBE 2991 computerized centrifuge system (**A**). A doughnut-shaped bag is placed in the centrifuge (**B**) and then loaded with either continuous (*1*) or discontinuous (*2*) gradients. Continuous gradients are obtained using a gradient mixer (*1*), followed by top loading of the pancreatic digest in preservation solution using an infusion bag. When using discontinuous gradients, the pancreatic digest is resuspended in the denser gradient, and the lower densities are added on top with a peristaltic pump (*2*). After centrifugation, the hydraulic system of the centrifuge is activated, and different fractions are collected separately for assessment of purity (*3*).

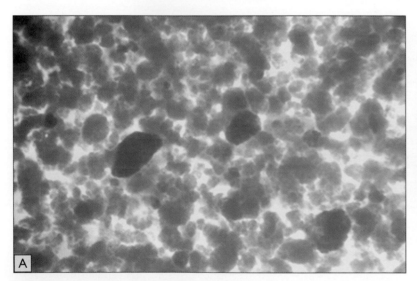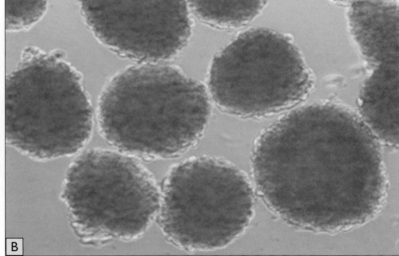

FIGURE 19-5. (See Color Plate) Assessment of islet cell purity. Islet cells can be recognized by dithizone staining that binds to the zinc present in the secretory granules of the endocrine cells, conferring a characteristic red color to the endocrine cell clusters. After purification, different degrees of islet purity can be obtained, which can be combined before transplantation. Assessment of an islet preparation shows the presence of islet cells of different sizes (red color) and acinar tissue (not stained) (**A**). **B,** A fraction with higher islet purity.

Pancreatic Islet Cell Assessment and Culture

After purification, islet cells can be transplanted immediately or cultured for a short period before implant. Before transplantation, assessment of sterility and *in vitro* function of the islet cell preparation is required for product release. Assessment includes gram staining to exclude bacterial contamination, assessment of endotoxin concentrations 5 EU/mL or greater of final product volume/kg recipient body weight), viability, and potency of the islet cell preparations.

Purity and Cell Identity

Islet purity is assessed by dithizone (DZT) staining to estimate the percentage of endocrine cell clusters in the final preparation [34]. Selective binding of DTZ to the zinc–insulin complex in β-cell granules results in a red staining of the islet cells (*see* Fig. 19-6) that can be observed using light microscopy. Purity of the islet preparation and size distribution of the islet cells is quantified using an ocular micrometer. Islet volume is calculated in islet equivalents (IEQs) using an algorithm, with 1 IEQ equal to 150 μm islet [31]. Fractions with different degree of purity (generally 30% or greater) can be pooled up to a volume of 10 mL or less to meet the minimal requirement for transplantation of greater than 5000 IEQ/kg of recipient body weight. Assessment of the cellular composition of final preparation by immunohistochemistry can also be used to further characterize the quality of the transplanted tissue [10, 40].

Cell Viability

The viability of islet cell preparations is assessed with the use of fluorescent compounds that are capable of binding to cell cytoplasm of viable cells (fluorescein diacetate [FDA]) and to nucleic acids by crossing cell membranes of necrotic cells (propidium iodide [PI]). Relative percentages of PI-positive over FDA-positive cells allows for a semiquantitative analysis of islet cell viability. Islet preparations with viability of 70% or above are generally considered suitable for transplantation. Novel methods able to quantify the viability of islet cell subsets and with higher sensitivity may be of assistance in the near future to assess the quality of islet preparation [40].

In Vitro Potency Assays

Islet cell function can be assessed in vitro by measuring the insulin release during a glucose challenge. This can be performed during a static incubation in which islet cells are exposed to sequential incubations in the presence of low and high glucose concentrations. Insulin output is measured by enzyme-linked immunoassay in the supernatant obtained after each of the incubation steps, and the ratio of stimulated insulin (high glucose) release over basal (low glucose) is calculated and expresses as stimulation index (*see* Fig. 19-7). Alternatively, a continuous perifusion method for islet assessment may be used, where islet cells are exposed to dynamic changes of glucose concentration. Measuring insulin output in the perifusate allows estimating the function of isolated islet cells.

Transplantation of human islet cells into chemically-induced diabetic immunodeficient mice (*see* Fig. 19-8) allows for the analysis of islet cell potency in vivo in a diabetic environment, measured as ability to correct diabetes [31]. Immunodeficient mice cannot reject tissues from other strains (allogeneic) or species (xenogeneic, including human), and therefore represent an invaluable tool for the study of islet function in the bsence of the confounding elements of rejection and autoimmunity.

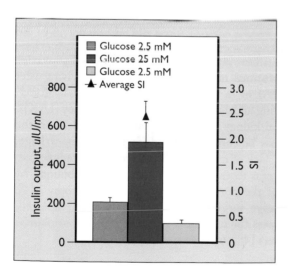

FIGURE 19-6. In vitro assessment of islet cell function. The quality of the isolated cells can be assessed in vitro by using static glucose stimulation. Islet aliquots are incubated sequentially in solutions containing low (2.5-mM), high (25-mM), and low (2.5-mM) glucose concentrations, and the amount of insulin release in the media is measured by enzyme-linked immunosorbent assay (*bars*). A stimulation index (SI) can be calculated by dividing the amount of insulin produced during the incubation in high glucose by that produced during the first incubation in low-glucose solution (*black triangle*).

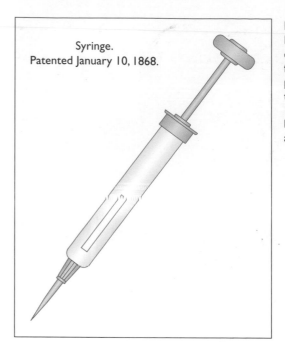

Syringe.
Patented January 10, 1868.

FIGURE 20-2.
Illustrated here is the earliest picture of the first syringe and needle patented in 1868. From the 1920s through the 1950s, insulin was given by reusable glass syringes and needles.

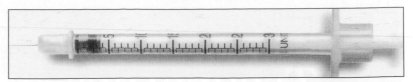

FIGURE 20-3. Current insulin syringe. These syringes are disposable, come in multiple sizes ranging from 0.25 cc to 1 cc, have half-unit and 1-unit measurements, and have needles that range in size from 29 to 32 gauge.

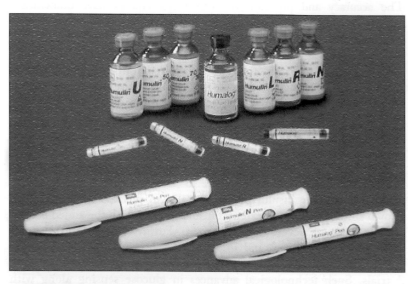

FIGURE 20-4. Insulin cartridges for reusable pens and disposable pens. Insulin has traditionally been given by vial and syringe. In the 1980s, insulin cartridges for reusable pens were developed along with disposable pens.

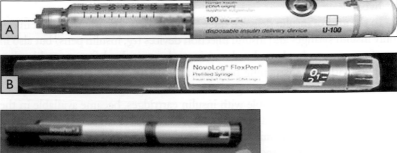

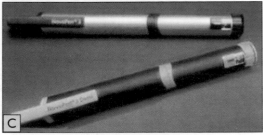

FIGURE 20-5. The first insulin pen was developed by NovoNordisk (Novo A/S, Bagsvaerd, Denmark) in 1926, but the first commercial pen was not available until 1985. Since then, numerous pens, both disposable and reusable, have been developed, adding to accuracy in dosing and convenience to insulin injection therapy. **A,** Disposable Lilly pen (Eli Lilly and Company, Indianapolis, IN). **B,** Disposable NovoNordisk pen. **C,** Reusable pen with disposable cartridge.

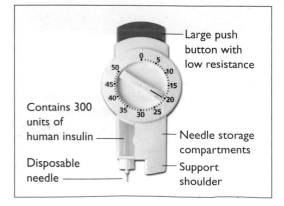

Large push
button with
low resistance

Contains 300
units of
human insulin

Disposable
needle

Needle storage
compartments

Support
shoulder

FIGURE 20-6. The Novo Innolet (Novo A/S, Bagsvaerd, Denmark) insulin pen. Other insulin pens have been developed to aid in convenience and accuracy in dosing for a variety of patient types. Pens such as the one shown here are easy to use, with large-scale numbers; audible clicks; and clear, uncomplicated dials.

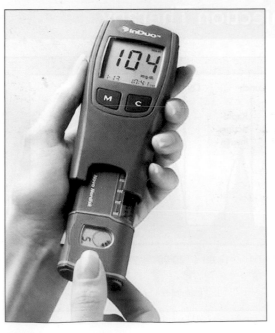

FIGURE 20-7.
Combined insulin pen and blood glucose monitor (InDuo by NovoNordisk [Novo A/S, Bagsvaerd, Denmark] and Lifescan [Milpitas, CA]). The benefits of integration are the convenience of self-monitoring of blood glucose when injecting as well as the convenience of injecting when testing blood glucose level or the level is not in range.

Insulin Pump Therapy

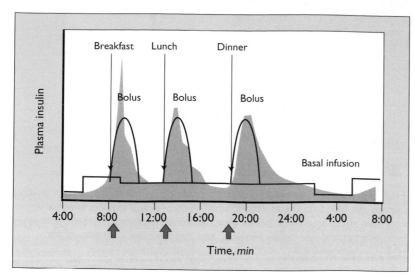

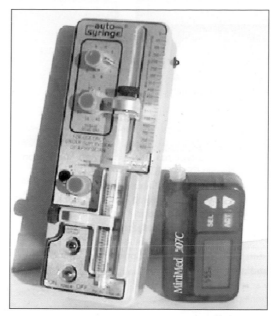

FIGURE 20-8. Insulin pump therapy. Insulin pump therapy has been the gold standard for basal bolus therapy. The basal rate can be varied to cover the dawn phenomenon and exercise, and boluses can be easily given to cover all meals and snacks as well as given over time to cover high-fat meals and slowly absorbing carbohydrates.

FIGURE 20-9. Pump therapy: older versus newer generation. Insulin pump therapy was first approved in the United States in 1979 using the Autosyringe (DEKA, Manchester, NH) 2-C pump, a bulky, rather complicated mechanical syringe. Multiple improvements in size, safety, software enhancements, durability, and ease of programming been made. Pictured here also is the 507C pump (Medtronic Diabetes, Northridge, CA), the first downloadable pump, launched in 1998.

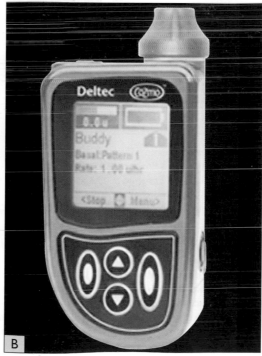

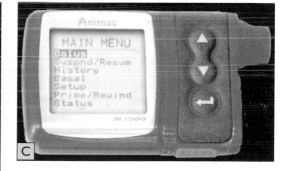

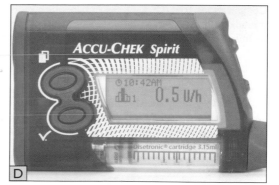

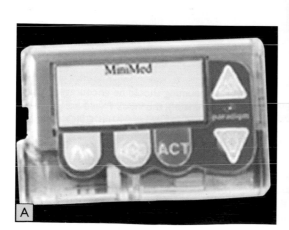

FIGURE 20-10. These are the most current models of insulin pumps approved by the US Food and Drug Administration for sale in the United States as of July 2004. **A,** The Medtronic MiniMed Paradigm pump. **B,** The Smiths Medical Deltec (St. Paul, MN) Cozmo pump. **C,** The Animas (West Chester, PA) IR 1200 pump. **D,** ACCU-CHEK (Roche, Basel, Switzerland) Spirit insulin pump. (*Panel A from* Medtronic; with permission.)

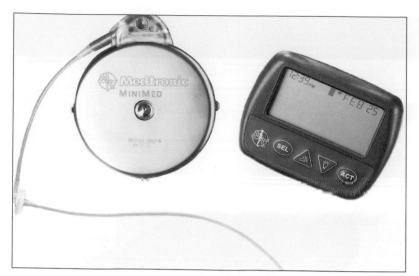

FIGURE 20-27. Implantable insulin pump. Medtronic's (Northridge, CA) implantable insulin pump delivers insulin into the peritoneal cavity, where it is more rapidly and predictably absorbed by the body, with fewer hypoglycemic episodes compared with external pump therapy or multiple daily injections. The pump holds 10 cc of 400 U insulin and needs refilling every 2 to 4 months. Catheter blockages are the main adverse event. This device is not yet cleared by the US Food and Drug Administration; it bears CE approval in Europe. (*From* Medtronic Diabetes; with permission.)

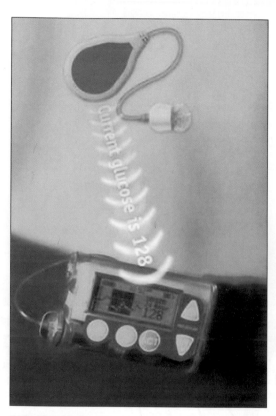

FIGURE 20-28. Sensor-augmented insulin pump system. A future-generation insulin pump and continuous glucose monitoring system are designed to be integrated to form a sensor-augmented pump system. Patients are expected to make immediate therapy adjustments based on real-time continuous glucose readings displayed every 5 minutes and by viewing a graph with 3- and 24-hour glucose trends. This device is not yet cleared by the US Food and Drug Administration or European health authorities. (*From* Medtronic Diabetes; with permission)

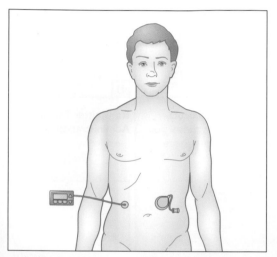

FIGURE 20-29. External artificial pancreas. A future closed-loop system is expected to integrate an external insulin pump and an external continuous glucose monitoring system, which uses a glucose sensor to record blood sugar readings from interstitial fluid. The external system will be designed to automatically integrate glucose levels and deliver insulin accordingly. This device is not yet cleared by the US Food and Drug Administration or European health authorities.(*From* Medtronic Diabetes; with permission)

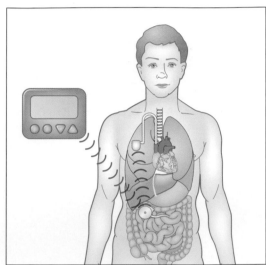

FIGURE 20-30. Implanted artificial pancreas. A future closed-loop system is expected to integrate an implantable insulin pump and an implantable long-term glucose sensor. The implantable sensor is inserted into the superior vena cava, where it is designed to continuously measure glucose levels using an enzyme-based electrode, which detects oxygen consumed in a glucose oxidase reaction. The sensor is designed to be replaced every year through a minor surgical procedure and is connected to an implantable insulin pump by an abdominal lead. This implantable system is designed to automatically record blood glucose levels and deliver insulin to patients with diabetes. This device is not yet cleared by the US Food and Drug Administration or European health authorities. (*From* Medtronic Diabetes; with permission)

References

1. Bode BW, Gross TM, Thornton KR, *et al.*: Continuous glucose monitering used to adjust diabetes therapy improves glycosylated hemoglobin: a pilot study. *Diabetes Res Clin Pract* 1999, 46:183–190.

2. Bode B, Weinstein R, Bell D, *et al.*: Comparison of insulin aspart with buffered regular insulin and insulin lispro in continuous subcutaneous insulin infusion: a randomized study in type 1 diabetes. *Diabetes Care* 2002, 25:439–444.

3. Davidson P, Hebblewhite H, Steed RD, Bode BW: Analysis: the suboptimal roadmap to he intensive therapy target. *Diabetes Technol Ther* 2004, 6:17–19.

Index

Color Plates

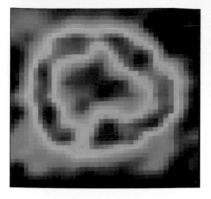

FIGURE 3-9A. Page 30

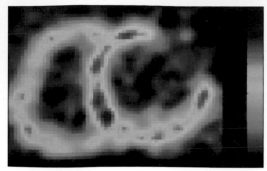

FIGURE 3-9B. Page 30

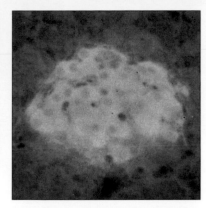

FIGURE 4-2A. Page 42

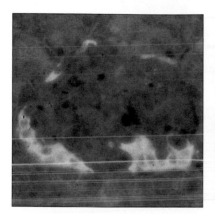

FIGURE 4-2B. Page 42

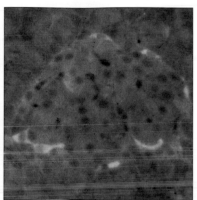

FIGURE 4-2C. Page 42

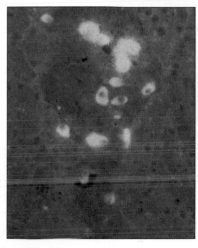

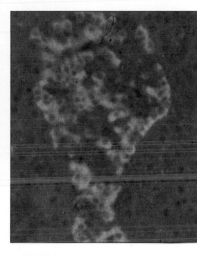

FIGURE 4-2D. Page 42

FIGURE 4-2E. Page 42

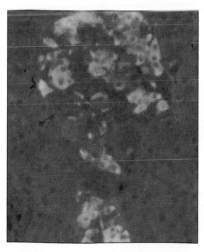

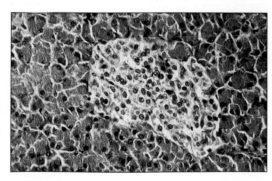

FIGURE 4-4A. Page 43

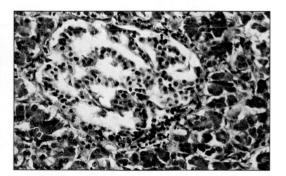

FIGURE 4-4B. Page 43

FIGURE 4-2F. Page 42

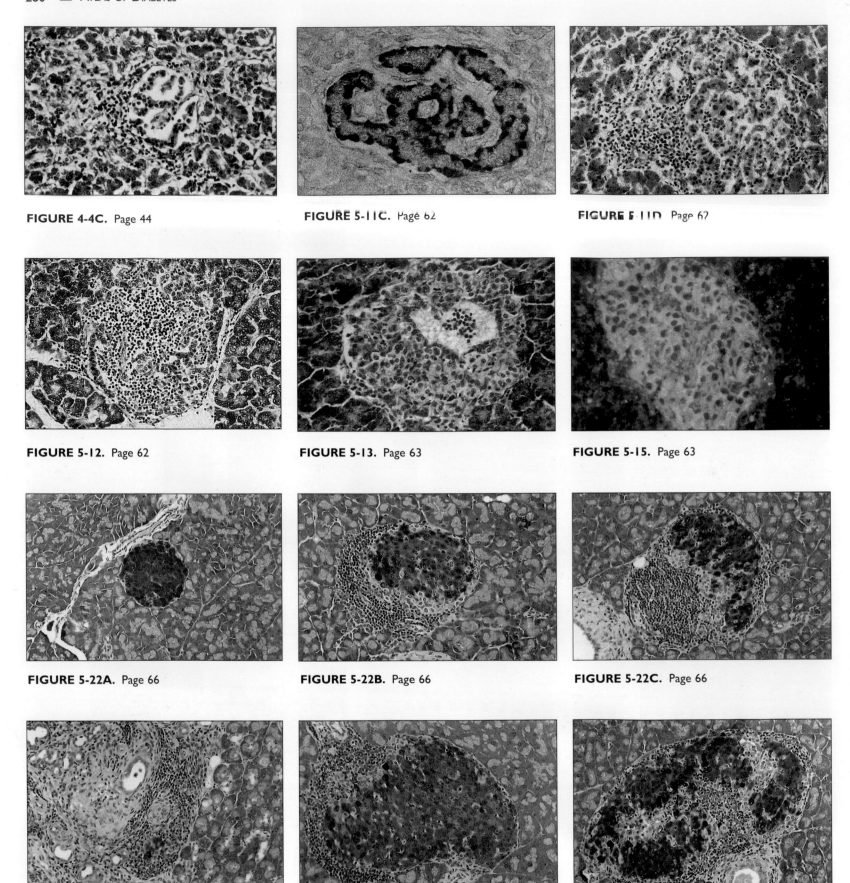

FIGURE 4-4C. Page 44

FIGURE 5-11C. Page 62

FIGURE 5-11D. Page 62

FIGURE 5-12. Page 62

FIGURE 5-13. Page 63

FIGURE 5-15. Page 63

FIGURE 5-22A. Page 66

FIGURE 5-22B. Page 66

FIGURE 5-22C. Page 66

FIGURE 5-22D. Page 66

FIGURE 5-22E. Page 67

FIGURE 5-22F. Page 67

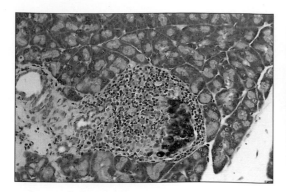

FIGURE 5-22G. Page 67

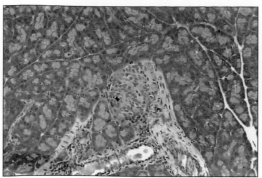

FIGURE 5-22H. Page 67

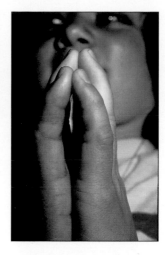

FIGURE 7-13A. Page 98

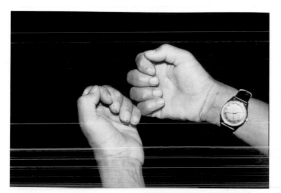

FIGURE 7-13B. Page 98

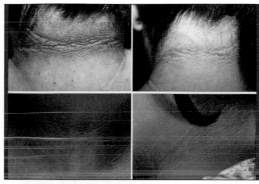

FIGURE 7-25. Page 105

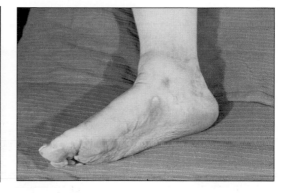

FIGURE 15-17. Page 211

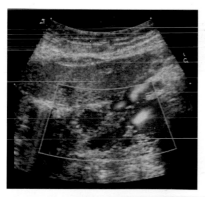

FIGURE 17-14. Page 236

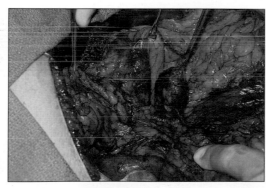

FIGURE 17-18. Page 237

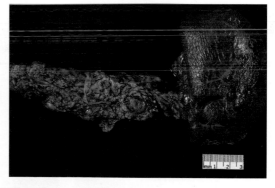

FIGURE 17-19. Page 237

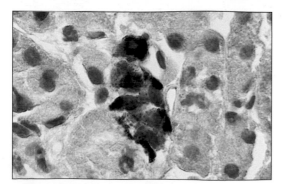

FIGURE 17-21A. Page 237

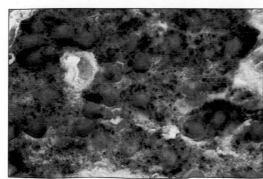

FIGURE 17-21B. Page 237

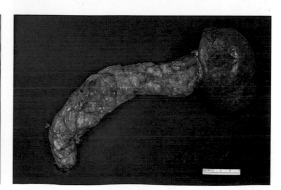

FIGURE 17-23. Page 238

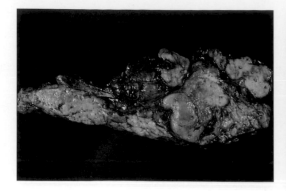

FIGURE 17-24. Page 238

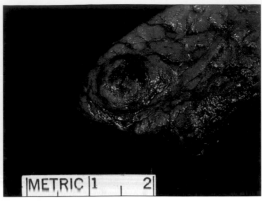

FIGURE 17-25. Page 238

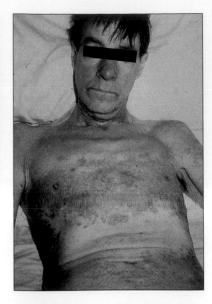

FIGURE 18-10A. Page 245

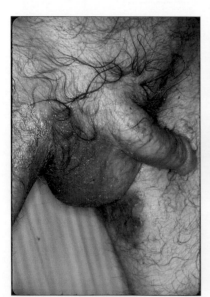

FIGURE 18-10B. Page 245

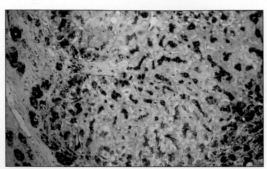

FIGURE 18-17A. Page 248

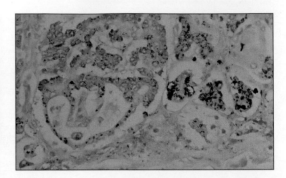

FIGURE 18-17B. Page 248

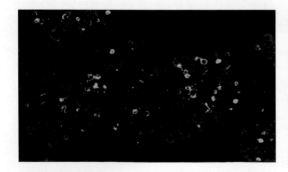

FIGURE 19-1. Page 254

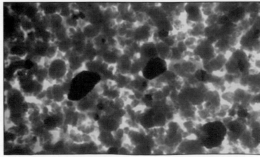

FIGURE 19-5A. Page 258

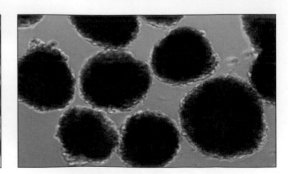

FIGURE 19-5B. Page 258